A P L S
The Pediatric Emergency Medicine Course

Third Edition

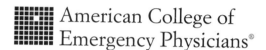 American College of
Emergency Physicians®

American Academy
of Pediatrics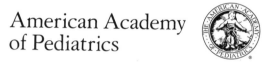

Editor

Gary R. Strange, MD, FACEP
The University of Illinois at Chicago
Department of Emergency Medicine
Chicago, Illinois

Associate Editors

Arthur Cooper, MD, FAAP, FACS, FCCM
College of Physicians and Surgeons of
Columbia University
Harlem Hospital Center
New York, New York

Marianne Gausche, MD, FACEP, FAAP
Harbor-UCLA Medical Center
Department of Emergency Medicine
Torrance, California

D. Anna Jarvis, MB, BS, FRCP(C), FAAP
University of Toronto
The Hospital for Sick Children
Toronto, Ontario, Canada

Cheri Nijssen-Jordan, MD, FRCP(C), FAAP
Alberta Children's Hospital
University of Calgary
Calgary, Alberta, Canada

Jonathan I. Singer, MD, FACEP, FAAP
Wright State University
Department of Emergency Medicine
Dayton, Ohio

Robert A. Wiebe, MD, FACEP, FAAP
University of Texas Southwestern Medical Center
Division of Pediatric Emergency Medicine
Children's Medical Center
Dallas, Texas

Advanced Pediatric Life Support Joint Task Force

American College of Emergency Physicians Representatives

Jonathan I. Singer, MD, FACEP, FAAP, Chair
Wright State University
Department of Emergency Medicine
Dayton, Ohio

Marianne Gausche, MD, FACEP, FAAP
Harbor-UCLA Medical Center
Department of Emergency Medicine
Torrance, California

American Academy of Pediatrics Representatives

Arthur Cooper, MD, FAAP, FACS, FCCM
Assistant Professor and Chief
Pediatric Surgery Critical Care
College of Physicians and Surgeons of Columbia University
Harlem Hospital Center
New York, New York

Robert A. Wiebe, MD, FAAP, FACEP
University of Texas Southwestern Medical Center at Dallas
Division of Pediatric Emergency Medicine
Children's Medical Center at Dallas
Dallas, Texas

Liaisons

Canadian Association of Emergency Physicians

Cheri Nijssen-Jordan, MD, FRCP(C), FAAP
Alberta Children's Hospital
University of Calgary
Calgary, Alberta, Canada

Canadian Paediatric Society

D. Anna Jarvis, MB, BS, FRCP(C), FAAP
University of Toronto
The Hospital for Sick Children
Toronto, Ontario, Canada

APLS: The Pediatric Emergency Medicine Course

3rd Edition, second printing, November 2000

3rd Edition, first printing, July 1998

2nd Edition, 1993

1st Edition, 1989

ISBN 1-58110-009-4

For more information on this manual, the additional course materials, and the course itself, contact:

American College of Emergency Physicians
Post Office Box 619911
Dallas, Texas 75261-9911
(800) 798-1822

American Academy of Pediatrics
141 Northwest Point Boulevard
Post Office Box 927
Elk Grove Village, Illinois 60009-0927
(800) 433-9016, ext. 6795

Contributors

The Editor and Associate Editors acknowledge with appreciation the contributions of the following individuals in the development of this manual.

William R. Ahrens, MD
Chicago, Illinois

Steven Baldwin, MD
Columbia, South Carolina

Barbara Barlow, MD, FAAP
New York, New York

E. Bradshaw Bunney, MD, FACEP
Chicago, Illinois

Richard M. Cantor, MD, FAAP, FACEP
Syracuse, New York

Wendy Coates, MD, FACEP
Torrance, California

Arthur Cooper, MD, FAAP, FACS, FCCM
New York, New York

Mary Ann Cooper, MD, FACEP
Chicago, Illinois

Timothy B. Erickson, MD, FACEP
Chicago, Illinois

Alexandra Fetter-Zarzeka, MD
Jacksonville, Florida

George L. Foltin, MD, FAAP, FACEP
New York, New York

Marianne Gausche, MD, FACEP, FAAP
Torrance, California

Michael Gayle, MD, FAAP
Jacksonville, Florida

Bruce M. Greenwald, MD, FAAP
New York, New York

Daniel Isaacman, MD, FAAP
Norfolk, Virginia

Niranjan Kissoon, MBBS, FRCP(C), FAAP
Jacksonville, Florida

Danielle Laraque, MD, FAAP
New York, New York

Steven Lelyveld, MD, FACEP, FAAP
Chicago, Illinois

Stephen Ludwig, MD, FAAP, FACEP
Philadelphia, Pennsylvania

Robert C. Luten, MD, FAAP
Jacksonville, Florida

Constance M. McAneney, MD, FAAP
Cincinnati, Ohio

Karin A. McCloskey, MD, FAAP
Dallas, Texas

James H. McCrory, MD, FAAP
Macon, Georgia

Arlene F. Mrozowski, DO
Bridgeport, Connecticut

Deborah A. Mulligan-Smith, MD, FAAP, FACEP
Coral Springs, Florida

Daniel A. Notterman, MD, FAAP
New York, New York

James A. O'Neill, Jr., MD, FAAP
Nashville, Tennessee

Linda Quan, MD, FAAP, FACEP
Seattle, Washington

Lou E. Romig, MD, FACEP, FAAP
Miami, Florida

Alfred D. Sacchetti, MD, FACEP
Voorhees, New Jersey

John P. Santamaria, MD, FAAP, FACEP
Tampa, Florida

Steven M. Selbst, MD, FAAP, FACEP
Wilmington, Delaware

Jonathan I. Singer, MD, FACEP, FAAP
Dayton, Ohio

Phyllis H. Stenklyft, MD, FAAP, FACEP
Jacksonville, Florida

Gary R. Strange, MD, FACEP
Chicago, Illinois

Joseph J. Tepas III, MD, FAAP
Jacksonville, Florida

Thomas E. Terndrup, MD, FACEP
Syracuse, New York

Michael G. Tunik, MD, FAAP
New York, New York

Tony Woodward, MD, FAAP
Philadelphia, Pennsylvania

Grace M. Young, MD, FAAP, FACEP
Baltimore, Maryland

Arno L. Zaritsky, MD, FAAP
Norfolk, Virginia

Staff

Rebecca Garcia, PhD
Michael M. Sheridan
American College of Emergency Physicians
Linda Lipinsky
Peggy Hecht
American Academy of Pediatrics

Acknowledgments

The Editor and Associate Editors acknowledge the work of previous APLS Joint Task Force members, as listed below. Their work resulted in the publication of the original manual for this course and served as the basis for the second and third editions.

Martha S. Bushore, MD, FAAP, FACEP, FCCM

Gary R. Fleisher, MD, FAAP, FACEP

Alex Haller, MD, FAAP

Carden Johnston, MD, FAAP, FACEP

Robert C. Luten, MD, FAAP

James Seidel, MD, PhD, FAAP

Benjamin K. Silverman, MD, FAAP

David Wagner, MD, FACEP

The Editor acknowledges the work of Susan M. Fuchs, MD, FAAP, FACEP, and Carden Johnston, MD, FAAP, FACEP, for their in-depth reviews on behalf of the American Academy of Pediatrics Committee on Pediatric Emergency Medicine.

Table of Contents

Foreword

After a long gestation, the American Academy of Pediatrics and the American College of Emergency Physicians delivered the first national course oriented toward initial assessment and early treatment of ill and injured children. Published in 1989, the *Advanced Pediatric Life Support* student manual and course curriculum were met with praise for their instructional value to the physician practicing in an emergency setting. The original APLS Joint Task Force framers were gratified by the content provided in the written documents and by the teachable moments delivered from the podium and interactive sessions.

Second editions of the course materials published in 1993 kept unaltered much of the established knowledge. New conclusions drawn from reason, fact, and experience of the second set of contributors were incorporated. To the benefit of sick and injured children, more courses were delivered nationally.

Readers of this new third edition and participants in the revised pediatric emergency medicine course will remain beneficiaries of the historical legacy established by a cadre of talented authors and contributors. The newest edition reminds us of the strength of our ancestors and perpetuates their lessons. The works maintain the original spirit of the APLS Joint Task Force and add accrued information and novel insight. The publications also project the developmental surveillance of a worthy third-generation APLS Joint Task Force.

Of greatest benefit, Dr. Gary Strange, editor of this student manual, and Dr. Marianne Gausche, editor of the instructor materials, looked back at previous task force efforts. They saw with new sets of eyes the potential for improvement and provided critical direction. Through their diligence and talents, we're proud to provide a more eloquent edition of *APLS: The Pediatric Emergency Medicine Course.*

Jonathan I. Singer, MD, FACEP, FAAP, Chair
Joint Task Force on
Advanced Pediatric Life Support
July 1998

Introduction

The initial moments of resuscitation for a child with a life-threatening illness or injury are the most important. Specialists in emergency medicine rely on an assessment-focused approach to initial management of life-threatening emergencies. The goal is rapid recognition and correction of life-threatening physiologic abnormalities, prior to establishing a working diagnosis. This assessment-focused approach, shown in Figure I-1, is characterized by an ongoing cycle of critical questions and critical actions guided by continuous assessment and reassessment of vital functions.

APLS: The Pediatric Emergency Medicine Course of the American Academy of Pediatrics and the American College of Emergency Physicians assumes a working knowledge of this assessment-focused approach. However, unlike the Pediatric Advanced Life Support (PALS) Course of the American Heart Association and the American Academy of Pediatrics, APLS does not concentrate on pediatric cardiopulmonary resuscitation. Rather, APLS concentrates on the initial management of illnesses and injuries that, if left untreated, could lead to life-threatening pediatric conditions requiring resuscitation. APLS emphasizes the key interventions that may prevent deterioration of illness or injury from an acute stage to a critical stage.

Physicians and other health care providers unfamiliar with the techniques used for the initial assessment of life-threatening illnesses and injuries in childhood may find it useful, prior to participation in APLS, to review the principles of pediatric cardiopulmonary resuscitation through participation in the PALS course. PALS stresses the fundamental elements of pediatric cardiopulmonary resuscitation, particularly rapid cardiopulmonary assessment and maintenance of ventilation, oxygenation, and perfusion. This is accomplished through stepwise evaluation and support of the airway, breathing, and circulation using the critical question/critical action format described above. At each step, focused assessment is followed by necessary interventions and subsequent reassessment to determine whether the intervention has repaired the derangement before proceeding to the next step.

The Pediatric Assessment Triangle (Figure I-2) is used as a model approach to initial assessment of the critically ill or injured child. It is used by the physician or other health care provider to quantify the initial impression of the child's condition and serve as a guide to further assessment and intervention. The Pediatric Assessment Triangle consists of systematic observation of the child's general appearance (mental status and muscle

---

FIGURE I-1.
Assessment-focused approach to recognition and treatment of life-threatening conditions.

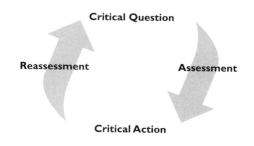

FIGURE I-2.
Pediatric Assessment Triangle.

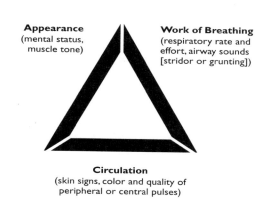

tone), work of breathing (respiratory rate and effort), and circulation (skin and mucous membrane color) and is used to form an initial impression of overall illness or injury severity.

The strategies used in the Pediatric Assessment Triangle are not new. They represent the observations that experienced physicians have long made "from the doorway" as they begin the assessment of acutely ill or injured children. However, presenting them in this format is a useful way of organizing these strategies so that they are more readily understood and incorporated into the daily practice of physicians and other health care providers unfamiliar with emergency management of pediatric patients. Use of this method also allows a maximum amount of information to be obtained in a minimum amount of time.

The systematic approach to the critically ill or injured child (Figure I-3) is the guiding principle of APLS. The initial impression is based on the Pediatric Assessment Triangle and leads either to rapid cardiorespiratory assessment and support, if the child's condition is urgent, or to a focused history and a detailed physical examination, if the child's condition is not urgent. In other words, the initial impression of the acutely ill or injured child forms a mental "snapshot" that leads the provider to rapid recognition of physiologic instability and immediate support of vital functions. The child's vital functions are therefore supported until a specific diagnosis can be made and appropriate therapy can be initiated to correct the underlying problem. The Pediatric Assessment Triangle model will be used to outline the approach to the initial management of a variety of acute pediatric conditions presented in the following chapters.

Gary R. Strange, MD, FACEP
Editor

ACKNOWLEDGMENT

The Editor gratefully acknowledges the contributions of Arthur Cooper, MD, FAAP, FACS, FCCM, and Marianne Gausche, MD, FACEP, FAAP, to this Introduction.

ADDITIONAL READING

Chameides L, Hazinski MF, eds. *Textbook of Pediatric Advanced Life Support*. Dallas, Tex: American Heart Association; 1994.

Dieckmann RA, Gausche M, Brownstein D, et al. *Pediatric Education for Paramedics Student Manual*. Sacramento, Calif: California EMS Authority; 1996.

Foltin G, Tunik M, Cooper A, et al. *Teaching Resource for Instructors in Prehospital Pediatrics (TRIPP)*. Washington, DC: Department of Health and Human Services; Health Resources and Services Administration; Maternal and Child Health Bureau; National Highway Traffic Safety Administration; 1997.

Gausche M, Henderson D, Brownstein D, et al. Education of out-of-hospital emergency medical personnel in pediatrics: report of a national task force. *Ann Emerg Med*. 1998;31:58-64.

FIGURE I-3.
Approach to the critically ill child.

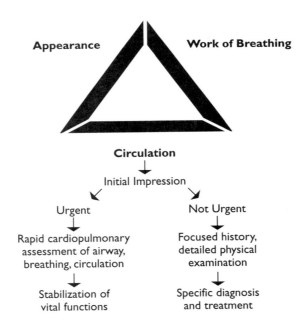

Cardiorespiratory Emergencies

Chapter 1

Respiratory Distress

OBJECTIVES

1. Recognize the infant or child who has respiratory distress or failure.

2. Differentiate between upper and lower airway obstruction.

3. Describe the differences between croup, epiglottitis, and foreign body airway obstruction, and describe the diagnostic tests used and the pitfalls in management that may occur.

4. Differentiate between asthma and bronchiolitis, and describe the appropriate treatment for each.

5. Explain the monitoring techniques used for patients in respiratory distress.

6. Discuss the indications for and use of pharmacologic agents in the treatment of acute airway distress.

Acute respiratory emergencies in the pediatric patient are common and if not properly treated can result in significant morbidity and mortality. Decisive intervention is mandatory to ensure the best outcome. The practitioner must understand the unique anatomic and physiologic characteristics of the respiratory tract in the growing infant and child. In addition, a knowledge of the most frequent types of airway problems encountered in children will assist in establishing a provisional diagnosis in the emergency setting. Most importantly, the ability to accurately assess the child in respiratory distress remains a most critical step in maintaining proficiency in patient care. The rapid, initial assessment of the child in respiratory distress includes elements of the Pediatric Assessment Triangle (Figure 1-1). Appearance reflects the adequacy of oxygenation (color) and ventilation (muscle tone and mental status). Increased work of breathing indicates areas of airway obstruction (lower: wheezes, retractions; upper: stridor) or lack of adequate oxygenation (grunting). Decreased work of breathing indicates respiratory failure (decreased tidal volume or respiratory rate). Typically, a child first develops respiratory distress and increased work of breathing. If this process is not interrupted by effective treatment, deterioration to respiratory failure may occur. This chapter is devoted to describing the pathophysiology, symptoms and signs, and management recommendations for the pediatric patient who presents with respiratory distress.

PATHOPHYSIOLOGY

Upper Airway Considerations

The small caliber of the upper airway in children makes it vulnerable to occlusion secondary to a variety of disease processes. The narrowness of the airway results in greater baseline airway resistance. Any process that narrows the airway further will cause an exponential rise in airway resistance and a secondary increase in the work of breathing. When the child perceives distress, the resultant increase in respiratory effort will further augment turbulence and raise resistance.

Because the neonate is primarily a nasal breather, any degree of obstruction of the nasopharynx may result in a significant increase in the work of breathing and present clinically as retractions. The tongue of infants and small children dominates the overall capacitance of the oropharynx, so any pediatric patient who presents with an altered mental status will be at risk for the development of upper airway obstruction secondary to a loss of muscle tone affecting the tongue. Occlusion of the oropharynx by the tongue is not uncommon in this setting, but tilting of the head, lifting the chin, or insertion of an oral airway may correct this obstruction.

Older children have tonsillar and adenoidal tissues that are large in proportion to available airways. Although these rarely are the cause of an upper airway catastrophe, they are vulnerable to traumatization and bleeding during clinical interventions such as insertion of an oral or a nasal airway. The pediatric trachea is easily distensible and compressible due to incomplete closure of semiformed cartilaginous rings. Any maneuver that overextends the neck will contribute to compression of this structure and secondary upper airway obstruction. The cricoid ring represents the narrowest portion of the upper airway in children younger than 7 to 9 years and often is the site of occlusion in tracheobronchial foreign body aspiration.

Lower Airway Considerations

The lower respiratory tract consists of all structures below the level of the midtrachea, including the bronchi, bronchioles, and alveoli. Developmental immaturity of these structures in infancy is reflected by a decreased number of subunits necessary for appropriate oxygenation and ventilation. In addition, the pediatric patient

FIGURE 1-1.
Pediatric Assessment Triangle in respiratory distress and failure.

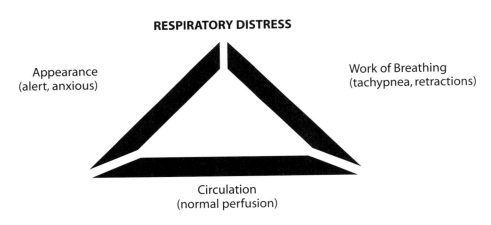

RESPIRATORY DISTRESS

Appearance
(alert, anxious)

Work of Breathing
(tachypnea, retractions)

Circulation
(normal perfusion)

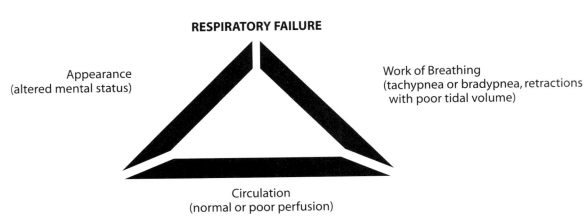

RESPIRATORY FAILURE

Appearance
(altered mental status)

Work of Breathing
(tachypnea or bradypnea, retractions
with poor tidal volume)

Circulation
(normal or poor perfusion)

possesses a diminished pulmonary vascular bed. The relatively small caliber of the pediatric lower airway predisposes it to occlusion. Even partial obstruction will result in an increased degree of airway resistance.

Immaturity of the musculoskeletal and central nervous systems of the pediatric patient also contributes to the development of respiratory failure. In infancy, the diaphragm remains the primary muscle of respiration, with only minor contributions provided by the intercostal musculature. Any degree of abdominal distention will provide significant interference to diaphragmatic function and secondary ventilatory sufficiency. The infantile diaphragm possesses muscle fibers that are more prone to fatigue than their adult counterparts. In addition, the chest wall of the pediatric patient is quite compliant, preventing adequate stabilization during periods of increased respiratory distress. Also, infants are less responsive to hypoxemia because of immature development of central respiratory control, placing them at risk for insufficient respiratory responses to disease states.

SIGNS OF DISTRESS AND IMPENDING RESPIRATORY FAILURE

Regardless of the specific disease process, abnormalities in respiratory function eventually are reflected in physical symptoms and signs ranging from subtle changes to obvious distress. Respiratory distress occurs when increased work of breathing is generated to maintain the respiratory function necessary to meet the requirements of the body. Respiratory failure ensues when respiratory efforts cannot maintain adequate respiratory function — either oxygenation or ventilation.

Tachypnea represents the most common response of the child to increased respiratory needs (Table 1-1). Central stimulation by the medullary respiratory center is predominantly responsible for this physiologic response. Although most commonly due to hypoxia and hypercarbia, tachypnea also may be a secondary response to metabolic acidosis, pain, anxiety, or central nervous system insult. Tachypnea and tachycardia represent protean signs of distress due to any etiology in the pediatric patient; this includes the patient with respiratory compromise.

Infants and children are quite adept in the recruitment of accessory muscles to augment the compensatory mechanism necessary to generate the increased work of breathing. Intercostal, subcostal, substernal and suprasternal, and supraclavicular retractions are common. In addition, the infant and child, if compromised further, will demonstrate nasal flaring.

Specific attention must be paid to the child who generates a grunting sound at the end of expiration. This response represents closure of the glottis at the end of expiration, generating additional positive end-expiratory pressure, which in many disease states is necessary to prevent compromised alveoli from collapse. Grunting usually is a sign of lower airway disease and represents an ominous sign.

Many infants and children, especially children with upper airway compromise, will assume a position of comfort, which represents the most adequate anatomic compensation they can generate relative to their disease state. Children with epiglottitis or severe croup often will assume the sniffing position, in which they maintain an upright position, lean forward, and generate their own jaw thrust maneuver to facilitate opening of the upper airway. Patients with lower airway disease, specifically those with reactive airway components, will assume a tripoding position consisting of an upright posture, leaning forward, and support of the upper thorax by the use of extended arms. This position allows full use of the thoracoabdominal axis for the work of breathing. Patients with upper airway compromise also may prefer to breathe through an open mouth, which suggests dysphagia with the inability to swallow secretions or the general presence of air hunger.

In situations in which significant excessive negative intrathoracic pressure is generated by

TABLE 1-1.
Normal resting respiratory rates.

Age	Rate (breaths/min)
Newborn	30-60
Infant (1-6 mo)	30-50
Infant (6-12 mo)	24-46
1-4 yr	20-30
4-6 yr	20-25
6-12 yr	16-20
>12 yr	12-16

marked respiratory effort, venous return will increase to the heart and left ventricular outflow may be compromised. These intracardiac phenomena result in the generation of a pulsus paradoxus of >20 mm Hg (normal is 0 to 10 mm Hg). The presence of an elevated pulsus paradoxus correlates well with severe respiratory distress. (Pulsus paradoxus is the difference in systolic blood pressure when measured during inspiration and again during expiration. It can be suspected by palpating the pulse and noting the marked diminution in pulse volume at the end of inspiration.)

The presence of cyanosis is an ominous sign in the pediatric patient with respiratory distress; it represents inadequate oxygenation within the pulmonary bed or inadequate oxygen delivery by the cardiovascular system. In the young infant, earlier signs and symptoms of hypoxemia include agitation, irritability, and failure to maintain feeding effort. In the older child, somnolence may develop, especially with accompanying hypercarbia.

The practitioner may be able to judge the respiratory status of a distressed patient using a standardized scoring system. The patient may be assessed using clinical or laboratory parameters. By far the most reliable sign of respiratory failure and impending respiratory arrest remains the generation of an ineffective respiratory effort by the infant or child. Auscultation of the chest may reveal decreased air entry, poor breath sounds, and bradypnea as the child progresses toward respiratory failure. Concomitant with hypoxia, infants may develop bradycardia. Although bradycardia may also be due to excessive vagal stimulation, hypoxemia should be ruled out in all cases of increasing anxiety and bradycardia with respiratory distress.

GENERAL MANAGEMENT PRINCIPLES

In general, any child with respiratory distress requires supplemental oxygen. Humidified oxygen may be delivered by mask, with or without a rebreather apparatus; nasal prongs; face tent; or oxyhood (Table 1-2). Infants and children who appear to be threatened by the use of equipment may be placed in the mother's arms and receive oxygen through tubing alone (at maximal flow) or through insertion of the end of the tubing through the bottom of a paper cup, with the cup then

placed on the child.

Further management is driven by whether the patient has respiratory distress due to an upper or a lower airway problem.

ASSESSMENT AND MANAGEMENT OF SPECIFIC CLINICAL CONDITIONS

Upper Airway Disorders

Stridor is a sign of upper airway compromise that results from the generation of inspiratory turbulence transmitted against a narrowed lumen in the subglottic region. In the young infant, stridor most often is the result of a congenital anomaly of the upper airway. When congenital abnormalities have gone unrecognized in the neonatal period, they may present emergently anytime during infancy.

In the emergency department, the most common causes of acute upper airway obstruction are croup and foreign body obstruction. Epiglottitis has become much less common with the increasing use of *Haemophilus influenzae* vaccine. Additional processes include bacterial tracheitis, retropharyngeal abscess, and peritonsillar abscess (Tables 1-3 and 1-4).

Epiglottitis (Supraglottitis)

Epiglottitis represents a true upper airway emergency with life-threatening complications if handled improperly. It may occur at any time of the year and, most importantly, in any age group. Traditionally, it involves children aged 2 to 7 years, but recently the age range appears to have widened. In some reviews, as many as 25% of patients are younger than 2 years, and many cases have been described in older individuals.

- The classic presentation is acute (several

TABLE 1-2.
Oxygen delivery techniques.

Device	Flow (L/min)	% Oxygen
Nasal prongs	2-4	24-28
Simple face mask	6-10	35-60
Face tent	10-15	35-40
Venturi mask	4-10	25-60
Partial rebreathing mask	10-12	50-60
Oxyhood	10-15	80-90
Nonrebreather mask	10-12	90-95

hours) onset of fever and dysphagia with progressive respiratory distress. The child often will assume a position of comfort, consisting of voluntary upper airway posturing (ie, sitting upright with mouth open and head, neck, and jaw extended). Drooling may be present. Children prefer not to speak, but when encouraged, their voices will be muffled. Stridor, if present, may progress with rapid intensity. The practitioner often will note that children with epiglottitis appear "toxic."

- Severe sore throat or dysphagia may be the dominant concern, and respiratory complaints may be absent. In the absence of signs of pharyngeal or tonsillar pathology, therefore, epiglottitis must be considered in this subgroup of patients. If the practitioner finds pharyngitis or uvulitis, this in no way excludes the possibility of epiglottic involvement as well.
- Young patients with croup-like presentations who fail to respond to traditional therapies should alert the practitioner to the possibility of epiglottitis or bacterial tracheitis.
- Patients younger than 2 years may present with fever for as long as 12 to 24 hours before

the development of abnormal vocalization, swallowing, or inspiratory complaints.

In the past, the vast majority of cases were caused by *H. influenzae* type B. Since the advent of *H. influenzae* type B vaccine, group A β-hemolytic streptococci are the most common cause. Uncommon but reported causative agents include *Streptococcus pneumoniae* and *Staphylococcus aureus*. Blood and epiglottic cultures will be positive in 80% to 90% of affected individuals.

Management. If the disease state goes unrecognized, airway obstruction with respiratory arrest and subsequent cardiac arrest usually occurs. Other factors contributing to airway and ventilatory deterioration include patient fatigue, aspiration of secretions, and sudden laryngospasm. Any and all maneuvers that agitate the child should therefore be avoided, including separation from parents, alteration of optimal airway posture, forced recumbency, fearful events (rectal temperatures, blood work, radiographs), and gagging (forcible tongue blade examination of the oral cavity, suctioning). In some instances with cooperative patients, tongue blade use may be performed to visualize the epiglottis, albeit with extreme caution.

A patient suspected to have epiglottitis should

TABLE 1-3.
Features of various upper airway disorders.

Entity	Usual Age Range	Mode of Onset of Respiratory Distress
Severe tonsillitis	Late preschool or school age	Gradual
Peritonsillar abscess	Usually >8 yr	Sudden increase in temperature, toxic appearance, unilateral throat pain, "hot potato" speech
Retropharyngeal abscess	Infancy to adolescence	Fever and toxicity after URI, pharyngitis, or penetrating injury
Epiglottitis	1-7 yr	Acute onset of hyperpyrexia, dysphagia, and drooling
Croup	3 mo to 3 yr	Gradual onset of stridor, barking cough, after mild URI
Foreign body aspiration	Late infancy to 4 yr	Choking episode resulting in immediate or delayed respiratory distress
Bacterial tracheitis	Infancy to 4 yr	Insidious onset of fever, toxic appearance, respiratory distress

have direct visualization of the supraglottic region in a controlled environment, such as the operating room. If radiographic evaluation is chosen as an alternate technique, this should be performed as an upright, portable lateral neck film. The patient should not be forced to lie down and should not be transported to the radiology suite to have this test performed. In summary, these management guidelines should be followed to avoid undue morbidity and mortality:

- Avoid agitating the child in any way.
- Provide supplemental oxygen as tolerated by the child, with the assistance of the caretaker.
- Allow the patient to assume a position of comfort.
- Prepare equipment for bag-valve-mask (BVM) ventilation, endotracheal (ET) intubation, and needle cricothyrotomy.
- Consult an expert in intubation and provision of a surgical airway and alert operating room personnel.
- Take the child to the operating room for direct visualization and culturing of the epiglottis and intubation.
- Provide appropriate intravenous antibiotics (cefotaxime 50 mg/kg every 6 hours).
- Transfer the patient to an intensive care unit for further treatment and monitoring.
- If the child has a respiratory arrest before stabilization:
    - Open the airway by positioning.
    - Ventilate by BVM (usually effective).
    - If unable to ventilate, intubate with an ET tube ≈1 mm smaller than that calculated.
    - If unable to intubate, perform needle or surgical cricothyroidotomy.

TABLE 1-4.
Clinical features of acute upper airway disorders.

	Supraglottic Disorders (Epiglottitis)	Subglottic Disorders (Croup)
Stridor	Quiet	Loud
Voice alteration	Aphonic, muffled	Hoarse
Dysphagia	+	−
Postural preference	+	±
Barky cough	−	+
Fever	+++	±
Toxicity	++	−

Croup (Viral Laryngotracheobronchitis)

Laryngotracheobronchitis (croup) is a respiratory infection that diffusely affects the upper respiratory tract. This entity accounts for 90% of stridor with fever and is the most common infectious cause of upper airway obstruction. The subglottic region is most commonly affected, resulting in edematous, inflamed mucosa with a fibrinous exudate. Agents responsible for croup are multiple, including parainfluenza types 1, 2, and 3 (most common); adenovirus; respiratory syncytial virus (RSV); and influenza. The seasonal predominance (winter) is related to the epidemiology of the most common causative agents.

Children aged 1 to 3 years are most commonly affected. They often present, after several days of nonspecific, upper respiratory tract infection symptoms, with a characteristic brassy or barking cough. Inspiratory stridor eventually develops, ranging in severity from mild (only when crying or agitated) to severe (present at rest). Temperatures may range from 38° to 40°C in the course of the disease. Higher temperatures (>40°C) or the presence of a toxic appearance should alert the practitioner to carefully consider other diagnoses (eg, atypical epiglottitis or bacterial tracheitis). The typical patient with croup worsens on the evening of the second day, followed by resolution over a period of days. Most children tolerate this common disease without significant morbidity; however, a small percentage may develop complete upper airway obstruction.

Croup scores have been developed that quantify and qualify a constellation of physical findings, assisting the practitioner in estimation of the severity of subglottic obstruction as mild, moderate, or severe (Table 1-5). Stridor at rest is an important hallmark of severe croup and should be assessed in all cases.

Croup most commonly presents as a mild obstruction that can be treated on an outpatient basis. If the child is taking liquids orally and is well hydrated and the practitioner is comfortable with parental reliability, cool-mist therapy may be suggested. Patients with mild to moderate croup can be discharged with adequate instruction if the child improves with cool, humidified oxygen therapy; the parents are reliable; and the child is older than 6 months.

Patients with a moderate croup score or stridor at rest may be treated as inpatients or treated and observed in the emergency department if extended observation is an option. The purpose of admission or extended emergency department observation is to provide continued pharmacologic therapy and observe the child who may be at risk for progression to severe airway obstruction. The use of oxygen, cool mist, and epinephrine delivered by nebulizer usually results in symptomatic improvement of the patient for up to 2 hours. The recommended dose for aerosolized epinephrine is 5 mL epinephrine of a 1:1000 solution prediluted with normal saline or 0.25 to 0.75 mL of racemic epinephrine diluted to 2 mL with normal saline. Peak effects have been demonstrated at 10 to 30 minutes, with a duration of action of up to 2 hours. Children may experience a return to a pretreatment level of obstruction at 1 to 2 hours after therapy. If aerosolized epinephrine is administered, observe the patient for 2 to 3 hours. If the patient's condition does not worsen, discharge may be accomplished after assurance that the caretaker has observational and communication skills and an understanding of transportation options if needed.

Corticosteroids in higher doses (dexamethasone, 0.6 mg/kg per dose intramuscularly or orally) appear to be of benefit in preventing the progression of croup to complete obstruction and may shorten the duration of illness. If corticosteroids are being considered (usually for the moderately or severely obstructed patient), they should be administered as soon as feasible.

If a child has severe croup (clinical croup score of ≥7 or a 2 in any category other than cough [Table 1-4]), it is prudent to admit the child to an intensive care setting. Treatment with oxygen, mist, epinephrine, and corticosteroids should be initiated as soon as possible. Children should be electively intubated for respiratory failure (lethargy, inability to maintain respiratory efforts, PO_2 of <70 on 100% oxygen, or PCO_2 of >60). Children who develop severe upper airway obstruction from this disease do not do so suddenly but rather progress gradually over time. If intubation must be performed in the emergency department, an ET tube that is 1 mm smaller than that calculated for age should be used to accommodate the subglottic edema and airway narrowing.

Management. The following regimen is suggested for managing the patient with croup:
- Avoid agitating the patient.
- Allow the patient to assume a position of comfort (usually in parent's arms or lap).
- Initially, provide cool, moist air; if distress is evident, provide humidified oxygen.
- If stridor is present at rest, both inspiratory and expiratory stridor are present, or the child

TABLE 1-5.
Clinical croup score.*

	0	1	2
Inspiratory breath sounds	Normal	Harsh with rhonchi	Delayed
Stridor	None	Inspiratory	Inspiratory and expiratory or stridor at rest
Cough	None	Hoarse cry	Bark
Retractions and flaring	None	Flaring and suprasternal retractions	Flaring and suprasternal retractions plus subcostal and intercostal retractions
Cyanosis	None	In room air	In 40% O_2

* A score of ≥4 indicates moderately severe airway obstruction. A score of ≥7, particularly when associated with $PaCO_2$ of >45 and PaO_2 of <70 (in room air), indicates impending respiratory failure.
From Downes JJ, Raphaely RC. Pediatric intensive care. *Anesthesiology.* 1975;43:238-250. Adapted with permission.

appears fatigued or in distress, administer aerosolized epinephrine at a dose of 5 mL of a 1:1000 solution prediluted with normal saline or 0.25 to 0.75 mL of racemic epinephrine diluted to 2 mL with normal saline. Patients who receive this intervention are candidates for possible admission, or, at a minimum, close observation for 2 to 3 hours before discharge is considered.

- Administer intramuscular or oral dexamethasone at 0.6 mg/kg.
- Intubate if clinically warranted.
- Upright anteroposterior (AP) and lateral neck radiographs may be considered to help rule out other causes of airway obstruction.
- Stridor at rest is a sign that prehospital personnel and parents can use as an indication to seek or provide therapy.

Foreign Body Obstruction

Most foreign body aspirations occur in children younger than 5 years, with 65% of deaths affecting infants younger than 2. Common offending agents are foods (eg, peanuts, hard candies, frankfurters) and items within the home (eg, disc batteries, coins, marbles). Symptoms range from mild (cough only) to full-blown upper airway obstruction. It is imperative that the practitioner maintain a high index of suspicion relative to the possibility of foreign body aspiration, especially in the afebrile child with a sudden onset of symptoms.

Most patients will present with symptoms of partial obstruction. Evaluation should include AP and lateral views of the upper airway extending from the nasopharynx to the carina. More extensive radiographic investigations include inspiratory and expiratory chest radiographs or bilateral decubital views. Both maneuvers may demonstrate the failure of the affected hemithorax to lose volume as a result of positioning. These examinations are of great value in diagnosing foreign bodies that are radiolucent. In any event, a high degree of suspicion dictates bronchoscopy as a definitive procedure to be certain no foreign body is present.

Esophageal foreign bodies, if the position is high or with prolonged retention, may impede the upper airway.

Management. Foreign body obstruction should be managed as follows:

- For incomplete obstruction (phonation, coughing present):
  –Provide supplemental oxygen.
  –Allow the position of comfort; avoid noxious stimuli.
  –Arrange for controlled airway evaluation and management.
- For acute complete obstruction:
  –Children aged <1 year: Five back blows followed by five chest thrusts
  –Children aged >1 year: Repetitive abdominal thrusts until clear or patient becomes unconscious
  –Attempt ventilation.
  –If unsuccessful, use Magill forceps under direct laryngoscopy in an attempt to remove the foreign body.
  –If unsuccessful, attempt vigorous BVM ventilation or, if necessary, intubation or cricothyrotomy.
  –If a mainstem foreign body can be pushed into a single bronchus, half of the respiratory tree will be supportive.
  –Prepare immediately for bronchoscopy.

Bacterial Tracheitis

Bacterial tracheitis, also referred to as membranous tracheitis, is an infection of the subglottic region. There is controversy about whether this entity exists alone or is a secondary bacterial colonization of a preexistent viral laryngotracheobronchitis. This entity occurs in the same age group as does croup; however, these children usually present atypically, with a toxic appearance and high fever. Pus may be produced during spasms of brassy or barking cough. In some cases, the stridor is sufficiently severe to be present during both inspiration and expiration.

Bacterial tracheitis represents a true upper airway emergency because, like epiglottis, progression to full airway obstruction is possible. The entity should be considered in the patient with stridor who has suddenly deteriorated or the hyperpyrexic or toxic child. The diagnosis should also be suspected if the subglottic air column on the radiograph has a shaggy or irregular border. Definitive diagnosis can be obtained at the time of airway control. On intubation, a normal epiglottis combined with the presence of pus, inflammation, and, in some cases, a pseudomembrane in the subglottic region confirms the diagnosis. Culture most commonly grows *S. aureus*, but *Streptococcus*, *H. influenzae*, and *S. pneumoniae* are possible. Meticulous ET suctioning in a pediatric intensive care unit usually will maintain artificial airway patency.

Retropharyngeal Abscess

Retropharyngeal abscess may occur de novo, probably secondary to suppurative extension from cervical lymphadenopathy, or it may follow penetrating trauma to the posterior oropharynx. Retropharyngeal abscesses are seen predominately in children younger than 3 years of age, but older individuals may be affected. Symptoms include muffled voice, difficulty in swallowing, drooling, and, less frequently, inspiratory stridor. Toxicity and a fixed upright posture are additional findings. Children with retropharyngeal abscess may exhibit neck stiffness, simulating bacterial meningitis. Patients are typically febrile, but afebrile patients with retropharyngeal abscess have been described.

Management. Given the potential overlap in presentation with supraglottitis, even if the diagnosis is suspected, it is prudent to first obtain a lateral neck film that will demonstrate swelling of the prevertebral soft tissue at the level of the pharynx and a normal epiglottis and aryepiglottic folds. Attempts to visualize the oral cavity and posterior pharynx wall may be made in an older cooperative child as long as agitation does not ensue. The posterior pharyngeal wall is edematous and bulges anteriorly.

In children with no evidence of airway obstruction, medical management without ET intubation may be carried out only if equipment and personnel are continuously on hand to perform emergency intubation. Patients who have evidence of partial airway obstruction should be intubated in a controlled environment under direct visualization to avoid rupture of the abscess. Intraoperative drainage of the abscess is an option but not mandated; successful outcome has been described with nonoperative intervention. The expectant antibiotic choice must cover a wide range of the aerobes as well as anaerobes that are associated with this condition (see "Bacterial Tracheitis").

Peritonsillar Abscess

Peritonsillar abscesses usually affect children older than 8 years. These abscesses are the most common deep infections of the head and neck, usually representing complications of bacterial tonsillitis or, in some cases, a superinfection of an existent Epstein-Barr infection.

These patients present with increasing dysphagia, ipsilateral ear pain, and progression to trismus, dysarthria, and toxicity. Drooling is common. Patients often will have a "hot potato" phonation, representing splinting of the palatine muscles during normal speech.

The pharynx is erythematous with unilateral tonsillar swelling, which in some cases may displace the uvula toward the unaffected side. The soft palate may be displaced medially. Fluctuation may confirm the presence of underlying purulent fluid. Reactive cervical adenopathy is common. Severe, although uncommon, complications have been reported, including sternocleidomastoid spasm and torticollis, fascitis, mediastinitis, and airway obstruction. There usually is an elevated white blood cell count.

Management. Throat cultures (superficial) should be obtained in all cases. Direct tonsillar needle aspiration should be performed by an experienced otolaryngologist after adequate sedation/analgesia has been administered. Serologic testing for Epstein-Barr virus infections also should be performed. Most infections are polymicrobial in origin, including group A streptococci (predominant), *Peptostreptococcus*, *Fusobacterium*, and other mouth flora, including anaerobes.

Drainage often can be accomplished on an outpatient basis, and the patient can be treated with oral antibiotics to cover Gram-positive cocci and anaerobes. Some patients will require admission for drainage, intravenous antibiotics, and hydration.

Lower Airway Obstruction

Asthma

Asthma is an intermittent, partially or completely reversible obstructive airway disease. The pathogenesis of asthma involves inflammation, bronchospasm, increased mucus production, and airway edema. It represents a chronic entity, with acute exacerbations. Precipitants are multifactorial, most commonly upper respiratory tract infections and environmental allergens.

The prevalence of asthma has increased in the past 10 years, as have hospitalizations for bronchospasm and overall mortality.

The small airway obstruction in asthma leads to distal air trapping with varying degrees of atelectasis. Patients will generate high negative intrathoracic pressure during inspiration, which may enhance their degree of hypoxemia. Increased venous return, combined with an overall fall in cardiac output, will result in a prominent pulsus paradoxus. As air trapping and expiratory effort increase, the development of a pneumothorax or pneumomediastinum is possible. Prolonged hypoxemia will result in metabolic and eventual respiratory acidosis, with the potential for eventual respiratory failure.

Asthmatic patients or their families should be interviewed for the following historical factors:

- Number, times, and severity of previous episodes of wheezing; school absence due to asthma and the number of emergency department visits also have been shown to be predictors of severity of disease.
- Age at first diagnosis
- Presence of other atopic diseases (eg, allergic rhinitis, eczema) in the patient or family members
- Any history of intensive care unit admission, respiratory failure, or intubation (imparts a more severe prognosis)
- Presence of underlying cardiopulmonary disease processes (eg, congenital heart disease, bronchopulmonary dysplasia)
- Current medications last used at home; specific attention should be directed to any recent theophylline use, especially long-acting preparations.
- Number of occasions on which corticosteroids were used in the preceding year.

After an initial assessment, patients with asthma should undergo repeated clinical evaluations to determine the overall status and response to pharmacologic interventions. One can correlate severity of disease with auscultation in the following manner:

- Mild: Tachypnea, moderate wheezing (often only end expiratory), peak expiratory flow (PEF) >80% predicted
- Moderate: Tachypnea, use of accessory muscles (suprasternal retractions), loud wheezing throughout expiration, tachycardia, pulsus paradoxus of 10 to 20 mm Hg, PEF of 50% to 80% predicted, oxygen saturation of 91% to 95% on room air
- Severe: Marked tachypnea, use of accessory muscles (suprasternal retractions), loud wheezing throughout expiration and inspiration, marked tachycardia, pulsus paradoxus of 20 to 40 mm Hg, PEF of <50% predicted, PaO_2 of <60 mm Hg, cyanosis possible, $PaCO_2$ of >42 mm Hg, oxygen saturation of <91%
- Imminent respiratory arrest: Drowsiness or confusion, paradoxical thoracoabdominal movement, absence of wheezing, bradycardia

Evaluation Adjuncts. Cooperative patients may be able to use a peak flow meter that will provide, if measured repeatedly, an objective parameter of therapeutic response. Arterial blood gas measurements, although not usually necessary, often will demonstrate hypocarbia initially when compensating mechanisms are effective. As severity increases, however, there may be progression to respiratory acidosis. Thus, absolute values of PCO_2 should be interpreted only in the context of the amount of respiratory effort necessary to generate them. Pulse oximeter monitoring of oxygen saturation is another important adjunct in the evaluation of the severity of the disease and response to treatment.

Chest radiographs are not indicated routinely; studies have shown that they rarely alter management. They should be reserved for patients suspected of having pneumonia, a pneumothorax, significant atelectasis, foreign body, or continued deterioration. It is also prudent to obtain a chest radiograph in infants who present with wheezing for the first time to exclude causes of wheezing other than asthma.

Management. Emergency management of the acutely ill asthmatic patient may include the following:

- Supplemental oxygen with attention to pulse oximetry
- Intravenous fluid replacement and maintenance hydration in patients with the inability to tolerate oral challenge
- Nebulized bronchodilators
  –Albuterol. Nebulizer solution available as 0.5% solution (5 mg/mL). Give 0.15 mg/kg to 0.3 mg/kg per dose (varying with the severity of the attack) diluted to 3 mL with

normal saline every 20 minutes, with a minimum dose of 2.5 mg and a maximum dose of 10 mg. (Note: Titrate dose to clinical effect and reevaluate patient for complications such as marked tachycardia for age.) Or, if indicated, give continuous nebulization of 0.5 mg/kg per hour (maximum of 15 mg/hr). In emergency situations, it is not necessary to fine tune the dosage of inhaled albuterol. It is acceptable to use albuterol as 0.25 mL of 0.5% solution in 2.5 mL of normal saline for younger children every 20 minutes and 0.5 mL in 2.5 mL of normal saline for older children and adolescents.

–Metaproterenol. Nebulizer solution available as 5% solution (50 mg/mL). Give 0.1 to 0.3 mL (5 to 15 mg) (maximum, 15 mg); or it is available as 0.6% unit dose vial of 2.5 mL (15 mg). Frequent high-dose administration has not been evaluated, but metaproterenol may be given every 20 minutes as 0.4 mL of 5% solution diluted in 4 to 5 mL of normal saline.

–Metered-dose inhalers (MDIs) used with spacers or holding chambers have been shown to be as effective as nebulized therapy for patients >6 years old. Four to eight puffs every 20 minutes for three doses is recommended for the initial treatment.

- Subcutaneous bronchodilators
–Epinephrine. Subcutaneous epinephrine, 1:1000, has been supplanted largely by the inhaled bronchodilators. It may still have a role in children who are unable to tolerate a respiratory treatment or where such treatment is unavailable. The dose is 0.01 mL/kg up to a maximum of 0.3 mL of the 1:1000 solution. Epinephrine has more side effects and is no more effective than the inhaled bronchodilators.
–Terbutaline. This is another agent that can be used subcutaneously (or by inhalation). The dose for subcutaneous use is 0.01 mg/kg up to a maximum of 0.25 mg. It is more β_2-specific and has fewer side effects than epinephrine.
- Ipratropium bromide is an anticholinergic agent that produces bronchodilatation. Its onset of action is slower than that of the β-agonists, but it has a longer duration of action. It is used mostly in combination with albuterol when patients are responding poorly to β-agonist therapy and should be used with caution in children younger than 5 years. The initial dose is 0.25 mg in 2 mL of saline (may be mixed in the same nebulizer with albuterol). This dose is repeated every 20 minutes for three doses. Ipratropium also can be administered by MDI (four to eight puffs as needed).
- Steroid use includes methylprednisolone (1 to 2 mg/kg intravenously) or prednisone (1 to 2 mg orally) to be followed by a 3- to 4-day course as the acute phase of the illness subsides. Tapering the dose is not necessary.
- Patients should be monitored for therapeutic side effects, including hypertension, vomiting, cardiac dysrhythmias, hypokalemia, gastric upset, and seizures.
- Rapid sequence intubation should be considered for the patient with impending respiratory failure. In this circumstance, ketamine is a good choice for the rapid sequence intubation sedative because it results in bronchodilation.

Admission of the asthmatic patient should be based on the following:

- Status asthmaticus unresponsive to therapy and with persisting oxygen requirement
- Failure to tolerate oral hydration
- Progressive respiratory failure, as demonstrated by worsening pulse oximetry or arterial blood gases and deteriorating clinical status
- Past history of severe, poorly responsive attacks
- In children old enough to cooperate with the procedure, a PEF rate persisting at <70% of known baseline level after therapy
- Parents or caretakers unable to cope or comply with instructions for care at home

Bronchiolitis

Bronchiolitis represents a viral inflammation of the lower respiratory tract and predominantly affects infants younger than 24 months. Causative agents include, most commonly, RSV but also influenza virus, parainfluenza virus, and adenovirus (a particularly severe form). Bronchiolitis occurs mostly during the early winter months. After a viral prodrome, the patient develops tachypnea, tachycardia, wheezing, retractions, marked coughing, and coarse rales. Younger infants are particularly susceptible to fatigue and eventual apnea. Children with a history of prematurity, congenital heart disease, bronchopulmonary dysplasia, underlying lung disease, and compromised immune function are at the highest risk for morbidity and mortality.

Bronchiolitis often presents as a cold, with rhinorrhea and a staccato cough. Non–toxic-appearing infants often present with mild temperature elevations. Infants with moderate distress may present with poor feeding and dehydration secondary to general fatigue. As mentioned, infants younger than 3 months may present with only apnea. Rales or wheezing will be diffusely audible. Prolongation of the expiratory phase is common, with many infants demonstrating variable degrees of decreased air entry. Hypoxemia is a common finding.

It may be difficult to distinguish bronchiolitis from asthma. Both may present during the first year of life, and they have common signs and symptoms. A history of wheezing as well as a family history of atopy points toward an asthmatic etiology. Fever is more consistent with bronchiolitis. Response to bronchodilators does not exclude bronchiolitis because many RSV infections are accompanied by varying degrees of reactive bronchospasm.

Management. The following initial management guidelines are recommended:

- Avoid agitation; provide supplemental oxygen as indicated by oximetry or arterial blood gas values.
- Provide hydration, either orally or intravenously (more likely to be necessary at respiration of >60 breaths/min).
- Provide a trial of inhaled bronchodilators. Some patients with bronchiolitis possess a reactive airway component and will demonstrate a significant clinical response.
- Consider admission if the following are present:
  –A history of prematurity, heart disease, or apnea
  –Persistent hypoxia in room air (or intermittent hypoxia in a child ≤6 months of age)
  –Failure to maintain hydration because of an inability to drink or vomiting

  –Evidence of potential respiratory failure, by both clinical evaluation and monitored parameters of arterial blood gases or pulse oximetry
  –Parents or caretakers unable to cope or comply with instructions for care at home

Pneumonia

Patients with pneumonia often will present with varying degrees of fever, toxicity, and distress. With the exception of the first 3 months of life, when fever may be absent, the cardinal triad for pneumonia includes fever, tachypnea, and cough.

The antecedent history of exposures in the household, day care, or school setting may provide useful information. The length of the illness, quality of the cough, or associated manifestations may further suggest a particular pathogen. In most cases in children, the etiology is a virus. RSV, influenza, parainfluenza, adenovirus, and rhinovirus are pathogens that typically cause an indolent illness. However, abrupt onset with respiratory failure or apnea may occur with these agents, particularly in children younger than 1 year of age. The bacterial agents causing pneumonia are numerous (Table 1-6). Disease caused by *S. pneumoniae* or *H. influenzae* may be clinically indistinguishable. Group A β-hemolytic *Streptococcus* may be a secondary invader after varicella or rubeola. *S. aureus* is notorious for its predilection for early infancy and for a rapid course over a number of hours. *Chlamydia* should be considered in the infant, and *Mycoplasma* should be considered in the older child. In the immunocompromised host, pneumocystis must be considered.

Patients younger than 1 year may present with nonspecific complaints such as anorexia, malaise, altered mental status, or isolated fever. Myalgia, abdominal pain, or vomiting may be predominant manifestations in older children. Further complicating the accuracy of diagnosis, even patients with tachypnea and cough have limited auscultatory findings.

Management. If the history of present illness and physical examination (tachypnea, altered percussion note, diminished air entry, or vocal fremitus and rales) suggest pneumonia, a chest radiograph is not mandated. Chest radiographs may be of assistance in defining pleural effusion or mediastinal lymphadenopathy or alerting the clinician to complications such as empyema or pneumatocele. The presence of consolidation supports a bacterial etiology; peribronchial infiltrates suggest viral etiologies. Measurements of the peripheral blood count or acute-phase reactants do not accurately predict causative organisms and need not be performed routinely. Blood cultures are of limited use because most pediatric patients with pneumonia are nonbacteremic. Patients with pneumonia, like those with any respiratory disease, may require monitoring of their respiratory and acid-base status.

Most children with pneumonia can be managed as outpatients. Admission is required for those who demonstrate hypoxia, respiratory distress, toxic appearance, or dehydration. In addition, infants under the age of 3 months and those with immune deficiency or significant comorbid disease or without adequate caregivers require admission. Antibiotic therapy guidelines are included in Table 1-6. The use of antiviral therapy (ribavirin) is controversial but may be considered as a part of inpatient management.

MONITORING THE PATIENT WITH RESPIRATORY DISTRESS

Pulse oximetry is noninvasive and provides useful information that may alert the practitioner to patient deterioration. It plays an important role in the monitoring of patients with respiratory complaints.

Arterial blood gases are required only for children with progressive deterioration or severe respiratory distress. Measurement of $PaCO_2$ provides the practitioner with an estimate of

TABLE 1-6.
Pathogens and empiric therapy in pediatric pneumonia.

Age	Bacterial Pathogens	Viral Pathogens	Other Pathogens	Empiric Therapy
<1 mo	Group B Streptococcus, Escherichia coli, Klebsiella, Pseudomonas, Listeria	Varicella, RSV	Chlamydia*	Ampicillin + aminoglycoside **or** ampicillin + cefotaxime*
1-3 mo	Haemophilus influenzae, Streptococcus pneumoniae, group A Streptococcus, pertussis, group B Streptococcus	RSV, parainfluenza, influenza, adenovirus	Chlamydia*	Ampicillin + cefotaxime*
3 mo to 5 yr	S. pneumoniae, H. influenzae, Staphylococcus aureus, group A Streptococcus, pertussis	RSV, parainfluenza, influenza, enterovirus, rhinovirus	Chlamydia*	Cephalosporin **or** ampicillin + chloramphenicol **or** antistaphylococcal rhinovirus agent if course indicates*
>5 yr	S. pneumoniae, H. influenzae, group A Streptococcus	Parainfluenza, influenza, adenovirus, rhinovirus	Mycoplasma	Penicillin **or** ampicillin **or** cephalosporin **or** antistaphylococcal agent if course indicates **or** erythromycin if course suggests Mycoplasma

*If Chlamydia is the suspected pathogen, erythromycin should be added to the treatment regimen.

alveolar ventilatory sufficiency. The absolute value must be interpreted in the face of the amount of respiratory effort the patient must generate to attain that particular $PaCO_2$. Therefore, a $PaCO_2$ of 40, although listed as within normal limits in most textbooks, is not acceptable when applied to an infant in distress with marked tachypnea. Any degree of fatigue in this patient will promote CO_2 retention and the rapid development of potentially irreversible respiratory failure. Tachypnea does not guarantee adequate ventilation because many patients, although breathing rapidly, will fail to generate adequate tidal volumes; in effect, they are hypoventilating and therefore retaining CO_2. PaO_2 provides an estimate of alveolar gas exchange and, to some degree, a measure of the balance between tissue perfusion and metabolic demand. The use of percutaneous oximetry reflects only oxygenation and may, in some circumstances, falsely depict the adequacy of ventilation. The use of oximetry should not replace physical examination in evaluation of the pediatric patient with respiratory distress. Arterial pH represents the balance between metabolic demand and respiratory expenditure. In patients with metabolic acidosis, the respiratory system represents the primary compensatory mechanism for overall balance. In patients with excessive work of breathing, the generation of lactate related to poor perfusion may remain uncompensated, resulting in profound acidemia.

SUMMARY

Competency in the management of the pediatric patient with respiratory distress is a necessary skill for the emergency practitioner. This chapter provides an overview of the most common upper and lower airway disorders encountered in clinical practice. Standardized therapeutic interventions will maximize overall clinical outcomes.

ADDITIONAL READING

American Academy of Pediatrics, Provisional Committee on Quality Improvement. Practice parameter: the office management of acute exacerbations of asthma in children. *Pediatrics.* 1994;93:119-126.

Bank DE, Krug SE. New approaches to upper airway disease. *Emerg Med Clin North Am.* 1995;13:473-487.

Brilli RJ, Benzing G, Cotcamp DH. Epiglottitis in infants less than two years of age. *Pediatr Emerg Care.* 1989;5:16-21.

Cruz MN, Stewart G, Rosenberg N. Use of dexamethasone in the outpatient management of acute laryngotracheitis. *Pediatrics.* 1995;96:220-223.

Custer JR. Croup and related disorders. *Pediatr Rev.* 1993;14:19-29.

Gorelick MH, Baker MD. Epiglottitis in children, 1979 through 1992. Effects of *Haemophilus influenzae* type B immunization. *Arch Pediatr Adolesc Med.* 1994;148:47-50.

Kairys SW, Olmstead EM, O'Connor GT. Steroid treatment of laryngotracheitis: a meta-analysis of the evidence from randomized trials. *Pediatrics.* 1989;83:683-693.

Kelley PB, Simon JE. Racemic epinephrine use in croup and disposition. *Am J Emerg Med.* 1992;10:181-183.

Larsen GL. Asthma in children. *N Engl J Med.* 1992;326:1540-1545.

Ledwith CA, Shea LM, Mauro RD. Safety and efficacy of nebulized racemic epinephrine in conjunction with oral dexamethasone and mist in the outpatient treatment of croup. *Ann Emerg Med.* 1995;25:331-337.

Maneker AJ, Petrack EM, Krug SE. Contribution of routine pulse oximetry to evaluation and management of patients with respiratory illness in a pediatric emergency department. *Ann Emerg Med.* 1995;25:36-40.

National Asthma Education and Prevention Program, National Heart, Lung and Blood Institute. Expert Panel Report II: Guidelines for Diagnosis and Management of Asthma. February 1997. JAMA Asthma. http://www.ama-assn.org/special/asthma/treatmnt/guide/guidelin/guidelin.htm

Panitch HB, Callahan CW, Schidlow DV. Bronchiolitis in children. *Clin Chest Med.* 1993;14:715-731.

Rothrock SG, Perkin R. Stridor in children: a review, update and current management recommendations. *Emerg Med Rep.* 1997;18:113-124.

Saipe C. Respiratory emergencies in children. *Pediatr Ann.* 1990;19:637-642.

Schuh S, Johnson DW, Callahan S, et al. Efficacy of frequent nebulized ipratropium bromide added to frequent high-dose albuterol therapy in severe childhood asthma. *J Pediatr.* 1995;126:639-645.

Schutze GE, Jacobs RF. Management of community-acquired bacterial pneumonia in hospitalized children. *Pediatr Infect Dis J.* 1992;11:160-164.

Singer JI, McCabe JB. Epiglottitis at the extremes of age. *Am J Emerg Med.* 1988;6:228-231.

Waisman Y, Klein BL, Boenning DA, et al. Prospective randomized double-blind study comparing L-epinephrine and racemic epinephrine aerosols in the treatment of laryngotracheitis (croup). *Pediatrics.* 1992;89:302-306.

Chapter 2

Advanced Airway Management: Rapid Sequence Induction for Emergent Intubation

OBJECTIVES

1. Compare the airway anatomies of the infant, child, and adult.

2. Recognize the indications for rapid sequence induction (RSI).

3. Describe the clinical pharmacokinetics of the essential medications.

4. Discuss the preferred sequence of RSI in a variety of clinical indications.

Emergency assessment and control of the airway represent the first and most important step in the management of any critically ill child. The methods of airway management, including bag-valve-mask (BVM) ventilation and endotracheal (ET) intubation, have been presented in the *Pediatric Advanced Life Support* textbook and should be reviewed in conjunction with this chapter. This chapter presents the evaluation and management of the pediatric patient requiring immediate intubation and the use of RSI.

The purpose of RSI is to rapidly induce anesthesia and neuromuscular blockade in preparation for intubation; this makes intubation easier, faster, and less traumatic. RSI also blunts the cardiovascular and intracranial pressure (ICP) responses associated with awake intubations.

Any patient requiring acute airway management who is fully or partially conscious is a candidate for RSI; this includes patients with full stomachs, combative behavior, seizures, increased ICP, drug overdoses, and trauma.

A thorough knowledge of the medications used in RSI, technique of ET intubation, and anatomy of the pediatric airway is essential before attempting intubation with RSI.

THE PEDIATRIC AIRWAY

To have successful advanced airway management skills, the practitioner must understand the normal airway anatomy, differences between adult and pediatric airways, and anatomic airway anomalies that occur in children. The infant airway differs most significantly from that of the adult; as a child becomes older, the airway becomes more comparable to the adult anatomy. By 8 or 9 years of age, the airway is considered similar to the adult airway, with the exception of size. Table 2-1 provides a comparison of infant and adult airways.

These anatomic differences affect all the steps involved in airway management. For example, small infants may need a towel placed under the backs to correct for too much of a "sniffing" position, or a straight blade may be preferred to a curved blade to accommodate the infant's anterior airway and large tongue. Certain conditions predispose the airway to difficult management; some of these conditions are listed in Table 2-2.

BASIC AIRWAY MANAGEMENT

Before the application of advanced airway techniques, the airway should be secured and the patient ventilated as needed. For the conscious, spontaneously breathing patient, it usually is appropriate to allow the child to assume the position of comfort and to supply enriched oxygen for inhalation via nasal cannula or mask. If the child resists, a blow-by technique usually is well tolerated. If the child is unconscious, the airway should be checked for obstruction. Noisy breathing and poor air flow result from obstruction, and the airway should be opened through either the chin lift/head tilt or jaw thrust maneuver. If cervical spine trauma is possible, a chin lift or jaw thrust maneuver is used, with great care taken to avoid

movement of the neck. If opening the airway does not restore adequate ventilation, the child can be ventilated with the mouth-to-mouth or mouth-to-mask technique. In health care settings or in the field when airway equipment is available, the child is ventilated with the BVM technique. An oral or a nasal airway will help to maintain the airway during BVM ventilation. Suctioning of the airway often is required to remove secretions, blood, or foreign material. Gastric inflation can be minimized by the use of cricoid pressure (Sellick maneuver) during ventilation and insertion of a nasogastric tube. Ventilation with the BVM technique using high-flow oxygen should always precede ET intubation to build up an oxygen reserve for the time required to place the ET tube and reinitiate ventilation.

EQUIPMENT

Equipment should be available for children ranging from premature newborns to large adolescents. Table 2-3 lists the necessary equipment for advanced airway management. Equipment should be carefully inventoried at regular times and checked for proper functioning. Alternative airway equipment should always be readily available, especially when neuromuscular blocking agents are used. Appropriate monitoring during airway management includes cardiorespiratory and blood pressure monitoring as well as continuous pulse oximetry and ongoing clinical assessment. Colorimetric end-tidal CO_2 detectors are available

TABLE 2-1.
Comparison of infant and adult airways.

	Infant	Adult
Head	Large prominent occiput resulting in sniffing position	Flat occiput
Tongue	Relatively larger	Relatively smaller
Larynx	Cephalad position, opposite C-2 and C-3 vertebrae	Opposite C-4 through C-6
Epiglottis	Ω Shaped, soft	Flat, flexible
Vocal cords	Short, concave	Horizontal
Smallest diameter	Cricoid ring, below cords	Vocal cords
Cartilage	Soft	Firm
Lower airways	Smaller, less developed	Larger, more cartilage

for verifying ET tube placement in infants and children. Quantitative end-tidal CO_2 detectors are used for ongoing monitoring and assessment.

Ideally, charts with age- and weight-related equipment sizes and dosages should be available. Because there is little time to guess weights and find the correct-sized equipment during a true emergency intubation, equipment should be stocked in an age- or a length-related manner with easy access. A pediatric resuscitation tape that relates patient length to dosages and equipment size can be helpful during the acute emergency when weight and age cannot be determined accurately.

PHYSIOLOGIC RESPONSES TO AIRWAY MANEUVERS AND INTUBATION

Mask Ventilation

BVM ventilation may rapidly distend the stomach, leading to difficult ventilation or emesis. The **Sellick maneuver (cricoid pressure)** may be used to occlude the esophagus and limit gastric distention. Insertion of a nasogastric tube will decompress the stomach but may induce emesis through stimulation of the oropharynx or keeping the lower esophageal sphincter open.

Laryngoscopy and Intubation

Direct laryngoscopy in a conscious patient is a noxious stimulus that may result in increased ICP, pain, emesis, hypoxemia, hypertension, and cardiac dysrhythmias. Bradycardia may develop due to a vagal reflex, as a direct effect of succinylcholine, or as a result of hypoxemia. Infants are much more likely to develop bradycardia than are adults.

All parts of the pediatric airway are very small and fragile. Intubation trauma can cause significant edema and obstruction. One millimeter of circumferential edema can result in a 16-fold increase in resistance in a 4-mm infant airway.

CONDITIONS FOR CONSIDERATION OF RAPID SEQUENCE INDUCTION

Nonfasting State

The obvious complications of intubating a patient with a full stomach are regurgitation and aspiration. Infants and young children are particularly susceptible due to air swallowing during crying, diaphragmatic breathing, and a short esophagus. Recent oral intake is one of many causes of increased risk for gastric aspiration (Table 2-4). A history of most recent oral intake should be elicited on all patients, if possible, before proceeding with intubation. This history may be unobtainable in the critically ill child. All patients should be assumed to be in a nonfasting state.

Head Trauma

Head-injured patients are at risk for increased ICP and often are in significant pain. RSI will blunt or decrease the rise in blood pressure and ICP associated with awake intubations. Victims of trauma often are at risk for aspiration secondary to

---

TABLE 2-2.
Selected conditions associated with difficult intubation.

Congenital Anomalies
Down's syndrome	Large tongue, small mouth, frequent laryngospasm
Goldenhar's syndrome	Mandibular hypoplasia
Pierre-Robin syndrome	Large tongue, small mouth, mandibular anomaly
Turner's syndrome	Short neck

Tumor/Mass
Cystic hygroma	Compression of airway
Hemangioma	Hemorrhage

Infection
Epiglottitis	Inability to visualize cords
Croup	Airway irritability, edema below cords

Cervical Spine Immobilization — Prevents optimal head and neck positioning
Upper Airway Obstruction
Angioneurotic edema	Difficulty visualizing cords
Peritonsillar abscess	

Facial Trauma — Difficulty opening mouth

a recent meal, swallowed blood, or crying. The use of RSI and the Sellick maneuver of cricoid pressure will decrease the likelihood of vomiting and aspiration, which could further increase ICP, causing more neurologic damage.

Other indications for RSI include combativeness, prolonged seizure activity, drug overdose, respiratory failure, near-drowning, burns, sepsis, and pneumonia with compromise of the airway and ventilation. In any child with progressive respiratory distress, RSI should be attempted before the child develops true respiratory failure. Early initiation of RSI permits the physician to complete the procedure while the child still has some physiologic reserve.

Contraindications

As mentioned, certain conditions are predictive of difficult intubation. RSI should be used very cautiously, under the following conditions: significant facial edema, trauma, or fractures; distorted laryngotracheal anatomy; or airway anomalies.

GENERAL ORDER OF RAPID SEQUENCE INDUCTION

The following sequence is recommended and is discussed in the order given. Many of the steps can be performed simultaneously by different health care personnel. A specific team leader must direct the sequence. All medications should be mixed and ready to administer before proceeding with step 4.

1. Brief history and anatomic assessment
2. Preparation of equipment and medications
3. Preoxygenation
4. Premedication with adjunctive agents (atropine, lidocaine, defasciculating agent)
5. Sedation and induction of unconsciousness
6. Cricoid pressure (Sellick maneuver)
7. Muscle relaxation
8. Intubation
9. Verification of ET tube placement
10. ET tube is secured; appropriate mechanical ventilation is begun; chest radiograph is ordered; nasogastric tube is placed.
11. Medical record documentation

Step 1, Brief History and Anatomic Assessment

The history of the acute illness plus the entire medical history influence the medications used in RSI. Frequently, emergency airway scenarios do not allow time for a detailed history. The mnemonic **AMPLE** has been used to direct the history needed for anesthesia and intubation:

A — Allergies
M — Medicines, drugs of abuse
P — Past medical problems, previous anesthesia
L — Last oral intake
E — Events, including prehospital course

It is assumed that a partial physical examination that focuses on airway, breathing, and circulation has been done before the decision to intubate was made. If time allows, a brief anatomic assessment of the head and neck should be done that includes the following considerations:

Neck/Cervical Spine. Check for tenderness, masses, short thick neck, signs of trauma,

TABLE 2-3.
Equipment for RSI.

Uncuffed ET tubes in sizes 2.5 to 8.5
Cuffed ET tubes in sizes 5.5 to 9
ET tube stylets
Laryngoscope handles in good working order
Laryngoscope blades
    Straight (Miller) in sizes 0 to 3
    Curved (Macintosh) in sizes 2 to 3
Oral airways
Nasal airways
Magill forceps
Nonrebreather oxygen masks (adult and pediatric)
Ventilation masks in all sizes for BVM ventilation
Self-inflating ventilation bags (250 to 1500 mL) with
    oxygen reservoir and positive end-expiratory pressure
    valve
Oxygen source
Suctioning source
Large-bore stiff suction tips (Yankauer)
Flexible suction catheters (French sizes 5 to 16)
Nasogastric tubes (French sizes 6 to 14)
Pulse oximeter
Cardiorespiratory monitor
Tracheostomy tubes
Tracheostomy surgical instrument set
14-Gauge needle catheter for needle cricothyrotomy
Cricothyrotomy tray
End-tidal CO_2 monitor or detector

hematoma, and tracheal shift.

Face/HEENT. Check for ability to open mouth, size and position of mandible, globe injury, burns, edema, anatomic variants, size of tongue, and crepitus.

Teeth. Check for fixed or loose teeth and dental appliances.

A **brief neurologic evaluation** should be documented before proceeding with the administration of paralytic agents.

Step 2, Preparation of Equipment and Medications

This step should begin as soon as intubation is anticipated. The mnemonic **SOAPME** can be used to complete the preparation phase, as follows:

S — Suction
O — Oxygen
A — Airway (laryngoscope, ET tube, stylet, BVM)
P — Pharmacology (mix, draw-up, and label all anticipated drugs)

TABLE 2-4.
Risks for aspiration of gastric contents.

Full Stomach
    Children, <6 hr
    Infants, <4 hr
Unknown History of Last Oral Intake
Trauma
    Elevated ICP
    Swallowed blood
Delayed Gastric Emptying
    Drugs
    Diabetes
    Infection/sepsis
Intestinal Obstruction
Esophageal Conditions
    Reflex
    Motility disorders
Obesity
Pregnancy
Pain

ME — Monitoring equipment (cardiorespiratory monitor, pulse oximeter, end-tidal CO_2 monitor)

Step 3, Preoxygenation

Preoxygenation is required before proceeding with sedation and paralysis. The purpose of preoxygenation is to cause a nitrogen washout in the lungs and create a functional residual capacity (FRC) that serves as an O_2 reservoir. A 95% nitrogen washout will occur within 2 minutes of administration of 100% O_2 to a spontaneously breathing patient. This O_2 reservoir will allow ≈3 to 4 minutes of apnea, without hypoxemia, in a normal patient. This may eliminate the need for BVM ventilation immediately after the neuromuscular relaxant is administered.

Spontaneously breathing children should be administered 100% O_2 for 2 to 5 minutes via an appropriately sized nonrebreather face mask. Manual ventilation is not warranted in those patients and will only lead to gastric distention. Patients with apnea or inadequate ventilation should be preoxygenated manually with a BVM apparatus for ≥1 to 2 minutes. The Sellick maneuver is performed during bagging to prevent gastric distention and emesis.

Step 4, Premedication with Adjunctive Agents

It is essential that physicians performing RSI know the mechanism of action, dosage, and contraindications of the pharmacologic agents used. All medications should be given intravenously, if possible. Intramuscular, intraosseous, or rectal administration can be used with certain medications in extreme circumstances.

Atropine

Atropine frequently is used as a premedication because it decreases secretions and vagal tone. During airway management, bradycardia may be caused by hypoxia, succinylcholine, or vagal stimulation during laryngoscopy. Bradycardia is more pronounced in infants and children. Indications for atropine include age of less than 1 year, succinylcholine (in children), a second dose of succinylcholine (in adolescents and adults), and bradycardia at the time of intubation. The dose is 0.02 mg/kg, with an initial minimum of 0.1 mg and a maximum of 0.5 mg for a child and 1 mg for an adolescent.

Lidocaine

Lidocaine often is administered before intubation to provide local airway anesthesia and blunt the ICP response to intubation. Maximum mucous membrane anesthesia is reached within 3 to 5 minutes and lasts 30 to 90 minutes. Lidocaine can be administered by aerosol, local injection, or intravenously. The optimal route of administration is unclear. Several studies support administration of lidocaine (1 mg/kg intravenously) 30 seconds before airway instrumentation. This regimen has been used primarily in cases of head trauma with increased ICP.

Step 5, Sedation and Induction of Unconsciousness

Sedatives are administered during RSI to eliminate the sensation of paralysis and decrease sympathetic tone. The ideal sedative should have a rapid onset, short duration, and minimal side effects. Sedative selection must be done on an individual patient basis with consideration given to the presence of hypovolemia, hypotension, or increased ICP; age; and underlying medical conditions. The most frequently used agents are summarized below and in Table 2-5.

Thiopental (Pentothal) is a short-acting barbiturate that produces rapid, deep sedation but not analgesia. The main advantage of thiopental is the cerebroprotective effect it provides. More specifically, thiopental attenuates the ICP response to intubation, reduces the cerebral metabolic rate and oxygen consumption, and acts as a free radical scavenger to decrease damage by toxic metabolites in the injured brain. This makes thiopental the drug of choice for anesthetizing children with head trauma and suspected ICP elevation. The major disadvantage is that thiopental acts as a myocardial depressant and may lower blood pressure. In the face of hypotension, hypovolemia, or suspected shock, thiopental should be avoided or used at a reduced dose (1 to 2 mg/kg).

Thiopental is available in several commercial preparations and involves mixing a sodium chloride diluent with the powdered drug. The 1-g kit is sufficient for use in RSI intubations and avoids wasting excess medication. Thiopental is alkaline and is incompatible with acidic drugs such as succinylcholine, vecuronium, and atropine. Intravenous tubing, therefore, should be flushed after thiopental is administered. Thiopental should be stored in a cool place and used within 24 hours of reconstitution.

Adverse effects include respiratory depression, apnea, decreased cardiac output, hypotension,

TABLE 2-5.
Agents for sedation and induction of unconsciousness.

Agent	Dose (IV)	Onset	Duration
Thiopental	4-6 mg/kg	10-30 sec	10-30 min
Ketamine	1-2 mg/kg	1-2 min	15-30 min
Diazepam*	0.1-0.3 mg/kg (maximum, 10 mg)	2-4 min	30-90 min
Midazolam*	0.05-0.2 mg/kg (maximum, 5 mg)	1-2 min	30-60 min
Fentanyl	2-10 µg/kg[†]	1 min	30-60 min
Propofol	2.5 mg/kg	20 sec	10-15 min
Etomidate	0.2-0.3 mg/kg	30-60 sec	3-10 min

*Administer slowly.
†Variable induction dose.

anaphylaxis, cough, and bronchospasm. Thiopental is contraindicated in patients with porphyria and sensitivity to barbiturates and should be used cautiously in patients with asthma or hypotension.

Ketamine (Ketalar), a derivative of phencyclidine, is a dissociative anesthetic agent. The dissociative anesthetic state is characterized by analgesia, amnesia, dissociation from the environment, maintenance of reflexes, and cardiorespiratory stability. The effects of ketamine are summarized in Table 2-6. Increases in ICP, blood pressure, airway secretions, intraocular pressure, and intragastric pressure may be detrimental in certain airway management situations. Ketamine is not recommended in adolescents and adults because it may cause hallucinations and nightmares known as emergence reactions. Children younger than 11 years have a low incidence (0% to 10%) of emergence reactions. The incidence of emergence reactions can be reduced by the use of a short-acting benzodiazepine, such as midazolam. Laryngospasm is another area of concern in the use of ketamine; the incidence of laryngospasm is increased in infants younger than 3 months and in patients of all ages with an active respiratory infection or a history of tracheal abnormalities.

The main advantages of ketamine over other sedative agents include rapid action, short duration, provision of sedation and analgesia, and preservation of respiratory drive and airway reflexes.

There are two clinical situations in which ketamine should be considered strongly; the first is in the child with asthma and respiratory failure. Ketamine possesses intrinsic bronchodilating activity. The second is in the patient with shock or hypovolemia. Because ketamine is a sympathomimetic agent, it produces no depression of cardiac output (Table 2-6). Contraindications include use in infants younger than 3 months, increased ICP (eg, head injury, mass lesions), globe injury, glaucoma, coronary artery disease, hypertension, active pulmonary infection, tracheal abnormalities, or psychosis.

The pharmacokinetics of ketamine are given in Table 2-5. When given for sedation, ketamine is administered intravenously in a dose of 1 to 2 mg/kg and should be given slowly over 1 minute to prevent respiratory depression. Rapid administration is used for RSI. Ketamine also is commonly given intramuscularly, but it has a wide dosing range. Adherence to a range of 4 to 7 mg/kg intramuscularly will provide adequate sedation and dissociation with a lower incidence of side effects.

Table 2-7 summarizes the clinical conditions in which particular indications for ketamine and thiopental are recommended.

Benzodiazepines are anxiolytic and provide sedation, amnesia, and anticonvulsant properties. They provide no analgesic properties. Adverse effects may include cardiovascular and respiratory depression. The most significant disadvantage of the use of a benzodiazepine for RSI is the broad dosing range and need for titration. Midazolam (Versed), lorazepam (Ativan), and diazepam (Valium) have all been used in RSI. See Table 2-5 for dosages and pharmacokinetic properties. Midazolam has gained popularity over the other benzodiazepines because it has a faster onset and a shorter duration.

Fentanyl (Sublimaze), a short-acting narcotic, has been used as both a premedication and a sedative in RSI. It often is used in combination with a benzodiazepine. The dose for induction of unconsciousness is variable and much higher than

TABLE 2-6.
Effects of ketamine.

Increased oral secretions
Increased intragastric pressure
Increased ICP
Increased blood pressure, heart rate, cardiac output
Increased intraocular pressure
Hypertonicity
Bronchodilation
Emergence reactions

TABLE 2-7.
Clinical conditions and commonly used sedation drugs.

Condition	Ketamine	Thiopental
Head injury	–	+ (And lidocaine)
Hypotension	+	– (Or cut dose)
Bronchospasm	+	–

the premedication dose. Chest wall rigidity has been reported with rapid injection and in doses of >15 µg/kg.

New Sedative Agents

Propofol (Diprivan) is a relatively new anesthetic induction and sedative agent. Propofol has several advantages for use in RSI, including a rapid onset, short duration of action, and cerebroprotective effects similar to those of thiopental (Table 2-5). Propofol can cause decreases in mean arterial blood pressure. The manufacturer currently recommends propofol only for children aged 3 years and older. However, there are a number of reports of the successful use in younger children.

Etomidate (Amidate) is a rapid-onset short-acting sedative-hypnotic agent approved for children older than 10 years. It has the advantage of causing less cardiovascular depression than thiopental or propofol, as well as having similar cerebroprotective qualities. A transient reduction in plasma cortisol and aldosterone levels has been reported after induction with etomidate. See Table 2-5 for pharmacokinetics and dosages. Etomidate also has been used successfully in younger children.

Step 6, Cricoid Pressure (Sellick Maneuver)

The Sellick maneuver was first reported in 1961 as a means to prevent aspiration by passive regurgitation during the intubation of patients with full stomachs. The maneuver consists of placing digital pressure over the cricoid cartilage to occlude the esophagus. A resuscitation team member should be assigned this maneuver as a sole task. Pressure is applied during bag ventilation of an apneic patient or after sedation of a spontaneously breathing patient. Overly vigorous pressure can distort the anatomy and make intubation more difficult. Cricoid pressure is released after intubation and verification of ET tube placement. If vomiting develops during the procedure, cricoid pressure should be released and the patient vigorously suctioned.

Step 7, Muscle Relaxation

Muscle paralysis usually allows easier intubation and ventilation. The muscle relaxant is given in rapid sequence with a sedative agent and can be administered before or after the sedative, depending on the onset of action. The ideal paralytic agent would have a rapid onset, short duration, and minimal side effects and be reversible. Unfortunately, none of the available relaxants meets all of these criteria. There are two categories of agents used for neuromuscular blockade. Table 2-8 provides a summary of the pharmacokinetics of muscle relaxants.

Depolarizing (noncompetitive, nonreversible) relaxants bind to the postsynaptic receptors, resulting in depolarization. Depolarization produces a brief period of repetitive excitation resulting in transient muscle fasciculations. This is followed by a block of neuromuscular transmission and flaccid paralysis. The mechanism is not completely understood.

Succinylcholine (Anectine) is a muscle relaxant commonly used for emergency RSI and the only drug to be discussed in the depolarizing class. A

TABLE 2-8.
Agents for muscle relaxation.

	Dose (IV)	Onset	Duration
Succinylcholine	1.0-2.0 mg/kg (>10 kg) 1.5-2.0 mg/kg (<10 kg)	30-45 sec	4-10 min
Vecuronium	0.2-0.3 mg/kg (RSI) 0.1 mg/kg (standard dose) 0.01 mg/kg (defasciculating dose)	60-90 sec 1.5-2.0 min	90-120 min 25-40 min
Pancuronium	0.1 mg/kg 0.01 mg/kg (defasciculating dose)	2-3 min	45-90 min
Rocuronium	0.8-1.2 mg/kg	45-60 sec	30-45 min

rapid onset of action and short duration are the main reasons for the popularity of this relaxant. Some of the physiologic effects of succinylcholine include increased ICP and intraocular and intragastric pressures; hyperthermia; release of potassium; and muscarinic stimulation of the sinoatrial node resulting in bradycardia (prominent in children). The release of potassium usually is clinically insignificant with the exceptions of patients with burns and massive muscle injury, who may develop significant hyperkalemia from 3 to 60 days after the trauma, and patients with upper motor neuron disease, who are at risk for hyperkalemia from 1 week to 6 months after the onset of illness. Patients also at risk for hyperkalemia are those with muscular dystrophy or a family history of muscular dystrophy.

Fasciculations caused by succinylcholine are seen mainly in muscular adolescents. Fasciculations can cause muscle pain, rhabdomyolysis, myoglobinuria, and increased ICP and intragastric pressure. A defasciculating dose (10% of paralytic dose) of a nondepolarizing muscle relaxant is recommended in children older than 5 years to prevent fasciculations. **Pancuronium** or **vecuronium** (0.01 mg/kg), given 2 to 3 minutes before succinylcholine, is the agent primarily used for this defasciculation step. Table 2-9 summarizes the age groups in which atropine or a defasciculation step is needed before the administration of succinylcholine.

Contraindications for the use of succinylcholine are controversial and include penetrating globe injury, glaucoma, neuromuscular disease, history of malignant hyperthermia, crush injuries, and trauma or burns that are >48 hours old. The rapid onset and short duration of succinylcholine are offset by possible adverse effects; recent recommendations have suggested that other agents are preferred for children.

Nondepolarizing (competitive, reversible) neuromuscular blockers compete with acetylcholine for the postsynaptic receptors but do not activate them. This group is characterized by the absence of muscle fasciculations at the onset of paralysis. Relaxants in this class generally have a slower onset and longer duration of action than succinylcholine (Table 2-8).

Rocuronium (Zemuron) is a relatively new nondepolarizing muscle relaxant with the advantages of rapid onset and vagolytic properties. Studies in which rocuronium was compared with succinylcholine have shown no differences in time to intubation. Many practitioners prefer the use of rocuronium to vecuronium for induction because of the more rapid onset. The dose is 0.8 to 1.2 mg/kg, and the duration is 30 to 45 minutes.

Vecuronium (Norcuron) has been used as an alternative to succinylcholine in emergency RSI. It has minimal cardiovascular effects and produces no histamine release. The duration of action is dependent on the dose given. The standard dose of vecuronium is 0.1 mg/kg; however, recent literature supports the use of a larger dose of vecuronium (0.2 to 0.3 mg/kg) in RSI. This dose produces a more rapid onset of action (60 to 90 seconds), which is advantageous for RSI, but the duration is prolonged to 90 to 120 minutes.

TABLE 2-9.
Paralysis with succinylcholine.

	Atropine	Defasciculation Dose of Nondepolarizer
Infant <1 yr	+	–
1-5 yr	± (Controversial)	–
>5 yr	–	+

FIGURE 2-1.
Flow diagram of suggested sequence for rapid induction in more common clinical situations.

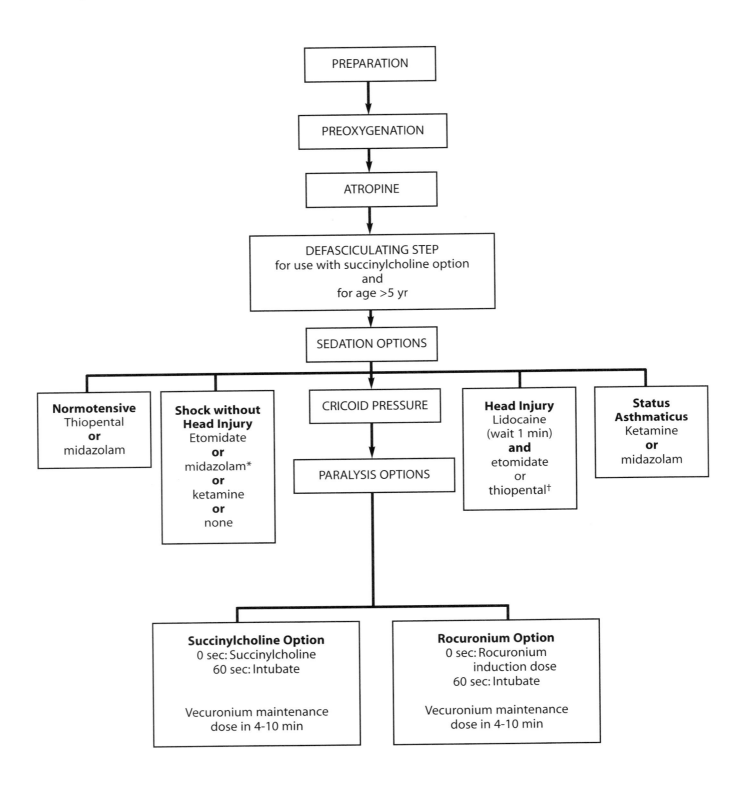

*Use midazolam only in mild shock.
†Decrease dose of thiopental or use none at all if hypotensive.

Nondepolarizing agents are reversible with **neostigmine, edrophonium,** or **pyridostigmine.** Reversal is rarely indicated in the emergency setting. Reversal agents have anticholinesterase activity and allow the concentration of acetylcholine to rise. Atropine usually is given before reversal agents to abort the muscarinic effects (eg, bradycardia, salivation, bronchospasm) of these agents. Reversal should not be attempted until some movement is noted or a peripheral nerve stimulator is used to demonstrate return of function. Depolarizing agents, such as succinylcholine, are not reversible.

There are many factors that influence neuromuscular blockade. Nondepolarizing agents are potentiated by respiratory acidosis, hypokalemia, magnesium, lidocaine, and aminoglycosides. The action of succinylcholine is prolonged by quinine, magnesium, hyperkalemia, alkalosis, hypothermia, decreased or atypical plasma cholinesterase, and aminoglycosides. Muscular stress, as occurs with seizures, shivering, and pronounced respiratory distress, will shorten the onset of action for all paralytics.

Steps 8 Through 10, Intubation, Verification of Placement, Security of Tube

The method of ET intubation is described in Chapter 5. Appropriate ET tube placement is verified with auscultation of bilateral breath sounds, observance for symmetrical chest rise, and chest radiography. Placement also should be confirmed through continuous capnometry. The ET tube is secured with tape.

Step 11, Medical Record Documentation

A detailed procedure note, including all agents used and any complications or injuries, should be added to the medical record.

SUMMARY

RSI should be performed only by physicians who have a complete knowledge of the medications used and are skilled in airway management procedures. Many controversies exist as to which medications should be used and in what order. The physician leader may elect to simplify medication selection by using a limited number of agents that are appropriate for most clinical scenarios. For example, etomidate or midazolam can always be used as the sedative agent, but the dose will need to be lowered in poor perfusion states. Premedications also can be simplified by using atropine for all children, lidocaine for all patients with head trauma, and a defasciculating dose for all children older than 5 years or weighing >20 kg who are receiving succinylcholine as a paralytic. In more emergent situations, certain premedications may be eliminated. A flow diagram summarizing RSI options is helpful in determining the best sequence for an individual patient (Figure 2-1).

ADDITIONAL READING

American Academy of Pediatrics, Committee on Drugs. Drugs for pediatric emergencies. *Pediatrics.* 1998;101:1-11.

Dailey RH, ed. *The Airway: Emergency Management.* St Louis, Mo: Mosby–Year Book; 1992.

Gerardi MJ, Sacchetti AD, Cantor RM, et al. Rapid-sequence intubation of the pediatric patient. *Ann Emerg Med.* 1996;28:55-74.

Gnauck K, Lungo JB, Scalzo A, et al. Emergency intubation of the pediatric medical patient: use of anesthetic agents in the emergency department. *Ann Emerg Med.* 1994;23:1242-1247.

Miller RD, ed. *Anesthesia,* 3rd ed. New York, NY: Churchill Livingstone; 1990.

Morris IR. Pharmacologic aids to intubation and the rapid sequence induction. *Emerg Med Clin North Am.* 1988;6:753-768.

Motoyama EK, Davis PJ, eds. *Smith's Anesthesia for Infants and Children,* 5th ed. St Louis, Mo: Mosby; 1990.

Yamamoto LG. Rapid sequence anesthesia induction and advanced airway management in pediatric patients. *Emerg Med Clin North Am.* 1991;9:611-638.

Yamamoto LG, Yim GK, Britten AG. Rapid sequence anesthesia induction for emergency intubation. *Pediatr Emerg Care.* 1990;6:200-213.

Chapter 3

Shock

OBJECTIVES

1. Explain the basic pathophysiologic mechanisms of shock.

2. Evaluate age-specific vital signs in relation to the stages and treatment of shock.

3. Describe the clinical presentations of the various types of shock.

4. Recognize the subtlety of early pediatric shock and rapid progression to later stages.

5. Discuss the principles and specifics of the management of the various types of shock.

Although the primary cause of infant mortality in the world, beyond the early neonatal period, is dehydration caused by infectious gastroenteritis, death is usually due to shock. Childhood mortality for diarrheal disease in the United States has stabilized at 300 to 400 cases per year since 1985 and principally occurs in infants (78% of cases). In the United States, trauma is the major killer of children older than 1 year, and in many instances, the cause of death is hemorrhagic shock.

The rapid, initial assessment of the child in shock includes elements of the Pediatric Assessment Triangle (Figure 3-1). Appearance reflects the adequacy of perfusion. As perfusion is compromised, the child may become combative and then lethargic, with poor muscle tone and inability to interact normally with parents or caretakers. The circulation to the skin shows overall decreased perfusion as demonstrated by coolness, diaphoresis and change in color (pale, mottled, or blue), and decreased pulses. A child in shock will have an abnormal appearance and decreased circulation to the skin, which reflects inadequate overall perfusion.

The physician must rapidly assess a child for shock and treat it aggressively before the child's condition deteriorates to cardiopulmonary failure. Resuscitative efforts should be directed at reversing the circulatory compromise rapidly and preserving vital organ function to prevent progression to irreversible shock or death. Early, aggressive resuscitation reduces the period of hypoperfusion and reduces the subsequent risk of multiple organ failure.

Types of shock include distributive, hypovolemic, obstructive, cardiogenic, and dissociative. Hypovolemic shock is the most common in children (Table 3-1). Shock also is classified according to the state of physiologic progression that has occurred. In **compensated shock**, vital organ perfusion is maintained via endogenous compensatory mechanisms. **Uncompensated shock** results when compensatory adjustments have failed; it is associated with hypotension and impairment of tissue perfusion. **Irreversible shock** occurs when there is multiple end-organ failure, and death occurs despite the occasional temporary return of spontaneous cardiorespiratory function. In children, arterial blood pressure often is preserved via compensatory vasoconstrictive mechanisms until very late in shock. Pediatric care providers who infrequently evaluate ill children may have difficulty in recognizing early shock. An overreliance on normal arterial blood pressure readings may delay recognition and timely treatment of shock in children.

PATHOPHYSIOLOGY

Shock is a state of circulatory dysfunction resulting in the failure to provide sufficient blood nutrients and oxygen to satisfy the needs of tissues. Less commonly, shock may occur due to the impaired use of these cellular substrates. As a result of the disruption of circulatory function, compensatory mechanisms may temporarily maintain arterial blood pressure at the cost of exacerbating inadequate tissue perfusion. Reduced tissue perfusion further worsens the shock state, ultimately leading to progressive organ failure unless it is rapidly reversed.

Oxygen delivery is a function of oxygen content and cardiac output, so any alteration in the factors that influence these two parameters may reduce tissue oxygenation.

Tissue Hypoxia

Tissue hypoxia results when arterial blood contains a lower-than-normal amount of oxygen. Hypoxia can result from any one or a combination of the following three mechanisms:

- Failure to completely oxygenate the blood in the lungs due to airway or breathing problems.
- Shunting of deoxygenated venous blood so it bypasses the alveoli of the lungs and remains deoxygenated when it reenters the systemic circulation; intracardiac shunting of blood is the mechanism by which cardiovascular

FIGURE 3-1.
Pediatric Assessment Triangle in compensated and decompensated shock.

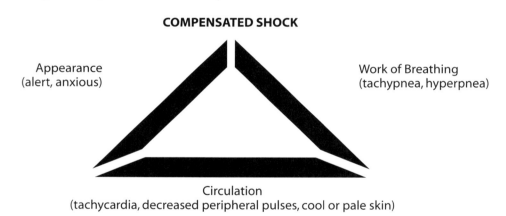

COMPENSATED SHOCK

Appearance
(alert, anxious)

Work of Breathing
(tachypnea, hyperpnea)

Circulation
(tachycardia, decreased peripheral pulses, cool or pale skin)

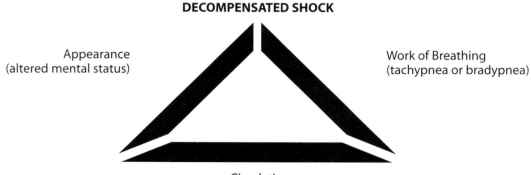

DECOMPENSATED SHOCK

Appearance
(altered mental status)

Work of Breathing
(tachypnea or bradypnea)

Circulation
(tachycardia or bradycardia, absent peripheral pulses, mottled or cyanotic skin)

disorders produce hypoxemia.
- Presence of a low concentration or an abnormal type of hemoglobin that reduces the amount of oxygen that can be carried by the blood.

Anemia can profoundly decrease the amount of oxygen carried to tissues. Transfusion with 10 mL/kg packed red blood cells will raise the hemoglobin level by 1 to 1.5 g/dL. In special circumstances, methemoglobin and carboxyhemoglobin levels are indicated to rule out toxicity from agents producing those compounds (see Chapter 9).

Cardiac Function

Cardiac output is the product of heart rate and stroke volume (Figure 3-2). Adequate cardiac output is required to meet the metabolic needs of the body and to carry away toxins.

Heart rate is determined by the intrinsic pacemaker located in the sinoatrial node and by neural and humoral modulators. Because infants and small children have a limited ability to increase stroke volume, they rely on changes in heart rate to adjust their cardiac output. Sinus tachycardia usually is the first response to most forms of stress. Low heart rates can be problematic because cardiac output decreases substantially.

Stroke volume is determined by preload, contractility, and afterload. It should be adequate to produce a readily palpable pulse in the wrists and ankles. Cold extremities and absent distal pulses are important signs of low stroke volume, poor contractility, and inadequate cardiac output.

Preload is defined by the diastolic pressure or volume or the fiber length of the heart muscle. Preload determines the amount of blood received by the heart. Decreasing the amount of blood flow into the heart lowers the cardiac output. Conversely, increasing the amount of blood flow into the heart increases the cardiac output until the point of maximal ventricular compliance is reached.

Afterload is defined as peak systolic or end-systolic wall stress in the heart. Afterload is best estimated on the basis of mean blood pressure or systemic vascular resistance. Arterial vasoconstriction and vasodilatation are the major determinants of afterload.

Contractility (inotropy) is the ability of the cardiac muscle to pump blood out of the heart; it determines the amount of work that the heart can perform. Increasing cardiac contractility tends to increase stroke volume. Inotropy is also modulated by neural and humoral mechanisms.

Poor coronary artery perfusion results in diminished cardiac performance; however, cardiac ischemia is rare in children. When it occurs, it is necessary to achieve and maintain an adequate mean blood pressure to ensure adequate coronary perfusion and cardiac performance. Signs of diminished coronary perfusion may include tachycardia, bradycardia, hypotension, dysrhythmias, or chest pain and may be associated with signs of impaired perfusion of other organs. Therapy can be titrated through frequent reassessment of these parameters. Vasoactive infusions with α-adrenergic agents, such as neosynephrine, norepinephrine, or epinephrine, can be helpful in raising diastolic pressure and increasing coronary perfusion. Invasive monitoring is indicated for severe, complex, or refractory problems.

THERAPEUTIC IMPLICATIONS

All medical approaches to increasing cardiac output involve modulation of heart rate, preload, afterload, or contractility or restoration of a normally perfusing rhythm.

Oxygen Delivery

Optimal contractility depends on a steady supply of oxygen being delivered to the myocardium during diastole. The factors important in ensuring myocardial oxygen supply are PO_2, hemoglobin (quantity and function), coronary artery perfusion, and cardiac output (Figure 3-2).

Heart Rate

Symptomatic bradycardias are treated with oxygenation, epinephrine or atropine, and, if necessary, a pacemaker. Symptomatic tachycardias must first be differentiated into sinus, supraventricular, or ventricular before specific therapy is initiated.

Preload

In most cases of shock, absolute or relative hypovolemia results in decreased preload. In congestive heart failure and cardiogenic shock, preload can be excessive. Diuretic agents can be

TABLE 3-1.
Common causes of shock in children.

Type	Primary Insult	Common Causes	Treatment
Hypovolemic	Decreased circulating blood volume	Dehydration	Oral rehydration IV or IO rehydration
		Hemorrhage (see Chapter 5)	Direct pressure IV or IO rehydration Stabilization of fractures Transfusion Surgical control of internal hemorrhage
Distributive	Vasodilation	Sepsis	IV or IO rehydration Antibiotic therapy (see Table 3-3)
		Anaphylaxis	Oxygen IV access and rehydration Cessation of antigen exposure Epinephrine SQ/IM/IV Steroids Antihistamines H_1 antagonists H_2 antagonists Pressors Inhaled β-agonists
		Drug intoxication (see Chapter 9)	Prevention or minimization of absorption Gastric lavage Activated charcoal Whole bowel irrigation Enhancement of excretion Ion trapping Urine acidification Urine alkalinization Neutral diuresis Multidose charcoal Hemodialysis Hemoperfusion Specific antidotes Supportive care
		Spinal cord injury (see Chapter 7)	Airway support Immobilization IV or IO rehydration Inotropic support Methylprednisolone

TABLE 3-1. (Continued)
Common causes of shock in children.

Type	Primary Insult	Common Causes	Treatment
Obstructive	Obstruction of cardiac filling	Cardiac tamponade (see Chapter 5)	Pericardiocentesis (see Appendix 5-2) Pericardial window Thoracotomy and pericardiotomy
		Tension pneumothorax (see Chapter 5)	Needle thoracostomy (see Appendix 5-5) followed by tube thoracostomy
		Pulmonary embolism	Oxygen Anticoagulation Embolectomy
Cardiogenic	Decreased contractility	Congenital heart disease (see Chapter 4)	Oxygen Fluid bolus Cardiology consultation Inotropic support Diuretic agents for congestive heart failure PGE_1 for shunt-dependent lesions
		Myocarditis (see Chapter 4)	Upright position Oxygen Fluid restriction Diuresis Inotropic support Antidysrhythmic agents Cardiology consultation
		Dysrhythmias (see Chapter 4)	Bradycardia Oxygen Epinephrine Atropine Pacer Tachycardia Cardioversion Antidysrhythmic agents
Dissociative	Oxygen not released from hemoglobin	Carbon monoxide intoxication (see Chapter 9)	Oxygen Hyperbaric oxygen
		Methemoglobinemia	Oxygen Cessation of exposure Methylene blue Exchange transfusion Hyperbaric oxygen

used cautiously to reduce preload in these situations.

Acidosis

At very low pH levels (<7.0), myocardial contractility may be adversely affected. For metabolic acidosis that persists after hypovolemia has been corrected, 1 to 2 mEq/kg sodium bicarbonate given slowly over several minutes can rapidly improve contractility. For respiratory acidosis, intubation and mechanical ventilation are useful for correcting hypercapnia and decreasing the metabolic demand generated by the patient's work of breathing.

Temperature

A markedly elevated temperature increases oxygen consumption significantly and may result in decompensation of an otherwise marginal cardiovascular system. Shivering also increases oxygen consumption by as much as two to three times that of normal. A neutral thermal environment must be maintained to avoid the stresses of hypothermia or hyperthermia.

Stress

With stable patients, parents can hold and comfort the child to minimize excess oxygen demand caused by agitation. The diagnostic work-up can proceed at a more leisurely pace, with invasive procedures, such as rectal temperature measurements and venipuncture, well timed and kept to a minimum. For intubated and ventilated patients, appropriate sedation, pain management, and neuromuscular blockade are necessary.

Hypoglycemia

Impairment of glucose metabolism frequently occurs during stressful situations and can further compromise myocardial contractility. A serum glucose level of <40 mg/dL is an indication for rapid correction with 2 to 4 mL/kg $D_{25}W$ for infants younger than 2 years. For neonates, 2 to 4 mL/kg, $D_{10}W$ is used. For patients older than 2 years, 1 to 2 mL/kg $D_{50}W$ can be used.

Electrolyte Abnormalities

Electrolyte abnormalities can cause or complicate both inotropic and chronotropic problems. During acute illnesses, routine screening of potassium,

FIGURE 3-2.
Determinants of cardiac function and oxygen delivery to tissues.

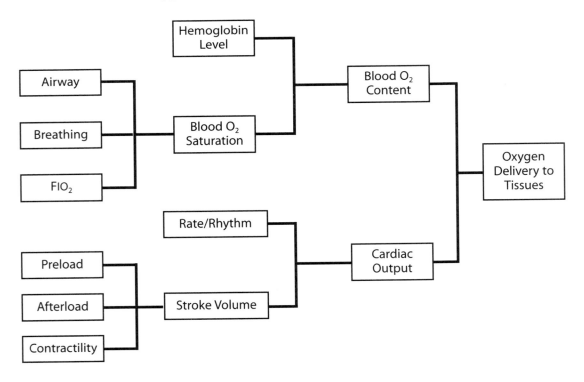

calcium, magnesium, sodium, chloride, bicarbonate, and phosphate levels is indicated.

HEMODYNAMICALLY UNSTABLE PATIENTS

The initial management of a child in shock follows certain priorities, regardless of the cause. Airway, breathing, cardiovascular, and neurologic parameters are evaluated rapidly to determine the patient's stability so those in impending arrest situations can receive prompt supportive care. Patency of the airway, adequacy of chest wall expansion, and breath sounds should be assessed and corrected if abnormal. High-flow oxygen in a concentration of 100% is initiated immediately and maintained until the child is stabilized. Pulse oximetry provides an instantaneous assessment of heart rate and oxygenation, but it requires a pulsatile vascular bed and may be unobtainable in patients in severe shock. Children in severe shock may require immediate endotracheal intubation to reduce the work of breathing and increase oxygen delivery. During the initial assessment, a cardiac monitor is placed to determine and monitor the cardiac rate and rhythm.

The next priority should be intravenous access or, failing that, intraosseous access for patients younger than 6 years. Current clinical data demonstrate widespread success with intraosseous fluid and drug administration in infants and young children by both in-hospital and out-of-hospital providers.

The rapid administration of 0.9% saline or lactated Ringer's at a dose of 20 mL/kg allows earlier assessment of response to therapy than when administration is by slower infusion. Children may require three or more rapid fluid pushes (≥60 mL/kg) to improve perfusion during hypovolemic shock. Traumatized children also may require the administration of packed red blood cells (initial dose, 10 mL/kg) if they do not respond adequately to 40 mL/kg fluid. Emerging evidence indicates little benefit and some risk of further hemorrhage when overzealous fluid resuscitation is used in trauma patients before definitive control of bleeding. There is no reason to delay initial fluid pushes to measure central venous or pulmonary artery wedge pressure. Isolated central venous pressure measurements are not predictive of the volume status of patients. The occasional child with congestive heart failure and cardiogenic shock will still benefit from increased left ventricular filling pressure as a result of a fluid bolus.

Clinical Signs of Inadequate Cardiac Output

Inadequate perfusion produces signs of dysfunction in one or more organ systems. The diagnosis of shock is based on an assessment of the patient's skin perfusion and mental status, followed by palpation of distal pulses. **Pallor, cyanosis**, and **mottling** are usually present. The **hands and feet are cold** and, with worsening perfusion, the coolness of the extremities progressively worsens and advances proximally. **Capillary refill** is a widely used initial physiologic parameter that in general can be assessed and repeated more often than other vital signs. A delay of palmar or dorsal foot refill of >2 seconds, after gentle pressure, may be consistent with shock. When assessed at the nailbeds, pressure just sufficient to remove coloration results in a mean capillary refill time of 1 second in newborns. It should be remembered that a delay in capillary refill time also may be seen under cool ambient

TABLE 3-2.
Estimation of blood loss in childhood hemorrhagic shock.*

	Stage			
	1	**2**	**3**	**4**
Blood loss (%)	<15	15-20	25-40	>40
Capillary refill (sec)	≤2	>2	>5	>5
Sensorium	Normal	Irritable	Lethargy	Unresponsive
Heart rate	Normal	Increase	Increase	±
Pulse pressure	Normal	Normal/decrease	Decrease	Decrease
Systolic blood pressure	Normal	Normal	Normal/decrease	Decrease
Urinary output	Normal	Normal/decrease	Decrease	Absent

*Assuming a blood volume of ≈80 mL/kg.

TABLE 3-3.
Most common pathogens in childhood bacterial sepsis.

Age Group	Pathogens (pending cultures)	Antimicrobial	Initial Dose (mg/kg)
0-1 mo	Group B *Streptococcus*, *Enterobacteriaceae*, *Staphylococcus aureus*, *Listeria monocytogenes*, *Staphylococcus epidermidis*	Ampicillin + gentamicin **or** ampicillin + cefotaxime	50-100 2.5 50-100 50
1-3 mo	Group B *Streptococcus*, *S. aureus*, *Streptococcus pneumoniae*, *Haemophilus influenzae*	Ampicillin + cefotaxime **or** ampicillin + ceftriaxone **or** ampicillin + chloramphenicol*	50-100 50 50-100 50-100 50-100 25
3-24 mo	*S. pneumoniae*, *Neisseria meningitidis*, *H. influenzae*, *S. aureus*	Cefotaxime **or** ceftriaxone **or** ampicillin + chloramphenicol*	50 50-100 50-100 25
>24 mo	*S. pneumoniae*, *H. influenzae*, *S. aureus*, *N. meningitidis*	Cefotaxime **or** ceftriaxone **or** ampicillin + chloramphenicol*	50 50-100 50-100 25
Immuno-compromised	*S. aureus*, *Proteus*, *Pseudomonas*, *Enterobacteriaceae*	Vancomycin + ceftazidime + ticarcillin	15 50 75

*Primarily used in parts of the world in which cephalosporins are unavailable.

temperature conditions or when excessive pressure is applied.

The measurement of **blood pressure** should be performed after the initial assessment. Normal values for children of varying ages are listed in Table 4-3. Hypotension in the setting of shock indicates decompensation.

Mental status may be only mildly impaired, with the child exhibiting apathy or lethargy but still recognizing the parents. As mental status impairment progresses, the child may fail to respond to venipuncture and other painful procedures. Movement is minimal or absent. Children with impaired mental status should be maintained in a supine position.

Urine output is closely correlated with renal perfusion and should be maintained at >1 mL/kg per hour.

Sinus tachycardia is an early compensatory mechanism. Hypotension occurs late in shock in infants and children. Laboratory findings initially may be normal but will demonstrate metabolic acidosis, as shock progresses.

HYPOVOLEMIC SHOCK

Hypovolemic shock results from decreased intravascular volume, which causes reduced venous return and preload. Loss of blood, plasma, and water may be responsible for this most common form of childhood shock. The percentage of blood loss from hemorrhage may be estimated (Table 3-2), although data to support this subcategorization in children are scant. A rapid head-to-toe survey is conducted to search for sites of bleeding. In the setting of trauma, hemorrhage into the chest, abdomen, or pelvis may be present.

Because the average blood volume in small children is 80 mL/kg, limited volumes of external or internal hemorrhage may result in shock. For example, a blood loss of only 200 mL in a 10-kg child (total blood volume, 800 mL) represents a 25% decrease in blood volume. Thus, rapid control of ongoing blood loss is vital to successful resuscitation of infants and children.

Recognition of the child in less severe stages of shock can be difficult. Typical early signs and symptoms of shock in infants are lethargy, poor feeding, decreased responsiveness, pale skin, delayed capillary refill, tachycardia, and oliguria. For children dehydrated as a result of

gastroenteritis, assessment of the extent of vomiting and diarrhea (frequency and amount of each) may raise or lower the level of suspicion for shock. Children with diabetic ketoacidosis frequently present with severe dehydration, often with volume deficits of ≥20%. They typically have a history of polydipsia and polyuria and findings of abdominal pain, tachypnea, lethargy, tachycardia, and an acetone-like odor.

DISTRIBUTIVE SHOCK

Distributive shock is caused by vasodilatation resulting in relative hypovolemia. The most common causes of distributive shock are sepsis and neurologic injury; other causes include anaphylaxis (Table 3-1), spinal cord injury (see Chapter 7), and some drug intoxications (eg, iron and cyclic antidepressants) (see Chapter 9).

Septic shock is caused by microorganisms or their products in the blood, which lead to decreased vascular resistance and relative hypovolemia. Gram-negative bacteria are the most common microorganisms associated with septic shock (Table 3-3), although Gram-positive bacteria, viruses, rickettsia, fungi, and protozoa also may be responsible. Invasive group A streptococcal infections, producing a toxic shock–like syndrome, have been described in children with varicella and cellulitis. Risk factors for septic shock include immunodeficiency, asplenia, sickle cell disease, and indwelling catheters.

Early in sepsis, a period of high cardiac output and low systemic resistance is associated with fever, tachycardia, bounding pulses, elevated cardiac index, mild confusion, normal capillary refill, warm extremities, respiratory alkalosis, and decreased systemic vascular resistance. During late septic shock, characteristics of severe shock develop that are largely indistinguishable from those of cardiogenic shock. Endotoxins are lipopolysaccharides that are released during septic shock, along with other vasoactive mediators. These products lead to systemic vasodilatation, myocardial depression, leaky capillaries, decreased oxygen extraction, cytokine activation, and derangement in intermediary metabolism. Rapid evaluation and treatment should include patient isolation, supportive measures for shock, blood culture, and antimicrobial coverage.

The rapid administration of empiric

antimicrobial therapy should not be delayed for complete diagnostic evaluation in children with suspected sepsis or meningitis. The initial antimicrobial agent chosen depends on age, suspected organism, and immunocompetency (Table 3-3). Resistance of invasive strains of *Streptococcus pneumoniae* to penicillin and cephalosporins has increased over the past few years. Because vancomycin is the only antibiotic to which all strains of *S. pneumoniae* are susceptible, vancomycin in combination with a broad-spectrum cephalosporin is recommended when resistant organisms are suspected. When possible, obtaining a blood culture before antimicrobial therapy is beneficial in determining subsequent treatment. Children should be stabilized, however, before undergoing any further diagnostic work-up. When stable, samples of spinal fluid, urine, and fluid from potentially infected sites (eg, indwelling vascular catheter) for Gram stain and culture should be obtained along with routine hematologic and chemistry tests. The presence of fever and petechiae (particularly when isolated to the trunk or lower extremities), even in well-appearing children, raises the issue of meningococcemia or other bacteremia or disseminated intravascular coagulopathy. Rapid evaluation and treatment should include patient isolation, supportive measures for shock, blood culture, coagulation studies, and antimicrobial coverage.

OBSTRUCTIVE SHOCK

Obstructive shock is caused by impairment of cardiac filling and may occur with pericardial tamponade, tension pneumothorax, or massive pulmonary embolus. When shock occurs suddenly and coincident with distended neck veins and cardiomegaly in a patient with a penetrating chest injury or a history of cardiac surgery, pericardial tamponade is likely. Rapid relief of severe shock from pericardial tamponade can be provided at the bedside with or without confirmation of excess pericardial fluid through echocardiography. With the subxiphoid approach, a long needle pointed at the left shoulder is advanced slowly during aspiration with a syringe. To relieve tension pneumothorax, an angiocatheter may be advanced over the second rib in the midclavicular line simultaneously with aspiration with a syringe. The patient should be carefully monitored during each

of these procedures, if time permits (see Chapter 5, Appendices 2 and 5).

CARDIOGENIC SHOCK

Cardiogenic shock (see Chapter 4) is uncommon in children. Although a variety of conditions may lead to cardiogenic shock, congestive heart failure secondary to congenital heart disease, myocarditis, or tachydysrhythmias, such as supraventricular tachycardia (SVT), is most common. In children who have ductal-dependent congenital heart disease, such as tricuspid atresia, aortic coarctation, and transposition of the great vessels, shock develops during the first few months of life. As the ductus arteriosus closes, the sudden increase in afterload elevates ventricular wall tension and reduces myocardial perfusion. Infusion of prostaglandin E_1 (PGE_1) vasodilates the ductus arteriosus, temporarily reversing the severe afterload caused by a closing ductus. The dosage of PGE_1 begins at 0.05 µg/kg per minute and then is titrated to a maximum of 0.2 µg/kg per minute.

Presenting signs and symptoms of cardiogenic shock are similar to those of other forms of shock, except that these children usually have hepatomegaly, jugular venous distention, cardiomegaly, and a gallop rhythm. Infants with congestive failure may present with poor feeding, failure to gain weight, sweating during feedings, and SVT in addition to signs of poor perfusion. A 12-lead ECG may demonstrate low voltage or diffuse ST-T wave changes in children with myocarditis or marked ventricular hypertrophy in congenital heart disease, and a chest radiograph may show cardiomegaly. Additional findings in children with aortic coarctation include a systolic ejection murmur, reduced femoral pulses, and upper extremity hypertension. For children with shock associated with tachydysrhythmias, differentiation of SVT from ventricular tachycardia and their treatments are discussed in Chapter 4.

Vasoactive drug therapy should not be initiated in the child with shock until the airway is controlled, the child is being ventilated and oxygenated, and intravascular volume has been replaced. After optimization of preload and metabolic parameters, patients with severe heart failure or cardiogenic shock require aggressive therapy with vasoactive infusions to enhance contractility and cardiac output.

Dopamine has been a first-line treatment for many years. At low doses (2 to 5 μg/kg per minute), dopamine enhances renal blood flow and urinary output and produces a small increase in cardiac output. At midrange doses (6 to 10 μg/kg per minute), its β-adrenergic effect improves contractility and increases heart rate. In high doses (>10 μg/kg per minute), its α-adrenergic effect produces vasoconstriction to correct hypotension.

Epinephrine has replaced dopamine as the initial infusion of choice in a crisis situation at many institutions. The β_1 and β_2 effects usually predominate at low doses (0.05 to 0.1 μg/kg per minute). For severe hypotension, α-adrenergic effects can be rapidly achieved by further increases in dosage.

Dobutamine is useful to increase contractility without increasing systemic vascular resistance. Its vasodilatory effects and lack of α-adrenergic effect limit its usefulness as a single agent to situations in which cardiac output is low but blood pressure remains normal.

Nitroprusside (0.5 to 5 μg/kg per minute) can be useful in increasing stroke volume through afterload reduction. It is necessary to monitor arterial pressure continuously to titrate and evaluate the effects of this medication, so its use is often reserved for the intensive care unit.

Rules of 6 and 0.6

The rules of 6 and 0.6 simplify the computation of dosage for vasoactive infusions and minimize the amount of fluid given to infants. For dopamine, dobutamine, nitroprusside, and lidocaine, a 6 mg/kg concentration of medication is mixed with D_5W to produce a final volume of 100 mL. An infusion at a rate of 1 mL/hr provides 1 μg/kg per minute. For epinephrine, isoproterenol, neosynephrine, norepinephrine, and PGE_1, a concentration of 0.6 mg/kg is diluted to 100 mL. An infusion rate of 1 mL/hr provides 0.1 μg/kg per minute.

DISSOCIATIVE SHOCK

Dissociative shock is caused by the inability of hemoglobin to carry or discharge oxygen to tissue, as occurs with methemoglobinemia or carbon monoxide poisoning. Methemoglobinemia should be considered in patients with no discernible heart disease who remain cyanotic in 100% oxygen.

Intoxication with carbon monoxide is suspected in patients with persistent shock after smoke inhalation. Treatment of carbon monoxide poisoning includes standard shock measures and hyperbaric oxygen when neurologic insults or cardiovascular compromise is present (see Chapter 9).

ADDITIONAL READING

American Academy of Pediatrics, Provisional Committee on Quality Improvement, Subcommittee on Acute Gastroenteritis. Practice Parameter: The management of acute gastroenteritis in young children. *Pediatrics.* 1996;97:424-435.

Atici A, Satar M, Alparslan N. Serum interleukin-1 beta in neonatal sepsis. *Acta Pediatr.* 1996;85:371-374.

Carcillo JA, Davis AL, Zaristky A. Role of early fluid resuscitation in pediatric septic shock. *JAMA.* 1991;266:1242-1245.

Inaba AS, Seward PN. An approach to pediatric trauma: unique anatomic and pathophysiologic aspects of the pediatric patient. *Emerg Med Clin North Am.* 1991;9:523-548.

Jacobs RF, Sowell MK, Moss MM, Fiser DH. Septic shock in children: bacterial etiologies and temporal relationships. *Pediatr Infect Dis J.* 1990;9:196-200.

Kallen RJ, Lonergan JM. Fluid resuscitation of acute hypovolemic hypoperfusion states in pediatrics. *Pediatr Clin North Am.* 1990;37:287-294.

Moses AE, Ziv A, Harari M, Rahav G, Shapiro M, Engelhard D. Increased incidence and severity of *Streptococcus pyogenes* bacteremia in young children. *Pediatr Infect Dis J.* 1995;14:767-770.

Perkin RM, Anas NG. Cardiovascular evaluation and support in the critically ill child. *Pediatr Ann.* 1986;15:30-41.

Press S, Lipkind RS. Acute myocarditis in infants. *Clin Pediatr.* 1990;29:73-76.

Saez-Llorens X, Vargas S, Guerra F, Coronado L. Application of new sepsis definitions to evaluate outcome of pediatric patients with severe systemic infections. *Pediatr Infect Dis J.* 1995;14:557-561.

Teach SJ, Antosia RE, Lund DP, Fleisher GR. Prehospital fluid therapy in pediatric trauma patients. *Pediatr Emerg Care.* 1995;11:5-8.

Wetzel RC. Shock. In: Rogers MC, ed. *Textbook of Pediatric Intensive Care.* Baltimore, Md: Williams & Wilkins; 1987;483-524.

Witte MK, Hill JH, Blumer JL. Shock in the pediatric patient. *Adv Pediatr.* 1987;34:139-174.

Zimmermann JJ, Dietrich KA. Current perspectives on septic shock. *Pediatr Clin North Am.* 1987;34:131-163.

Chapter 4

Cardiovascular Disorders

OBJECTIVES

1. Recognize previously undiagnosed congenital and acquired heart disease.

2. Anticipate acute medical problems associated with known cardiovascular disorders.

3. Rapidly evaluate the cardiac output and hemodynamic stability of infants and children.

4. Select appropriate agents for increasing cardiac output by modulating heart rate, preload, afterload, and contractility.

5. Optimize metabolic parameters in patients with acute cardiac compromise.

Cardiovascular dysfunction in infants and children may result from a primary cardiac disorder or be a secondary effect of a noncardiac problem. Unlike adults, children rarely present with emergencies due to primary cardiovascular disorders. Cardiovascular embarrassment in children is much more commonly a result of other insults, such as trauma, respiratory disorders, infections, and poisonings.

Emergency and primary care providers are challenged with timely recognition, stabilization, and referral of infants and children with cardiovascular disease. Problems encountered range from the asymptomatic, such as discovery of a murmur, to the life threatening, such as cardiogenic shock.

Traditionally, cardiovascular disorders of infants and children are classified according to etiology (congenital versus acquired), anatomy (shunt, obstruction, transposition, or complex), and physiology (cyanotic versus noncyanotic, with or without persistent fetal circulation). This chapter classifies pediatric heart diseases according to their clinical presentation. There are two broad categories of patients: those with previously undiagnosed cardiovascular disease (Table 4-1) and those with known heart problems.

The **previously undiagnosed** category is subdivided into four groups. The **hemodynamically unstable** group requires immediate supportive care, even before a definitive diagnosis can be established. The **stable symptomatic** group requires optimization of metabolic parameters before hospitalization. The **stable asymptomatic** group has problems, such as murmurs, that are discovered on routine examination and can be referred to a pediatrician or pediatric cardiologist for elective outpatient evaluation. Finally, **sudden death** from heart disease is rare in children. Family counseling should include reassurance that resuscitative attempts were timely and appropriate, that efforts will be made to determine the cause, and that follow-up counseling will be available.

Children with known heart disease present with routine illnesses and trauma, as well as with acute cardiovascular complications. Once parents notify medical personnel that their child has a heart problem, the physician can anticipate a set of special problems, which are discussed below. Most children in this category have normal immune systems and tolerate common childhood infectious illnesses quite well. Children with severe cardiac disease, such as uncorrected cyanotic heart lesions, are less resilient and can decompensate during an otherwise minor illness.

Adequate cardiovascular function is required for circulation and delivery of oxygen to the tissues of the body. In periods of stress, increased cardiac output is required. The myocardium of the neonate and infant is less efficient than that of the child or adult, and therefore major increases in cardiac output depend on increasing rate rather than stroke volume. For a more extensive discussion of determinants of cardiac function, see Chapter 3.

HEMODYNAMICALLY UNSTABLE PATIENTS

The initial approach to the hemodynamically unstable patient with a cardiovascular disorder is the same as that for patients with other forms of shock (see Chapter 3). Airway, breathing, circulation, and neurologic parameters are evaluated, in that order, and resuscitative measures are immediately taken as indicated. Intravenous or intraosseous access and fluid resuscitation are initiated. The occasional child with congestive heart failure and cardiogenic shock will still benefit from increased left ventricular filling pressure as a result of a fluid bolus.

Shunt-Dependent Congenital Lesions

Immediately after delivery, flow ceases through the umbilical arteries and veins. As the lungs inflate, pulmonary vascular resistance decreases and pulmonary blood flow increases. Immediately after birth, pulmonary vascular resistance is at or near systemic resistance, but it rapidly falls to near adult levels by 2 months of age. The ductus arteriosus and foramen ovale close; both, however, are capable of reopening under stressful conditions until they permanently seal.

As many as 1% of babies are born with one or more congenital heart anomalies. Many of these lesions are trivial, but a few are severe enough to become incompatible with life once the ductus arteriosus begins to close. With pulmonary atresia, for example, blood will be prevented from reaching

the lungs. With severe coarctation of the aorta, critical aortic stenosis, and hypoplastic left ventricle, on the other hand, blood will be prevented from reaching the systemic circulation. Both cyanotic and acyanotic lesions can present in this fashion within the first 2 weeks of life. Chapter 23 includes a discussion of cardiac diseases of the neonate that are likely to present in the first few weeks of life. Infants may present with hypotension, poor distal pulses and perfusion, decreased renal function, and severe metabolic acidosis. Cardiogenic shock is an ominous finding.

All shunt-dependent lesions require immediate surgical intervention for definitive repair or a palliative shunt. Infusions of **prostaglandin E₁** (**PGE₁**) are successful in reopening the ductus arteriosus in a large number of these patients, so repair can be postponed for several days, or even weeks if necessary. PGE_1 is initially infused at a rate of 0.05 to 0.1 µg/kg per minute. If there is no

---

TABLE 4-1.
Classification of pediatric cardiovascular disorders: new presentation of previously undiagnosed cardiovascular disease.

Unstable
  Shunt-dependent lesions
  Acquired cardiogenic shock
  Shock due to left heart obstruction
  Tachycardia
  Bradycardia
  Myocarditis/pericarditis*
Stable Symptomatic
  Cyanosis
  Congestive failure
  Febrile illness
  Chest pain
  Syncope
Stable Asymptomatic
  Growth failure
  Heart murmur
  Congenital syndromes
  Hypertension
  Abnormal pulses
Sudden Death/Syncope
  Prolonged QT syndrome
  Hypertrophic cardiomyopathies
  Coronary abnormalities (Kawasaki disease)
  Congenital heart disease
  Pulmonary hypertension
  Postoperative cardiac patients

*Presentation is variable and may range from stable to sudden death.

improvement within several minutes, the rate is increased progressively to 0.2 µg/kg per minute. The minimal effective dosage is used to minimize the risk of adverse effects, which include apnea, hypotension, fever, flushing, diarrhea, and seizures. Intubation and ventilatory support often are necessary.

Cardiogenic Shock from Acquired Cardiomyopathies

Cardiomyopathies are uncommon disorders but noteworthy because they may cause severe disability or death. Most cases are idiopathic, but a specific cause can sometimes be determined (Table 4-2).

Cardiomyopathies in children are usually classified into two groups: **dilated** and **hypertrophic**. Presentation varies from asymptomatic (cardiomegaly discovered on chest radiograph) to congestive heart failure, cardiogenic shock, or sudden death. Often, the child restricts his or her activity for a period of time. Then, during a febrile illness, there is an acute decompensation in cardiac output, and the child presents in extremis.

Dilated cardiomyopathies are discussed in more detail in "Congestive Heart Failure." Hypertrophied cardiomyopathies are described in "Sudden Death."

Dysrhythmias

Dysfunction of the electrical activity of the heart is suspected when an abnormality of the cardiac rate (Table 4-3) or rhythm is noted. Dysrhythmias often are paroxysmal with an abrupt onset and offset; they may interfere with cardiac output in an insidious or abrupt manner. Depending on the severity of the cardiac compromise, signs of congestive heart failure, low cardiac output, or sudden cardiovascular collapse may be seen.

Tachydysrhythmias

The heart rate of the normal newborn is 85 to 205 beats/min while awake and 80 to 160 beats/min during sleep. The most common rhythm disturbance in children is **sinus tachycardia**. Rates of 200 beats/min occur frequently in children up to age 5 years. Tachycardia usually results from benign causes such as exercise, crying, anxiety, or fever. Less common but more serious causes that should be considered are hypovolemia, pain, poisons, sepsis, and anemia.

The ECG demonstrates the usual sinus morphology: all P waves are normal in configuration (upright in lead II), QRS complexes are preceded by a P wave, and the QRS and T-wave characteristics are unaltered. Sinus tachycardia usually does not exceed 220 beats/min, even in small infants. Sinus tachycardia usually abates once the stress ceases. Sinus tachycardia that persists with no apparent inciting cause may be indicative of occult cardiac dysfunction, as occurs with myocarditis or an unrecognized noncardiac problem such as hypovolemia.

Supraventricular tachycardia (SVT) refers to a group of dysrhythmias caused by dysfunction of the cardiac conduction system at the level of the atria or the atrioventricular node. Abnormal conduction pathways that cause persistent retransmission of the

---

TABLE 4-2.
Causes of cardiomyopathy.

Autoimmune disorder
Collagen vascular disorder
Drugs and toxins
Endocrine disorder
Genetic disorder
Granulomatous disorder
Idiopathic
Infection
Inflammatory disorder
Metabolic disorder
Neoplasm
Neuromuscular disorder
Nutritional disorder

TABLE 4-3.
Usual ranges for awake heart rate and blood pressure for children.

Age	Heart Rate (beats/min)	Blood Pressure (mm Hg)
Neonate	85-205	60-80 by palpation
1 yr	100-130	80/40 to 105/70
5 yr	80-110	80/50 to 110/80
10 yr	70-100	90/55 to 130/85
15 yr	60-80	95/60 to 140/90
Adult	60-80	100/60 to 140/90

same electrical signal back and forth between the atria and the ventricles (reentry) are probably the most common cause of SVT in children. SVT can also occur when an abnormal site in the atrium begins to generate electrical signals on its own (automaticity). This latter phenomenon is less common but is frequently associated with structural heart defects and previous cardiac surgery. The site and mechanism of the conduction disturbance are used to subclassify SVTs. Distinguishing the subtypes may be useful to guide therapy, as with the selection of agents for Wolff-Parkinson-White (WPW) syndrome, or to determine the prognosis, but such differentiation is not usually possible before restoration of normal rhythm with rapidly acting pharmaceutical agents or cardioversion.

Differentiation of sinus rhythm from SVT can be difficult. The following features favor SVT:

- Nonvarying heart rate of >220 beats/min
- Abnormal P-wave axis (ie, inverted in leads II, III, and aVF and upright in leads I and aVL)
- Structural heart disease
- History of WPW syndrome

Patients with SVT usually have a sudden onset of tachycardia that may produce anxiety, irritability, pallor, or chest pain. Cessation of the dysrhythmia usually produces rapid resolution of the symptoms. Persistent or severe tachycardia can cause progressive cardiac dysfunction and ultimately lead to death.

Continuous ECG monitoring is necessary for all patients with SVT. A 12-lead ECG recording is made before and after therapeutic interventions.

If the infant is hypotensive and unresponsive to pain, emergency **synchronized cardioversion** is indicated. An initial energy dose of 0.5 to 1.0 J/kg is administered. The dose is doubled if the initial attempt at cardioversion is unsuccessful. Most infants with SVT are sufficiently stable to tolerate initiation of a peripheral intravenous line in preparation for administration of adenosine. The first dose is 0.1 mg/kg, with repeat doses of 0.2 mg/kg as necessary, to a maximum dose of 12 mg. Because the half-life is <10 seconds, adenosine is administered by rapid push, followed immediately by a rapid bolus of at least 2 to 5 mL of normal saline. Adenosine transiently impairs atrioventricular nodal conduction and slows sinus nodal automaticity via a direct cellular effect, producing a brief pause or bradycardia before there

is a return of normal sinus rhythm.

Failure of SVT to resolve with adenosine suggests a dosing error, slow administration, or refractory SVT. Failure to convert, however, must be differentiated from immediate recurrence. Administration of digoxin before repeating the dose of adenosine may prevent recurrence. Rarer forms of SVT and other dysrhythmias that can mimic SVT (eg, ventricular tachycardia [VT]) may not respond to adenosine. The ECG must be reviewed to ensure the diagnosis is correct. Certain medications, such as theophylline, can also affect the activity of adenosine and require substantial modification of the dosage.

Alternate therapies include vagal stimulation, digoxin, esmolol, neosynephrine, and verapamil. In the stable child, initial therapy can be vagal maneuvers, which include the application of ice water to the face with the use of a towel or plastic bag for <30 seconds. This technique tends to be more effective in infants who are already receiving digoxin, propranolol, or other long-term therapy. In older children, 5 to 10 seconds of unilateral carotid pressure can be effective. Repeated vagal maneuvers may be required. Ocular pressure is contraindicated because of the risk of retinal detachment. Verapamil is not used in infants under the age of 2 years, and esmolol should be used with caution in infants. Conversion with an overdrive pacemaker also is safe and effective.

For many years, digoxin was the medication of choice for SVT in pediatric patients. The onset of action for digoxin is 4 to 6 hours. Verapamil has a rapid onset of action but is contraindicated in children younger than 2 years because it can produce hypotension, ventricular fibrillation, or asystole and is a significant negative inotrope. Neither verapamil nor digoxin is recommended for use in WPW syndrome.

Atrial flutter and **atrial fibrillation** are uncommon dysrhythmias in children even in the presence of underlying heart disease. Atrial flutter is characterized by sawtooth-appearing flutter waves on the ECG. Atrial fibrillation produces an irregular rhythm with no discernible P waves. Both can interfere with cardiac output by interfering with blood flow from the atria to the ventricles and inducing rapid ventricular rates. Immediate cardioversion is indicated for patients with serious symptoms. Digoxin or procainamide can be used to treat stable patients.

A wide QRS tachycardia (>0.14 second) in children indicates ventricular tachycardia until proved otherwise. Usually, the T waves are in the opposite direction from the QRS complexes. VT can sometimes mimic SVT.

Findings in VT range from minimal to pulselessness. If the patient has a good pulse, satisfactory blood pressure, and no signs of serious compromise, drug therapy with lidocaine (1.0 mg/kg) is administered as an intravenous bolus. The initial dose of lidocaine can be repeated in 5 to 10 minutes and again in another 5 to 10 minutes if VT persists. The total of all lidocaine boluses should not exceed 3.0 to 5.0 mg/kg. If lidocaine is effective, a maintenance infusion is initiated at a rate of 20 to 50 µg/kg per minute. Procainamide and then bretylium can be used as further therapy. Patients who are unresponsive or hypotensive require immediate synchronized cardioversion, beginning with 0.5 J/kg. Repeated attempts at cardioversion with a dose of 1 J/kg may be required. If cardioversion is unsuccessful, lidocaine, procainamide, and bretylium are indicated, followed by additional cardioversion attempts.

Defibrillation is indicated for **pulseless VT** or **ventricular fibrillation**. The initial dose for defibrillation is 2 J/kg, with doubling if necessary. If the arrest is witnessed, defibrillation can be instituted before advanced airway and other life support techniques are begun.

Bradydysrhythmias

The deleterious effects of **bradycardia** are a result of decreased cardiac output. Older children and adults can compensate for bradycardia by increasing stroke volume; infants and young children are unable to appreciably increase stroke volume.

Asymptomatic **sinus bradycardia** can be seen normally during deep sleep and in highly trained athletes. An ECG will demonstrate sinus bradycardia and normal P-, QRS, and T-wave morphology. No diagnostic testing or treatment is necessary for conditions that produce physiologic asymptomatic bradycardia.

The most common causes of **symptomatic bradycardia** are hypoxemia and vagal stimulation (Table 4-4). Most vagally induced bradycardia resolves rapidly once the stimulus is withdrawn.

Symptomatic bradycardia due to hypoxemia in pediatric patients is a sign of impending cardiopulmonary arrest. In this situation, a patent airway is established and breathing is assisted, with the use of 100% oxygen, while the cause is sought.

Bradycardia that does not respond to oxygenation requires pharmacologic intervention. The initial approach is the use of epinephrine (0.01 mg/kg; 1:10,000 dilution) intravenously or intraosseously. Epinephrine also may be instilled via an endotracheal tube at a dose of 0.1 mg/kg (1:1000 dilution). In neonates, the dose is 0.01 to 0.03 mg/kg (0.1 to 0.3 mL/kg; 1:10,000 solution) intravenously or endotracheally. If the endotracheal route is used, the minimum volume for instillation is 3 to 5 mL.

If epinephrine is not effective, atropine (0.02 mg/kg; minimum dose, 0.1 mg) intravenously, endotracheally, or intraosseously is administered rapidly. Atropine is ineffective for hypoxic-ischemic injury at any age; it is most effective when used prophylactically before vagal stimuli such as laryngoscopy and endotracheal intubation in the hemodynamically stable infant or child. The total of all doses of atropine should not exceed 1 mg in children and 2 mg in adult-sized adolescents.

Transcutaneous, transvenous, or transesophageal pacing can be helpful in the management of refractory bradycardias. Chest compressions are indicated if the heart rate is so low that the patient

TABLE 4-4.
Significant causes of bradycardia.

Respiratory
  Hypoxemia
  Improper endotracheal tube placement
  Inadequate ventilation
  Persistent airway obstruction
  Pneumomediastinum
  Pneumothorax
Cardiovascular
  Acute hypertension
  Cardiac tamponade
  Cardiomyopathy
  Complete heart block
  Hypovolemia
  Severe anemia
Other
  Central nervous system insults
  Metabolic abnormalities
  Poisoning

remains flaccid and unresponsive and cardiac arrest is imminent (<80 beats/min in neonates and <60 beats/min in infants and children).

SUDDEN DEATH

When a previously healthy child or adolescent presents in cardiac arrest, physician attention is first directed to supervision of the technical aspects of resuscitation. The family must be notified of the child's condition and queried regarding any preexisting illnesses. Many centers allow parents to be with their child at this point, so they can see the reality of the situation and be assured of the maximum effort being expended to save the child. If resuscitation fails, an important first step in grieving is being allowed to hold the child after resuscitative efforts are discontinued.

Efforts to determine the cause begin in the emergency department and end at autopsy. A rectal temperature is determined to rule out heat stroke and to point to infectious etiologies. Blood and urine samples are obtained for toxicology studies. A family history of cardiac syncope indicates prolonged QT syndrome. A recent febrile illness suggests myocarditis. Coronary artery thrombosis as a sequela of Kawasaki disease is another possibility. An autopsy is helpful to relieve as much of the family's guilt as possible.

Hypertrophic cardiomyopathies can present as sudden death in children and adolescents. Dysrhythmias, myocardial ischemia, and acute severe subaortic obstruction to blood flow have been proposed as possible causes. Sudden death can occur after vigorous activity or at rest. Clinical manifestations can develop at any age. When symptomatic, dyspnea and exercise intolerance are common complaints and are due to elevated left atrial pressure. Chest pain, syncope, or near-syncope can occur during activity or at rest.

Hypertrophic cardiomyopathy is a primary cardiac disorder that is often associated with an autosomal dominant inheritance pattern. The primary abnormality in this condition is left ventricular hypertrophy, which often is irregular and may involve portions or all of the left ventricle. A minority of patients have hypertrophy involving the interventricular septum, which can cause the septal muscle to interfere with blood flow from the left ventricle into the aorta (subaortic obstruction). Hypertrophy can vary from mild to severe and can begin at any time during infancy, childhood, or early adulthood. Clinical symptoms and findings tend to correlate with the degree of ventricular hypertrophy.

Unlike dilated cardiomyopathies, the hypertrophy does not impair myocardial contractility. The primary cardiac impairment results from diastolic dysfunction. The left ventricle becomes stiff and noncompliant. Left atrial pressure rises as a result of diastolic filling difficulty.

The goal of therapy is to improve left ventricular filling during diastole. Increased blood volume increases ventricular preload. Reduced heart rate allows more time for diastolic filling. Decreased myocardial muscle tension improves ventricular compliance and results in easier filling. Oral β-blockers (starting dose: propranolol, 0.5 mg/kg per day) and calcium channel blockers (verapamil, 4 mg/kg per day; nifedipine, 0.6 mg/kg per day) are the agents most commonly used to treat hypertrophic cardiomyopathy, but they should be used with caution and in consultation with a pediatric cardiologist whenever possible. Both types of medication relieve symptoms and improve subaortic stenosis and diastolic dysfunction. Unfortunately, the risk of sudden death does not appear to change significantly with therapy. Diuretics and inotropes are contraindicated because they reduce blood volume, increase heart rate, and increase myocardial contractility. Afterload-reducing agents also are contraindicated because the increased contractility aggravates diastolic dysfunction and the lower blood pressure can result in coronary insufficiency.

STABLE SYMPTOMATIC PATIENTS

Patients presenting with cyanosis, congestive heart failure, hypertension, febrile illnesses, syncope, or chest pain usually do not require immediate intervention, but consultation often is indicated for patients in this category for definitive diagnostic studies and specialized therapies.

Cyanosis

Cyanosis occurs when >5 g/dL deoxygenated hemoglobin is present in the circulation. **Acrocyanosis** (restricted to the hands and feet) is a normal variant that is common in newborns. **Central cyanosis** is caused by respiratory, cardiac, or hemoglobin disorders. The presence of hypoxemia is confirmed by measurement of a low oxygen saturation level or a low arterial PO_2. However, hypoxemia can be present even in the absence of cyanosis.

Congenital heart defects produce cyanosis by shunting deoxygenated blood from the venous system into the arterial system, a right-to-left shunt. Although tachypnea frequently occurs, significant respiratory distress is usually absent. Close inspection will reveal that hyperpnea is present with both increased rate and tidal volume. The cyanosis can be subtle or inapparent at rest but more obvious during crying or sucking. In the past, these lesions have usually been diagnosed in the hospital shortly after birth. *With trends toward earlier discharge from the newborn nursery, however, infants may now present to the emergency department or pediatrician's office within the first few weeks of life with previously unrecognized cyanotic congenital heart disease.*

A **hyperoxia test** can be very helpful in distinguishing cyanotic heart disease from respiratory and hemoglobin disorders. Babies with right-to-left shunts have a low PaO_2 (25 to 45 mm Hg) when breathing room air. Although tachypneic, they have minimal to no respiratory distress. When placed on 100% oxygen, their PaO_2 fails to rise to >100 mm Hg.

Abnormalities on the chest radiograph and ECG often help confirm the presence of cyanotic congenital heart disease. A 13-lead ECG, which includes lead V_3R, may be useful. The chest radiograph may demonstrate an abnormal cardiac silhouette, abnormal cardiac position, or decreased pulmonary vascular markings. The ECG may show an abnormal axis, abnormal QRS morphology, or abnormal ST segments. Detection of an infant with cyanotic heart disease warrants immediate referral to a pediatric cardiology service for definitive diagnosis with echocardiography or cardiac catheterization.

Congestive Heart Failure

Congestive heart failure occurs when elevated preload produces symptoms of fluid retention (Table 4-5). As a result, blood backs up to produce venous congestion. **Tachypnea** develops, followed by **rales** and **wheezes** as late signs of left-sided heart failure. Systemically, **hepatomegaly** is the first sign of elevated venous pressure, followed by peripheral edema. **Cardiomegaly** and **tachycardia** are adaptations for a failing heart. A **gallop rhythm** may be heard. Constitutional symptoms such as **poor feeding, fatigue, irritability**, and **lethargy** become more prominent as congestive heart failure becomes more severe. A history of **sweating during feedings** is equivalent to dyspnea on exertion and is a sign of compensatory sympathetic overload.

Congestive heart failure can be the result of congenital or acquired heart disease or systemic disorders, such as severe anemia. The age of the child at the onset of heart failure is helpful in establishing a differential diagnosis. Premature infants in the neonatal intensive care unit are predisposed to heart failure from **patent ductus ateriosus** and persistent fetal circulation. Children with large **ventricular septal defects**, on the other hand, usually go into heart failure in the third or fourth week of life, when pulmonary vascular resistance falls and the amount of left-to-right shunting increases. These lesions overload the pulmonary circulation and then the left ventricle. Ultimately, cardiac output and myocardial perfusion become impaired.

TABLE 4-5.
Recognition of serious cardiovascular disease in infants and children.

	Right-Sided Failure	Left-Sided Failure	Right- or Left-Sided Failure
Common signs	Hepatomegaly	Dyspnea and sweating on feeding, tachypnea	Cardiomegaly, cyanosis, failure to thrive, shock, tachycardia
Less frequent signs	Ascites, jugular venous distention, peripheral edema	Rales	

Dilated Cardiomyopathies

Impaired cardiac contractility and ventricular dilatation are the universal hallmarks of dilated cardiomyopathies. Most cases are idiopathic. Those with underlying inflammation demonstrable by biopsy and suggested by clinical signs are classified as **myocarditis**. A history of a recent febrile illness is common. For cases with an identifiable cause, Coxsackie enterovirus is the most common agent. Children with myocarditis generally are acutely ill and may be unstable, requiring aggressive management. The mortality rate may exceed 30%.

Infants and toddlers with cardiomyopathy often present with respiratory symptoms. A chest radiograph will usually demonstrate an enlarged heart, with or without pulmonary venous congestion. Careful physical examination will reveal subtle signs of congestive failure. If pulmonary edema is present, it usually causes wheezing in infants and rales in older children.

Patients with dilated cardiomyopathy may present with acute cardiovascular collapse from severe congestive failure or dysrhythmia. The disease may have been present for some time, with the child remaining relatively asymptomatic due to compensation. Patients become overtly symptomatic or critically ill when their disease worsens or they are stressed by an intercurrent minor illness.

ECG abnormalities are variable and nonspecific. Tachycardia, abnormal QRS axis, Q waves, ST changes, flattened or inverted T waves, and left ventricular hypertrophy are common abnormal findings. Creatine phosphokinase levels may be elevated.

The diagnosis of dilated cardiomyopathy is usually confirmed with echocardiography, and usually both ventricles are affected. Markedly decreased myocardial contractility (often 25% to 50% of normal) and substantial ventricular dilatation are readily apparent. Echocardiography also can rule out other causes for an enlarged heart, such as pericardial effusion and anatomic defects.

Initial Therapy

The infant is kept comfortable and quiet, in an upright position in an infant seat if available. Oxygen is administered in a nonthreatening fashion. Pulse oximetry is assessed on a continuous basis. A neutral thermal environment is established to avoid any additional stress from hypothermia or hyperthermia. Continuous monitoring for dysrhythmias is initiated, and the family is counseled about the possibility of sudden death.

If pulmonary edema is a problem, 1 mg/kg furosemide intravenously is administered. Diuretics must be administered with caution to prevent intravascular volume depletion or electrolyte problems. Patients with low cardiac output states generally should not receive diuretics acutely because they usually do best with high intravascular volumes. For patients with low cardiac output states, infusions of crystalloid or colloid should be tried first.

Further Therapy

These infants require management by a pediatric cardiologist, usually in a pediatric intensive care unit or other closely monitored environment. **Digoxin** therapy may be initiated on the advice of a pediatric cardiologist.

Severe cases require vasoactive infusions and ventilatory support. Generally, a mean blood pressure of >50 to 60 mm Hg is satisfactory. If heart failure is refractory to supportive therapy, heart transplantation may be possible.

Febrile Illnesses

Fever can be the initial presentation of a child with serious infectious or autoimmune cardiovascular disorders. Children with known heart disease may develop fever due to routine infections, but consideration also must be given to the possibility of subacute bacterial endocarditis.

Acute Rheumatic Fever

Care must be taken in the initial diagnosis of acute rheumatic fever because of the need for long-term penicillin prophylaxis to prevent the development of serious valvular disease. When suspected, hospitalization usually is indicated to clarify and confirm the diagnosis. In addition to the demonstration of a recent streptococcal infection on the basis of an elevated antibody titer and to the presence of nonspecific signs of inflammation, two of the major Jones criteria or one major and two minor criteria must be present. The major criteria are carditis, migratory polyarthritis, chorea, erythema marginata, and subcutaneous nodules.

The minor criteria are arthralgia, fever, elevated acute-phase reactants (erythrocyte sedimentation rate, C-reactive protein), and prolonged PR interval.

Kawasaki Disease

Kawasaki disease is a systemic vasculitis of unknown cause. The disease occurs mostly in younger children. The presentation consists of an ill-appearing, irritable child with prolonged fever (5 to 14 days), inflamed conjunctivae, anterior uveitis, cervical lymphadenopathy, strawberry tongue, cracked red lips, and an erythematous rash involving the palms and soles. Frequently, there is associated edema of the dorsum of the hands and feet (Table 4-6). Children usually develop an elevated platelet count. After several days, peeling of the erythematous skin occurs.

All patients diagnosed with Kawasaki disease should be hospitalized immediately for the administration of intravenous γ-globulin, aspirin therapy, and cardiac evaluation. A pediatric cardiologist should be consulted immediately.

Occasionally, other organs can be involved, resulting in serious complications, including hydrops of the gallbladder, meningoencephalitis, and potentially fatal myocarditis. There is a marked predilection for inflammation of the coronary arteries. From 20% to 25% of untreated children develop serious coronary artery aneurysms. Coronary artery damage can lead to thrombosis or sudden death long after the acute symptoms have resolved. With acute thrombosis, thrombolytic therapy may be effective. Sequential echocardiographic examinations are necessary for the assessment of coronary artery involvement.

The administration of intravenous γ-globulin reduces the number of children who develop severe coronary artery damage and usually shortens the hospitalization stay by rapidly reversing many of the acute inflammatory signs. There is evidence that the sooner γ-globulin is administered, the less risk there will be of serious coronary artery disease. *A single dose of intravenous γ-globulin (2 g/kg) is administered over 10 to 12 hours.* Aspirin usually is administered in large doses (100 mg/kg per day) for its anti-inflammatory action; after the acute phase of the illness, a low dose is used for anticoagulation (3 to 5 mg/kg per day). Children with a history of serious coronary aneurysms may be receiving treatment with aspirin, persantine, and coumadin; these children may return with symptoms of myocardial infarction. Empiric treatment with tissue-type plasminogen activator (0.5 mg/kg intravenously over 1 hour) can be considered if the patient is >1 hour from cardiac catheterization. Steroids are contraindicated because of their association with an increased incidence of coronary complications.

Chest Pain

The most common causes of chest pain in children are trauma, costochondritis, esophageal reflux, and pleuritis. Scoliosis in teenaged girls is another important consideration. Exercise-induced chest pain may be due to exercise-induced asthma. Children and teenagers with SVT can present with chest pain and palpitations. There are very rare case reports of infants presenting with fists clenched over their chests and ST-segment depressions, secondary to anomalous coronary arteries originating from the pulmonary artery.

Pericarditis

If a child presents with chest pain and fever, pericarditis must be considered. Manifestations of pericarditis include dyspnea, chest pain, and fever.

TABLE 4-6.
Diagnostic criteria for Kawasaki disease.

1. Fever persisting for 5 or more days and

2. At least four of the following five findings:
   a. Bilateral painless bulbar conjunctival injection without exudate
   b. Mucous membrane changes of the upper respiratory tract, including injected dry, fissured lips, oral mucosal and pharyngeal injection, and "strawberry tongue"
   c. Changes in peripheral extremities, including erythema and edema of the hands and feet in the acute phase and periungual and generalized desquamation in the convalescent phase
   d. Polymorphous truncal exanthem
   e. Acute, nonpurulent cervical lymphadenopathy

3. Findings that cannot be explained by some other known disease process

From Jain S. Kawasaki syndrome. In: Strange GR, Ahrens W, Lelyveld S, et al, eds. *Pediatric Emergency Medicine: A Comprehensive Study Guide.* New York, NY: McGraw-Hill; 1996:270. Adapted with permission.

The chest pain can be precordial or referred to the left shoulder and is typically aggravated by lying flat and alleviated by leaning forward. Impaired venous return from pericardial effusion produces venous distention and hepatomegaly. A friction rub can be audible on auscultation. Heart sounds are distant. Small effusions can cause exercise intolerance, whereas large effusions produce symptoms at rest. In severe cases, cardiac tamponade can occur. The chest radiograph demonstrates a large heart. Echocardiography is essential for distinguishing pericardial effusion from cardiomyopathies.

Many disorders can cause a pericardial effusion. Infectious diseases are responsible for most cases in children. If the effusion is sufficiently large, a specimen of pericardial fluid is obtained through pericardiocentesis for diagnostic studies. Treatment involves drainage of the effusion if it is causing hemodynamic compromise. For purulent pericarditis, surgical drainage is indicated with a subxiphoid pericardial window or pericardotomy via a median sternotomy, in addition to antibiotic therapy.

Syncope

The sudden loss of consciousness in a child is usually due to a seizure or vasovagal reflex and seldom due to a cerebrovascular accident or dysrhythmia. An accurate history from a reliable witness is essential to establish cardiac syncope as the working diagnosis. If the person who brings the child in for care did not see the episode, that person can usually locate a primary witness for a telephone interview. A cardiac cause for syncope is suggested by a history of color change and a controlled fall, followed by loss of consciousness. Some form of bystander resuscitation often is given.

The differential diagnosis includes critical aortic stenosis, hypertrophic cardiomyopathy, pulmonary hypertension, tetralogy of Fallot, prolonged QT syndrome, sick sinus syndrome, and VT.

Sick Sinus Syndrome

Children with cardiac problems associated with enlarged right atria, such as Ebstein's anomaly, may present with episodes of sinus arrest alternating with tachydysrhythmias. The ECG shows a wandering atrial pacemaker. Referral to a pediatric cardiologist who specializes in electrophysiologic studies is indicated.

Prolonged QT Syndrome

Some inherited disorders, such as Romano-Ward syndrome and Jervell-Lange-Nielsen syndrome, are characterized by a prolonged QT interval and syncopal episodes that develop during childhood or early adulthood. These patients are at risk for serious cardiac dysrhythmias producing syncope or sudden death.

Because the QT interval of the ECG varies inversely with heart rate, QT interval measurements must be divided by the square root of the RR interval to correct for the heart rate. The normal corrected QT is <0.45 in infants, <0.44 in children, and <0.43 in adolescents. The administration of β-blockers and activity restriction represent the primary treatment for congenital prolonged QT interval syndromes.

Acquired causes of prolonged QT interval include toxicity due to quinidine, procainamide, phenothiazines, cyclic antidepressants, organophosphates, and lithium. Electrolyte abnormalities are associated with this problem, especially hypokalemia, hypomagnesemia, and hypocalcemia. Low-energy liquid protein diets and catastrophic central nervous system damage also can produce a prolonged QT interval.

ASYMPTOMATIC PATIENTS

During the examination of infants and children, incidental findings may be noted that indicate cardiovascular disease. The major findings are discussed below.

Growth Failure

Most infants gain 0.5 to 1 oz/day, so they double their birth weight at 5 months and triple it at 1 year. Average weights for age are 10 kg for 1 year and 40 kg for 10 years. Infants with heart lesions may demonstrate failure to thrive.

Heart Murmur

Innocent flow murmurs are common in infants and children, especially during hyperdynamic states, such as fever or anemia. Pathologic murmurs are caused by turbulent blood flow through a shunt or a stenotic valve or regurgitation through an incompetent valve. Referral as an outpatient to a pediatrician or pediatric cardiologist is indicated for

the following types of murmurs:
- Diastolic
- Holosystolic
- Those that produce a thrill or click
- Those that radiate to the axilla, neck, or back
- Those that augment with Valsalva maneuver

Congenital Syndromes

Many genetic disorders are associated with congenital heart lesions. For example, half of infants with Down syndrome, the most common genetic disorder, have associated congenital heart lesions. The discovery of dysmorphic features associated with one of these syndromes should be followed by a careful cardiovascular examination, with the signs of associated congenital heart lesions sought.

Hypertension

Coarctation of the aorta is the primary cardiovascular anomaly that produces hypertension. It can be present at any age. The diagnosis can be confirmed through documentation of a discrepancy in blood pressure between the upper and lower extremities. Blood pressure also should be measured in both upper extremities to detect an anomalous right subclavian artery arising below the coarctation site.

Abnormal Pulses

Pulses are rated clinically on a scale of 0 to 4+. Normal distal pulses can be readily palpated on the first attempt (rated 2 to 3+). Bounding pulses are 4+. The most common cause for bounding pulses is high cardiac output due to fever. Cardiovascular causes include aortic insufficiency, patent ductus arteriosus, and arteriovenous malformation.

Absent pulses are designated by 0+; this refers to the situation in which the first impression is one of absent pulses, but with additional palpation, a weak pulse is discovered. The differential diagnosis of 0 to 1+ pulses includes shock, hypoplastic left ventricle syndrome, and coarctation of the aorta.

ANTICIPATING PROBLEMS IN CHILDREN WITH KNOWN HEART DISEASE

Children with known heart disease often present for routine childhood illnesses and injuries, as well as for acute cardiovascular complications. A significant number of these children are treated with diuretics, digoxin, anticoagulants, and other medications, all of which can cause acute problems. Not every caretaker volunteers the information that the child has a preexisting heart disease. Heart murmurs and surgical scars on the chest suggest the possibility of preexisting heart disease. Once preexisting heart disease is confirmed, the physician is in a position to anticipate a special set of complications (Table 4-7).

Air Embolism

During the administration of intravenous infusions to patients with right-to-left shunts or to any newborn, it is important to prevent the passage of air bubbles into the circulation. *A small air bubble introduced into the vein of a patient with cyanotic congenital heart disease can cause a cerebrovascular accident or myocardial infarction.*

Hypoxemic (Tet) Spells

Tet spells are less common now that early surgical correction of heart defects is common. Infants with uncorrected tetralogy of Fallot and other cyanotic lesions can have spells characterized by acutely increased cyanosis and rapid respirations. Decreased mental status and altered muscle tone often accompany these spells. The mechanism is not totally clear. Some spells are thought to result from acute obstruction of pulmonary blood flow due to sudden increases in tone or spasm of the cardiac muscle near the origin of the pulmonary artery. Another potential cause is acute worsening of right-to-left shunting caused by

TABLE 4-7.
Anticipating problems in patients who have known heart disease.

Air embolism
Anemia
Anticoagulation problems
Artificial pacemakers
Digoxin toxicity
Diuretic complications
Fever
Hypoxemic spells
Pulmonary hypertension
Resuscitation
Subacute bacterial endocarditis
Surgical shunt malfunction

suddenly increased pulmonary vascular resistance, suddenly decreased systemic vascular resistance, or both. Regardless of the mechanism, pulmonary blood flow decreases and oxygenation decreases. Breathing becomes more rapid as the body senses and tries to compensate for worsening hypoxemia. Oxygen consumption increases further, and as the hypoxemia worsens, cyanosis becomes more profound and loss of consciousness may occur.

Treatment consists of calming the child while administering 100% oxygen. Simultaneously, the legs are flexed and pressed into the abdomen (knee-chest position) to increase resistance to blood flow in the systemic circulation. Spells that do not rapidly abate are treated with morphine (0.1 mg/kg) followed by a 10 mL/kg bolus of normal saline if necessary.

Hypercyanotic spells that persist despite these measures can be treated with the ultrashort-acting β-blocker **esmolol**. Esmolol is administered as a loading dose of 0.5 to 0.6 mg/kg over 1 to 2 minutes, followed by a constant infusion begun at 0.2 mg/kg per minute and increased slowly every few minutes until the heart rate and blood pressure begin to decrease. Another β-blocker, such as **propranolol** (0.01 to 0.02 mg/kg), can be substituted for esmolol. Some practitioners have used up to 0.15 to 0.25 mg/kg of propranolol for the treatment of refractory cases. (All intravenous doses of β-blockers must be administered slowly to avoid bradycardia and hypotension.) β-Blockers increase pulmonary blood flow by directly reducing cardiac rate and muscle tone. Alternative agents are **neosynephrine** and **ketamine**. Patients with severe hypercyanotic spells can benefit from endotracheal intubation, mechanical ventilation, general anesthesia, and neuromuscular blockade to reduce oxygen consumption due to their increased breathing efforts. The acid-base status is monitored closely, and abnormalities are corrected aggressively. Emergency cardiac surgery is necessary for patients with spells that persist despite the use of β-blockers.

Critical aortic stenosis can produce similar episodes of extreme irritability with poor perfusion but without systemic desaturation.

Surgical Shunt Malfunction

Surgical correction of some complex cyanotic lesions is not always possible in the neonatal period. Some infants require a shunt to facilitate blood flow from the systemic vessels to the pulmonary circulation as a temporary, palliative procedure. These infants often are critically dependent on the shunt.

Shunt malfunction is suspected when these infants develop signs of acute distress and increasing cyanosis. Usually, after several months of age, a continuous murmur is heard over the site of a shunt. In early infancy, the murmur may be heard in systole only. Disappearance of the murmur suggests occlusion. Other important signs are an increase in heart rate and respiratory rate and a decrease in PaO_2 and oxygen saturation levels compared with baseline values. The infant is placed in 100% oxygen. Blood is drawn for electrolyte and arterial blood gas determination, and chest radiography is indicated. Hospitalization is arranged for further evaluation by a pediatric cardiologist and possible surgery.

Pulmonary Hypertensive Crises

Children with heart or lung disease that causes increased pulmonary artery pressure or flow can have episodes of elevated pressure in their pulmonary arterial circulation. These patients develop pulmonary artery vasospasm, either spontaneously or as a response to stress. Pulmonary infections, acidosis, hypoxemia, pain, endotracheal intubation, tracheal suctioning, and perioperative stress are common antecedents. Profound decreases in oxygen saturation and cardiac output rapidly ensue. Bradycardia can occur within 1 or 2 minutes. Death will occur if the problem is not rapidly corrected.

Alkalinization and 100% oxygen are the principal approaches to bring about pulmonary vasodilation. Hyperventilation and sodium bicarbonate are used to induce and maintain alkalosis (pH >7.5 to 7.55). Sedative and analgesic agents are administered to prevent agitation and stress.

Fever

Children with cyanotic congenital heart disease are more fragile and less resilient. Illnesses that are usually mild in normal children can be severe in children with cyanotic heart lesions. The threshold for hospitalization for these patients should be relatively low. Even though supplemental oxygen does not produce a large change in PaO_2, it does result in an increase in the oxygen content of the blood and therefore can produce substantial clinical benefit.

Within reason, these children must be protected from exposure to contagious diseases. Measures to induce passive immunity and appropriate antimicrobial therapy deserve consideration when exposures or infections occur.

Subacute Bacterial Endocarditis

Children with congenital heart defects, valvular disease, hypertrophic cardiomyopathy, or mitral valve prolapse are susceptible to subacute bacterial endocarditis (SBE). Transient bacteremias produced by dental or gastrointestinal procedures can seed a nidus for continued growth within these lesions. The American Heart Association recommendations for prophylaxis depend on the location of the procedure (Tables 4-8 and 4-9).

The use of empiric antibiotic therapy for febrile children who are at risk of developing SBE should

be avoided. If a child is suspected of having SBE, is only mildly ill, and has an identifiable source of infection, such as otitis media, at least two blood cultures are drawn to rule out SBE before starting routine oral antibiotics and discharging the child. The toxic child deserves hospitalization. Once the diagnosis is established, treatment consists of 3 to 6 weeks of intravenous antibiotics.

Diuretic Complications

An incorrect diuretic dosage can lead to congestive failure or dehydration. Even proper doses can produce dehydration during times of diarrhea or poor feeding.

Hypokalemia is usually due to diuretic-induced losses combined with poor intake. A critically high potassium level can occur due to overdose with potassium supplements. Hypokalemia and hyperkalemia are confirmed through the detection of ECG abnormalities and measurement of serum potassium levels.

Digoxin Toxicity

There is only a narrow margin between the therapeutic and toxic doses of digoxin, and absorption and elimination can vary over time. Diagnosis relies on finding cardiac conduction system abnormalities on the ECG. Digoxin levels are not always a reliable index of toxicity but may help to confirm the diagnosis. Digoxin toxicity in infants and children is most often manifested by dysrhythmias, usually bradycardias. The adolescent is more likely to develop adult toxicity patterns of atrial tachycardia and VT. Concomitant electrolyte abnormalities will potentiate the toxicity of digoxin.

Therapy is based on the patient's condition. In most patients, withholding one or two doses of the drug, while carefully monitoring the ECG, is all that is necessary. Atropine can be of value in patients with sinus bradycardia. For patients with ventricular dysrhythmias, lidocaine or phenytoin can be helpful.

For the severely compromised child, an infusion of **antibody (Fab) fragments active against digoxin** (Digibind) will usually reverse toxic manifestations within 30 minutes. The dosage is calculated as follows:

Fab dose (mg) = serum digoxin level (μg/L) x body weight (kg) x 0.4

Although Fab fragment administration is the

TABLE 4-8.
Selected procedures for which endocarditis prophylaxis is recommended.*

Dental
Extractions
Implants and reimplantation of avulsed teeth
Initial placement of orthodontic bands
Intraligamentary local anesthetic injections
Periodontal procedures
Prophylactic cleaning of teeth
Root canal instrumentation
Subgingival placement of antibiotic fibers or strips
Respiratory Tract
Rigid bronchoscopy
Surgery involving respiratory muscosa
Tonsillectomy/adenoidectomy
Gastrointestinal Tract
Biliary tract surgery
Endoscopic retrograde cholangiography
Esophageal stricture dilation
Sclerotherapy for esophageal varices
Surgery involving intestinal mucosa
Genitourinary
Cystoscopy
Prostatic surgery
Urethral dilation

*This table includes selected procedures from the American Heart Association recommendations and is not meant to be all inclusive. See editor's note on page 56.

From Dajani AS, Taubert KA, Wilson W, et al. Prevention of bacterial endocarditis: recommendations by the American Heart Association. *JAMA.* 1997;277:1794-1801. Adapted with permission.

TABLE 4-9.
Endocarditis prophylaxis regimens.*

Situation	Agent	Regimen
Dental, Oral Respiratory Tract, or Esophageal Procedures		
Standard general prophylaxis	Amoxicillin	50 mg/kg orally 1 hr before procedure
Unable to take oral medications	Ampicillin	50 mg/kg IM or IV within 30 min before procedure
Allergic to penicillin	Clindamycin	20 mg/kg orally 1 hr before procedure
	or cephalexin or cefadroxil†	50 mg/kg orally 1 hr before procedure
	or azithromycin or clarithromycin	15 mg/kg orally 1 hr before procedure
Allergic to penicillin and unable to take oral medications	Clindamycin **or** cefazolin	20 mg/kg IV within 30 min before procedure 25 mg/kg IM or IV within 30 min before procedure
Genitourinary or Gastrointestinal (Excluding Esophageal) Procedures		
High-risk patients	Ampicillin plus gentamicin	Ampicillin 50 mg/kg IM or IV (not to exceed 2 g) plus gentamicin 1.5 mg/kg within 30 min of starting the procedure; 6 hr later, ampicillin 25 mg/kg IM or IV or amoxicillin 25 mg/kg orally
High-risk patients allergic to ampicillin/amoxicillin	Vancomycin plus gentamicin	Vancomycin 20 mg/kg IV over 1-2 hr plus gentamicin 1.5 mg/kg IV or IM; complete injection/infusion within 30 min of starting the procedure
Moderate-risk patients	Amoxicillin **or** ampicillin	50 mg/kg orally 1 hr before procedure 50 mg/kg IV or IM within 30 min of starting the procedure
Moderate-risk patients allergic to ampicillin/amoxicillin	Vancomycin	20 mg/kg IV over 1-2 hr; complete infusion within 30 min of starting the procedure

*See editor's note on page 56.
†Cephalosporins should not be used in individuals with immediate-type hypersensitivity reaction (urticaria, angioedema, or anaphylaxis) to penicillins.

From Dajani AS, Taubert KA, Wilson W, et al. Prevention of bacterial endocarditis: recommendations by the American Heart Association. *JAMA.* 1997;277:1794-1801. Adapted with permission.

primary therapy for patients with serious digoxin toxicity due to therapeutic use or acute poisoning, antidysrhythmic agents or a pacemaker may be necessary. Gastric lavage and activated charcoal may reduce absorption of digoxin that is present in the gastrointestinal tract.

Anticoagulation Problems

Some children with congenital heart disease are placed on low-dose aspirin or warfarin therapy, usually to prevent thrombosis of a surgically implanted artificial valve or graft. The risk of serious bleeding is small but always present. Careful monitoring of coagulation tests may be required in some patients. Care must be taken when performing invasive procedures on patients receiving anticoagulants; a number of antibiotics and other drugs can affect the degree of anticoagulation. Coagulopathy may require correction before major procedures can be safely performed.

Anemia in Children with Persistent Cyanotic Heart Defects

Children with cyanotic defects often require increased hemoglobin levels to help compensate for hypoxemia. Tachycardia, tachypnea, decreased activity, difficulty in feeding, irritability, lethargy, and acidosis can occur when hemoglobin is at "normal" levels. Transfusions and iron supplements are necessary when significant blood losses occur. Relative anemia can precipitate hypercyanotic spells.

Polycythemia in Children with Persistent Cyanotic Heart Defects

Progressive worsening of severe polycythemia in children who have cyanotic congenital heart disease suggests the need for surgical repair or palliation. Hyperviscosity due to extreme polycythemia can result in symptoms of decreased organ perfusion. Worsening congestive heart failure and cerebral ischemia are particularly serious. The acute management of hyperviscosity involves phlebotomy or partial-exchange transfusion to acutely lower the hemoglobin level sufficiently to restore perfusion. Cardiac surgery, if possible, should be considered to ameliorate the chronic hypoxemia.

Artificial Pacemakers

Some children with congenital or postoperative complete heart block have artificial pacemakers. During assessment of the patient's circulation, it is critical to ensure the pacemaker is producing an appropriate heart rate. Pacemaker spikes on the ECG should be followed immediately by a QRS complex. It is important to compare the child's distal pulse rate with the pacemaker rate on the ECG. If the pulse is too slow, too fast, or not concordant with the pacemaker spikes, the pacemaker may not be functioning properly. Discrepancies are reported to the child's pediatric cardiologist. Strong electromagnetic fields, such as those associated with magnetic resonance imaging equipment, can affect pacemakers and should be avoided by patients with pacemakers in place.

Cardiopulmonary Resuscitation

Major noncardiac emergencies can occur in children with congenital heart defects. In such situations, resuscitation efforts do not require modification. Once the patient is stabilized, consultation with a pediatric cardiologist is obtained to assist with the postresuscitation care.

SUMMARY

Many advances that have occurred in pediatric cardiology over the past two decades are available only at regionalized centers, yet when an infant or child develops an acute complication, parents often seek help at the nearest emergency department. The assessment done during this initial patient encounter is essential in establishing the level of care needed and in diagnosing previously unrecognized congenital and acquired heart disease.

ADDITIONAL READING

Fyler DC, ed. *Nadas' Pediatric Cardiology*. Philadelphia, Pa: Hanley and Belfus; 1992.

Gewitz MH, Vetter V, Silverman BK. Cardiac emergencies and the patient with a heart murmur. In: Fleisher G, Ludwig S, eds. *Textbook of Pediatric Emergency Medicine*, 3rd ed. Baltimore, Md: Williams & Wilkins; 1993:533-572.

Long WA, ed. *Fetal and Neonatal Cardiology*. Philadelphia, Pa: WB Saunders; 1990.

Silverman BK. Patients with heart murmurs. In: Fleisher GR, Ludwig S, eds. *Textbook of Pediatric Emergency Medicine*, 3rd ed. Baltimore, Md: Williams & Wilkins; 1993:233-243.

EDITOR'S NOTE

Table 4-8 and Table 4-9 are used with permission from the American Medical Association. They are based on recommendations from the American Heart Association, which cites the following sources:

Baskin G. Prosthetic endocarditis after endoscopic variceal sclerotherapy: a failure of antibiotic prophylaxis. *Am J Gastroenterol.* 1989;84:311-312.

Bender IB, Naidorf IJ, Garvey GJ. Bacterial endocarditis: a consideration for physicians and dentists. *J Am Dent Assoc.* 1984;109:415-420.

Berger SA, Weitzman S, Edberg SC, Coreg JI. Bacteremia after use of an oral irrigating device. *Ann Intern Med.* 1974;80:510-511.

Botoman V, Surawicz C. Bacteremia with gastrointestinal endoscopic procedures. *Gastrointest Endosc.* 1986;32:342-346.

Bryne W, Euler A, Campbell M, Eisenach KD. Bacteremia in children following upper gastrointestinal endoscopy or colonoscopy. *J Pediatr Gastroenterol Nutr.* 1982;1:551-553.

Child JS. Risks for and prevention of infective endocarditis. In: Child JS, ed. *Cardiology Clinics—Diagnosis and Management of Infective Endocarditis.* Philadelphia, Pa: WB Saunders Co; 1996;14:327-343.

Cohen L, Korsten M, Scherl E, et al. Bacteremia after endoscopic injection sclerosis. *Gastrointest Endosc.* 1983;29:198-200.

Dajani AS, Bawdon RE, Berry MC. Oral amoxicillin as prophylaxis for endocarditis: what is the optimal dose? *Clin Infect Dis.* 1994;18:157-160.

Dajani AS, Bisno AL, Chung KJ, et al. Prevention of bacterial endocarditis. *JAMA.* 1990;264:2919-2922.

Durack DT. Prevention of infective endocarditis. *N Engl J Med.* 1995;332:38-44.

Felix JE, Rosen S, App GR. Detection of bacteremia after the use of oral irrigation device on subjects with periodontitis. *J Periodontol.* 1971;42:785-787.

Fluckiger U, Franciolo P, Blaser J, Glauser MP, Moreillon P. Role of amoxicillin serum levels for successful prophylaxis of experimental endocarditis due to tolerant streptococci. *J Infect Dis.* 1994;169:397-400.

Guntheroth WG. How important are dental procedures as a cause of infective endocarditis? *Am J Cardiol.* 1984;54:797-801.

Ho H, Zuckerman M, Wassem C. A prospective controlled study of the risk of bacteremia in emergency sclerotherapy of esophageal varices. *Gastroenterology.* 1991;101:1642-1648.

Hunter KD, Holborrow DW, Kardos TB, Lee-Knight CT, Ferguson MM. Bacteremia and tissue damage resulting from air polishing. *Br Dent J.* 1989;167:275-277.

Logan R, Hastings J. Bacterial endocarditis: a complication of gastroscopy. *BMJ.* 1988;296:1107.

Low D, Shoenut P, Kennedy J, et al. Prospective assessment of risk of bacteremia with colonoscopy and polypectomy. *Dig Dis Sci.* 1987;32:1239-1243.

Low D, Shoenut P, Kennedy J, et al. Risk of bacteremia with endoscopic sphincterotomy. *Can J Surg.* 1987;30:421-423.

Niv Y, Bat L, Motro M. Bacterial endocarditis after Hurst bougienage in a patient with a benign esophageal stricture and mitral valve prolapse. *Gastrointest Endosc.* 1985;31:265-267.

Norfleet R. Infectious endocarditis after fiberoptic sigmoidoscopy. *J Clin Gastroenterol.* 1991;13:448-451.

Pallasch TJ, Slots J. Antibiotic prophylaxis and the medically compromised patient. *Periodontol 2000.* 1996;10:107-138.

Pritchard T, Foust R, Cantey R, Leman R. Prosthetic valve endocarditis due to *Cardiobacterium hominis* occurring after upper gastrointestinal endoscopy. *Am J Med.* 1991;90:516-518.

Raines DR, Branch WC, Anderson DL, et al. The occurrence of bacteremia after oesophageal dilatation and oesophagogastroscopy. *Aust N Z J Med.* 1977;7:22-35.

Rigilano J, Mahapatra R, Barnhill J, Gutierrez J. Enterococcal endocarditis following sigmoidoscopy and mitral valve prolapse. *Arch Intern Med.* 1984;144:850-851.

Rodriguez W, Levine J. Enterococcal endocarditis following flexible sigmoidoscopy. *West J Med.* 1984;140:951-953.

Roman AR, App GR. Bacteremia, a result from oral irrigation in subjects with gingivitis. *J Periodontol.* 1971;42:757-760.

Rouse MS, Steckelberg JM, Brandt CM, Patel R, Miro JM, Wilson WR. Efficacy of azithromycin or clarithromycin for the prophylaxis of viridans streptococcal experimental endocarditis. *Antimicrob Agents Chemother.* In press.

Shull H, Greene B, Allen S, et al. Bacteremia with upper gastrointestinal endoscopy. *Ann Intern Med.* 1975;83:212-214.

Stephenson PM, Dorrington L, Harris OD, Rao A. Bacteraemia following oesophageal dilatation and oesophagogastroscopy. *Aust N Z J Med.* 1977;7:32-35.

Sugrue D, Blake S, Troy P, MacDonald D. Antibiotic prophylaxis against infective endocarditis after normal delivery: is it necessary? *Br Heart J.* 1980;44:499-502.

Sullivan N, Sutter, V, Mims M, Marsh V, Finegold S. Clinical aspects of bacteremia after manipulation of the genitourinary tract. *J Infect Dis.* 1973;127:49-55.

Tseng C, Green R, Burke S, et al. Bacteremia after endoscopic band ligation of esophageal varices. *Gastrointest Endosc.* 1992;38:336-337.

Watanakunakorn C. *Streptococcus bovis* endocarditis associated with villous adenoma following colonoscopy. *Am Heart J.* 1988;116:1115-1116.

Welsh JD, Griffiths WJ, McKee J, et al. Bacteremia associated with esophageal dilation. *J Clin Gastroenterol.* 1983;5:109-112.

Yin T, Dellipiani A. Bacterial endocarditis after Hurst bougienage in a patient with a benign oesophageal stricture. *Endoscopy.* 1983;15:27-28.

Yin TP, Dellipiana AW. The incidence of bacteremia after outpatient Hurst bougienage in the management of benign esophageal stricture. *Endoscopy.* 1983;31:265-267.

Traumatic Emergencies

Chapter 5

Trauma

OBJECTIVES

1. Describe unique anatomic/physiologic characteristics of the pediatric age group.

2. Define concepts of the primary and secondary survey.

3. Establish and discuss management priorities based on life-threatening injuries identified in the primary survey.
   - Airway
   - Breathing
   - Circulation
   - Disability (neurologic)
   - Environment/exposure

4. Discuss the identification and initial treatment of life-threatening injuries to major organ systems.
   - Head/neck
   - Chest
   - Abdomen

More than half the deaths of US children result from serious injuries. A child often is affected much differently from an adult by the same type of injury. The inability of the young child to describe symptoms and localize pain makes pediatric trauma care a special challenge that requires experience and great patience on the part of the examining physician. The frequent occurrence of head trauma, often associated with altered consciousness, greatly increases the difficulty of initial evaluation and subsequent resuscitation of children with multiple injuries. Although blunt impact is responsible for 80% of multisystem trauma in young children, associated soft-tissue disruption or penetrating injury always must be considered.

Serious injury may have disastrous effects on a child's emotional well-being and disrupt normal development. Even seemingly minor injuries can have lasting effects as functional impairment that may emerge as subtle cognitive or behavioral deficits long after the acute process has healed.

This chapter addresses the initial assessment and management of the seriously injured child. The principles presented are vitally important because outcome often depends on the care given during the first critical minutes and hours after injury.

PATHOPHYSIOLOGIC AND ANATOMIC CONSIDERATIONS

Children clearly are not just small adults. They differ from adults in size but also in anatomy and physiology. A child's head occupies a larger relative body surface area and mass than does the head of an adult. Not surprisingly, head injuries in children are extremely common and account for a great percentage of the serious morbidity and mortality. The head is a major source of heat loss and contributes to the child's increased sensitivity to thermoregulatory stress. The occiput is more prominent in the young child and decreases in prominence from birth until ≈10 years of age. Head shape has significant implications for the care of the airway (see Chapter 6). The cranial sutures are open at birth and gradually fuse by 18 to 24 months of age; palpation of the anterior and posterior fontanels therefore can be an important source of information. A child's brain has a higher percentage of white matter than gray matter and is more susceptible to injuries that shear these layers.

A child's neck is shorter and supports a relatively greater mass than does the neck of an adult. Distracting forces frequently disrupt upper cervical vertebrae or their ligamentous attachments. Active growth centers and incomplete calcification make radiologic assessment especially challenging. Because the young child has a short, fat neck, evaluation of neck veins and the tracheal position also may be difficult.

The larynx in a child is located in a more cephalad and anterior position than the larynx of an adult. The epiglottis is tilted nearly 45 degrees in a child and is more floppy than that of an adolescent or adult (see Table 2-1). In an adult patient, the glottis (or the level of the true vocal cords) is the narrowest portion of the upper airway and therefore the limiting factor in endotracheal (ET) tube size. In the pediatric patient younger than 8 years, however, the cricoid cartilage is the narrowest portion of the airway and also the site of abundant loose columnar epithelium. This epithelium is more susceptible to pressure necrosis, which may stimulate exuberant scar tissue.

In children, the thorax is more pliable than in adults. The ribs are more cartilaginous and therefore more flexible. There is much less overlying muscle and fat to protect the ribs and underlying structures, so it is common for blunt force applied to the chest to be more efficiently transmitted to underlying tissues. The diaphragm inserts at a nearly horizontal angle in a newborn and maintains this angle of insertion until ≈12 years of age. This is in contrast to the oblique insertion of the diaphragm in an adolescent or adult. Children are diaphragmatic, or "belly breathers," which means they are dependent on effective diaphragmatic excursion for adequate ventilation. In addition, the diaphragmatic muscle is much more distensible in the child. A child's mediastinum is very mobile and therefore subject to sudden, wide excursions, as seen, for example, in tension pneumothorax.

A child's abdomen is less well protected by overlying ribs and muscle. The spleen and liver are more exposed to injury; as a result, seemingly insignificant forces can cause serious internal injury. Although the connective tissue and suspensory ligaments of the child are more elastic and can absorb more energy, the paucity of insulating fat allows more potential motion of these organs at impact. Significant internal injury therefore may be manifest by minimal external evidence.

Bone growth in children occurs at the epiphyses or growth plates of the long bones. Those areas and the epiphyseal-metaphyseal junction are sites of relative weakness. In most cases, the ligamentous structures near the epiphyseal region actually are stronger than the growth plate itself; this explains the frequency of epiphyseal fractures seen in children. Because of the implications of disturbances of the growth plate, a separate classification (Salter-Harris) has evolved for these injuries. In addition to the potential impact of fractures of the growth plate on long-term bony growth, changes in blood flow to the extremity can result in significant inequality of limb length.

ASSESSMENT AND MANAGEMENT

Because blunt injury in childhood so frequently involves the head, neuroventilatory impairments are far more common than hemodynamic impairments. Data from the National Pediatric Trauma Registry confirm that among children with trauma triage scores indicative of significant mortality risk (Pediatric Trauma Score of <8 or Injury Severity Score of >10), 30% to 40% have abnormalities in the respiratory rate and Glasgow Coma Scale score, among whom 25% will die, whereas only 7% to 8% are hypotensive, among whom 50% to 60% will die. Aggressive management of the airway and breathing therefore is the foundation of pediatric trauma resuscitation and is required in most children with serious head injuries. If serious truncal injuries also are present, vigorous support of the circulation may be required.

Management begins with the same rapid, initial assessment of the child presented in the Introduction and described in Chapters 1 and 3. It includes all of the elements of the Pediatric Assessment Triangle (Figure 5-1):

- Appearance (mental status and muscle tone) suggests the level of consciousness.
- Work of breathing (increased, labored, or

decreased) indicates the adequacy of ventilation and oxygenation.

- Circulation (skin and mucous membrane color) reflects the adequacy of oxygenation and perfusion.

A child with single-system injury involving the head would likely demonstrate abnormalities in appearance and breathing. A child with multisystem injury would likely demonstrate abnormalities in both of these parameters as well as additional abnormalities of the circulation.

Priorities for care of the seriously injured child are as follows:

- Determine whether there are any life-threatening disturbances and provide immediate appropriate treatment.
- Identify any injuries requiring surgical intervention and expedite this process.
- Examine the patient for non–life-threatening injuries and initiate therapy for those

conditions.

Although the process by which these goals are achieved is continuous, it can be divided conceptually into three phases: **assessment, stabilization,** and **initiation of definitive management.** The primary survey and initial resuscitation usually require the first 5 to 10 minutes and focus on treating immediate threats to life. The secondary survey continues and broadens the scope of treatment based on a more thorough process of physical examination and appropriate diagnostic testing. Ideally, this phase should be completed within the first hour so definitive care or preparation for safe transport can begin. Life-threatening disorders must be recognized promptly and corrected before treatment of less-threatening problems. The sequence for evaluation is always the same. If sufficient expert personnel are available for assistance, many of these tasks will be done simultaneously.

FIGURE 5-1.
Pediatric Assessment Triangle in isolated head or multisystem injury.

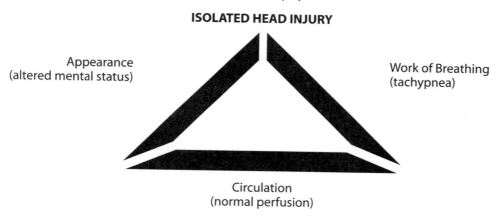

ISOLATED HEAD INJURY

Appearance
(altered mental status)

Work of Breathing
(tachypnea)

Circulation
(normal perfusion)

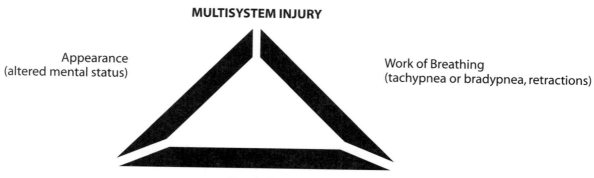

MULTISYSTEM INJURY

Appearance
(altered mental status)

Work of Breathing
(tachypnea or bradypnea, retractions)

Circulation
(tachycardia or bradycardia, poor perfusion to skin and vital organs)

The **primary survey** is an initial assessment of the status of the patient's airway, oxygenation, ventilation, circulation, and overall neurologic status. It primarily is a physiologic survey of the patient's vital systems. Because it is not uncommon to encounter serious physiologic alterations in the course of the primary survey, it frequently is necessary to interrupt the course of the survey to perform resuscitative phases of care. In contrast, the **secondary survey** is a timely, directed evaluation of each body area, usually performed in a head-to-toe fashion; the secondary survey is an anatomic survey in which the physician attempts to define the presence, type, and severity of injury to each anatomic area. The secondary survey essentially begins the definitive care of the patient. It is important to understand that children with multiple injuries require continual reassessment. The secondary survey must be performed while continuously reevaluating elements of the primary survey. As part of this reevaluation, vital signs must be reevaluated continuously on all seriously injured pediatric patients at least every 5 minutes during the course of the primary survey and every 15 minutes during the remainder of the evaluation.

Primary Survey

The steps in the primary survey include assessment of:

- Airway with cervical spine stabilization
- Breathing and emergency treatment of immediately life-threatening chest injuries
- Circulation with external control of hemorrhage
- Disability (neurologic screening examination)
- Exposure and thorough examination

The most important goals during the primary survey and resuscitative phase should be accomplished wthin 5 to 10 minutes (for a summary, see Table 5-1).

Airway and Cervical Spine

The highest priority is establishment of a patent airway with adequate ventilation. Until cervical spine injury is excluded, the cervical spine must be protected, especially during airway manipulation. Lateral cervical spine radiographs must be obtained as rapidly as feasible (see Chapter 7).

Some children with cervical spinal cord injury have symptoms of transient paresthesia, numbness, or paralysis but show no radiographic abnormality. This may occur in any patient with a significant injury above the level of the clavicles (which includes all patients with head injuries), any patient struck by a motor vehicle, any child who was involved in a high-speed motor vehicle crash or was an unrestrained passenger, and any unconscious patient who has sustained significant trauma. Adequate stabilization can be accomplished with gentle but firm longitudinal support until a cervical immobilization device or semirigid collars can be provided. Even in cases in which the initial cervical radiographs are normal, stabilization must be maintained if neurologic injury is suspected on the

TABLE 5-1.
Goals of the primary survey and resuscitative phase.

ASSESSMENT
Airway
   Obstruction
Breathing and ventilation
   Decreased rate
   Decreased breath sounds
   Decreased excursion
Circulation
   Neck vein distention
   Distant heart sounds
   Tachycardia
   Hemorrhage

THERAPY
Airway
   Relieve obstruction with jaw thrust
   Use of oral airway
   Endotracheal intubation
   Needle cricothyroidotomy
Ventilation
   Provide 100% oxygen
   Treat apnea with intubation/ventilation
   Stabilize flail thorax with positive pressure
      ventilation
   Aspiration of tension pneumothorax
   Nasogastric tube to relieve gastric dilatation
   Chest tube insertion for
      hemothorax/pneumothorax
Circulation
   Apply pressure to control hemorrhage
   Two large-bore (14- to 18-gauge) intravenous
      catheters
   Intraosseous infusion if needed
   Normal saline or lactated Ringer's at 20 mL/kg for
      volume replacement
   Relieve pericardial tamponade
   Thoracotomy when indicated (rare)

basis of the history or physical examination. If three views of the cervical spine are normal; the child is awake, reliable, and asymptomatic; and there is no evidence of a neurologic abnormality, spinal precautions may be discontinued (see Chapter 7).

Airway. To open the airway of a child with no neck or spine injury, place the child in the "sniffing" position, with the neck slightly flexed on the chest and the head slightly extended on the neck (Figure 5-2). This positioning is easily accomplished by placing a folded towel or the rescuer's hand under the victim's neck. In infants and young children, the prominence of the occipital region may actually provide this position without further assistance. To open the airway of a child with possible neck or spine injury, place the child in the neutral position, with cervical spine elements fully aligned, using bimanual cervical spine stabiliztion. In infants and young children, the prominence of the occipital region may force the neck into slight flexion when the patient is placed supine, so it may be necessary to place a thin layer of padding beneath the torso to account for this. Maintain cervical spine stabilization during the course of any airway maneuvers if cervical injury or neurologic abnormality has not been ruled out and immobilize the neck with an extrication collar once the airway is controlled. Because the mandible is relaxed in the unconscious patient, posterior displacement of the tongue will occur and can produce airway obstruction. This is treated with the jaw thrust maneuver, which should cause sufficient extension of the head on the neck to clear the airway. It is accomplished by placing hands at the angles of the mandible and applying gentle forward pressure. Remove any foreign matter present in the airway quickly with gentle suction. Neonates are obligate nasal breathers, so relieve nasal obstruction quickly through gentle suction to allow spontaneous ventilation.

Endotracheal Intubation. Indications for ET in the trauma patient are:

- Inability to ventilate the child by bag-valve-mask (BVM) methods
- Need for prolonged control of the airway, including prevention of aspiration in a comatose child
- Need for controlled ventilation in a patient with a serious head injury
- Flail chest
- Shock unresponsive to volume infusion

When intubation is necessary, preparation is an absolute requirement (see Chapter 2). The critical first step is preoxygenation using BVM ventilation with 100% oxygen. Clear the oropharynx of secretions and foreign matter through gentle suction. Unless contraindicated, emergency intubation of the child should always be accomplished using the oral approach (Figure 5-3). The acute angle of the posterior nasopharynx, necessity for additional tube manipulation, and probability of causing or increasing pharyngeal

FIGURE 5-2.
"Sniffing" position.

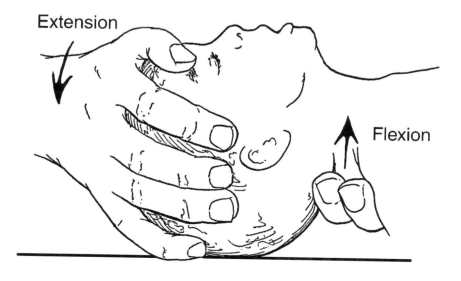

Extension

Flexion

bleeding make nasotracheal intubation unacceptably hazardous in emergency situations.

Oral ET intubation begins by maintaining in-line stabilization of the cervical spine with the head and neck in neutral position. Gentle pressure on the cricoid cartilage (**Sellick maneuver**) should be applied by an assistant so that the cricopharyngeus is compressed and the larynx is displaced posteriorly and brought into better view. If an oral tube cannot be placed within 30 seconds, resume ventilation for several minutes before making a second attempt at intubation. There are many age- and size-related protocols available to predict correct tube size; a time-honored indicator is equation of the diameter of the child's naris or fifth fingertip with the diameter of the tube. It is prudent, however, to have available a one-size-larger and a one-size-smaller tube due to the variations in children's sizes.

After the tube has been placed, assess its position by observing improvement in the patient's condition and the presence of bilateral symmetric chest wall expansion. Auscultate both lungs. Breath sounds are readily transmitted in the pediatric patient, however, and it is not uncommon to hear bilateral breath sounds, even when the ET tube is in a mainstem bronchus. Continue ventilation with 100% oxygen using a pediatric BVM ventilator at appropriate rates and with sufficient tidal volume to produce full chest wall expansion.

If airway obstruction prevents adequate BVM ventilation, there may be a direct injury to the larynx or trachea. In this unusual circumstance or in any situation in which effective ventilation is impossible, the preferred method for airway control is needle cricothyroidotomy. Using a 14-gauge needle and O_2 flow of $\geq$15 L/min, this approach can provide 30 to 40 minutes of temporary oxygenation (Appendix 5-1).

Breathing and Emergency Treatment of Immediately Life-Threatening Chest Injuries

Because the signs and symptoms of potentially serious airway and chest injury may be subtle and

FIGURE 5-3.
Insertion of laryngoscope.

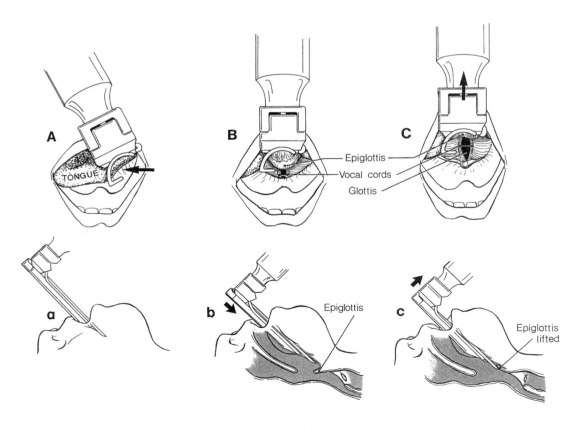

children may deteriorate rapidly after injury, administer supplemental oxygen to all pediatric major trauma victims in the initial stages of care even if they have no apparent airway or breathing difficulty. Supplemental oxygen given via face mask at a flow rate of 12 L/min is well tolerated by most children.

In assessing the adequacy of the pediatric airway, remember the adage, "**Look, listen, and feel.**" Once the airway has been opened, look at both sides of the thorax to determine whether there is symmetric chest wall rise. Because children have small tidal volumes, chest wall movement may be subtle. Carefully note suprasternal, intercostal, or subcostal retractions that may indicate respiratory distress. After ET tube insertion, listen for breath sounds on both sides of the chest. Because breath sounds can be transmitted easily through the chest wall and adjacent structures in small children, it is dangerous to rely solely on breath sounds to determine the adequacy of ventilation.

In addition to assessing the adequacy of bilateral chest wall movement, it is important to recognize that the patient's respiratory rate must be sufficient to provide oxygenation and ventilation. Any child who is hypoxic (SaO_2 <90%) or tachypneic needs additional respiratory support. A child in respiratory distress with absence of breath sounds and tracheal deviation should be suspected of having a tension pneumothorax. Thoracentesis and tube thoracostomy are indicated without a preliminary chest radiograph. The unstable child with an open pneumothorax should have a dressing with three sides occluded placed directly over the wound. Cardiac tamponade is associated with penetrating trauma to the parasternal area. Signs of cardiac tamponade include hypotension, distended neck veins, and muffled heart sounds. Children suspected of having cardiac tamponade should undergo immediate pericardiocentesis (Appendix 5-2). A child with penetrating injury to the chest who develops cardiac arrest may benefit from an emergency thoracotomy if a physician trained in the procedure is present.

Circulation

During the primary survey, the major goals of circulatory assessment and treatment are:

- To assess the overall circulatory status (pulse and perfusion) of the injured patient and provide appropriate intervention when necessary.
- To diagnose and control both external and internal hemorrhage.
- To obtain large-bore venous access.

Circulatory assessment should include palpation of the pulse for quality (ie, weak or strong), rate, and regularity. Tachycardia followed by hypotension is a normal homeostatic response to hypovolemia in both adults and children. Tachycardia is more prolonged in children; without adequate resuscitation, hypotension eventually will occur, followed rapidly by cardiac arrest.

The younger the child, the more fixed is the stroke volume and the more dependent is cardiac output on heart rate. Be familiar with the usual heart rates by age for children (Table 4-3). A weak and thready pulse is an indication of cardiovascular instability and impending collapse.

The **assessment of perfusion** is the basis for the early diagnosis and recognition of shock. Measures of circulatory adequacy include assessment of central nervous system status as a relative indicator of brain perfusion and urine output as an indicator of renal perfusion. Because central nervous system injuries are common in children, traumatic coma may cloud assessment of perfusion. Urine output is an accurate measure of renal perfusion, but it is of little benefit in very early patient assessment. Output should be maintained at 1 mL/kg per hour. Capillary refill is another adjunct used in the assessment of circulation. It is performed through the application of pressure on the skin or nail bed for 5 seconds and then observance of the time required for return of normal skin color. Under normal circumstances, the color should return within 2 seconds; prolongation beyond 2 seconds indicates relative hypovolemia. If the child has been in a cold environment, capillary refill of the extremities may be prolonged even in normovolemic patients.

Vascular Access. While the circulatory status is being assessed, reliable venous access must be established. The choices for vascular access include the following:

- Percutaneous peripheral venous cannulation with large-bore lines placed at one or two sites
- Intraosseous infusion
- Peripheral venous cutdown

Percutaneous central venous access is reserved

for situations in which other routes have failed. In the setting of trauma, the femoral approach is preferred.

Intraosseous fluid infusion (Appendix 5-3) is a valuable method for providing temporary circulatory access in children younger than 6 years when a peripheral line cannot be placed. The anterior tibial marrow can be cannulated quickly and used as an infusion site for fluids and medications. Complications are rare and usually involve subcutaneous infiltration of fluid or leakage from the puncture site after the needle has been removed, but more serious complications, such as compartment syndrome and tibial fracture, are known to occur. Although osteomyelitis and subcutaneous infections have been reported, these occur mainly when the intraosseous infusion is maintained for extended periods of time or when hypertonic fluids are infused. Intraosseous infusion must never be used in a fractured extremity. Whenever this means of access is used, it is to be regarded as a temporizing measure while attempts at direct vascular access are continued.

The best sites for **peripheral venous cutdown** (Appendix 5-4) are the saphenous vein at the ankle, the saphenofemoral junction at the groin, and the basilic vein near the antecubital fossa. The lower extremity and groin sites have the advantage of being distant from the sites of airway manipulation and cardiopulmonary resuscitation. In patients with major intra-abdominal vascular injury or hemorrhage, an upper extremity vein is preferred. Because the external jugular vein may be inaccessible as a result of airway manipulation and cervical spine stabilization, the basilic vein at the elbow should be used. This vein lies lateral and superior to the medial epicondyle of the elbow.

Hemorrhage Control. Systematic assessment of the entire body surface is necessary to ensure that all areas of **external hemorrhage** are evaluated and treated. Obtain information regarding the magnitude of blood loss at the scene of the injury from family, companions, or paramedical personnel. Any laceration may result in significant bleeding, but scalp and facial wounds are particularly prone to profuse hemorrhage. Begin measures to decrease external bleeding by applying direct pressure over bleeding sites with sterile dressings. Once pressure has been applied, maintain it with either manual pressure or pressure dressings. Ensure that pressure dressings do not occlude distal pulses. Elevate the bleeding areas to decrease the amount of blood loss. In most cases, the combination of direct pressure and elevation will arrest external hemorrhage.

In virtually every area of the body except the scalp, major nerves are in proximity to major blood vessels, and blind clamping of those vessels may result in peripheral nerve damage. Hemostats can be used to clamp spurting vessels on the hair-bearing areas of the scalp only.

Recognition of **internal bleeding** requires astute observation, a thorough physical examination, and attention to the subtle changes that sometimes occur with major internal hemorrhage. Life-threatening internal hemorrhage may occur in five body areas: chest, abdomen, retroperitoneum, pelvis, and thigh. Be alert to pain or swelling in any of those areas; this may be the first objective indication of internal hemorrhage.

Shock and Circulatory Failure. During the initial phase of care of the trauma patient, shock nearly always is hypovolemic in nature. Other causes of shock include hypoxia, cardiac tamponade, tension pneumothorax, and spinal cord injury.

Monitoring. Even when as much as 25% of a child's total blood volume has been lost, changes in heart rate or sensorium may be the only indicators of evolving shock. When blood loss exceeds 25% to 30% of total blood volume, compensatory vasoconstriction may fail abruptly and catastrophically. Hypotension, confusion, decreased urine output, and acidosis may emerge rapidly. At that point, irreversible vascular collapse may be imminent. Urine output, as a reflection of renal perfusion, thus becomes an important indicator of physiologic status. If there are signs of urethral injury, such as blood at the meatus, a quick retrograde urethrogram should be done before passing an indwelling bladder catheter. Urine present in the bladder at the time of the insertion usually was produced before injury and does not reflect current output.

All patients who have sustained significant trauma will benefit from an initial fluid infusion of 20 mL/kg. Patients with cool, pale extremities, tachycardia, and narrow pulse pressure may have lost up to 15% to 25% of their total blood volume and require immediate volume expansion with 20 mL/kg normal saline (approximately one fourth of their total blood volume, with blood volume calculated as 80 mL/kg) infused as rapidly as possible. If the patient does not respond rapidly to such fluid infusion, administer a second bolus of 20 mL/kg and prepare to administer blood.

Because patients with hypotension have lost ≥25% of their total blood volume and losses may well continue, they usually require multiple boluses of fluid. Although these boluses may transiently restore circulating volume, they add red cell dilution to exsanguination and soon undermine rather than improve oxygen delivery. When more than three crystalloid boluses are required, transfusion therapy usually is necessary.

Fluid Resuscitation. It is critical to assess and record accurately the initial indicators of circulatory status (pulse, respirations, blood pressure, pulse pressure, and mental status). Follow these findings closely to determine response to intervention.

Volume Replacement. Normal saline (NS) or lactated Ringer's (RL) is the fluid of choice for initial resuscitation of the pediatric trauma victim. Because the vast majority of severely injured children have sustained primary or secondary brain injury, it is logical to assume that the blood-brain barrier is compromised. In the face of evolving cerebral edema, excess free water is to be avoided. Fluid replacement is divided into two phases: **initial therapy** and **total replacement**. Fluids are administered rapidly via intravenous push with a 60-mL syringe. Three-way stopcocks should be in line so larger volumes of fluid can be administered in as short a period of time as possible. Vital signs are evaluated carefully before and after bolus therapy. If vital signs do not improve immediately, more volume is given.

The guidelines below are for initiation of therapy. If a child does not respond appropriately, suspect continued bleeding and look for other causes of refractory shock.

- All patients who have sustained significant trauma
  –Initial volume: 20 mL/kg NS or RL
- Mild shock (15% to 25% of blood volume loss)
  –Initial volume: 20 mL/kg NS or RL. If no improvement, repeat 20 mL/kg NS or RL.
  –Total volume: If improved, run NS or RL at 5 mL/kg per hour for several hours. If child remains stable, adjust intravenous rate down

toward maintenance levels.
  –Maintenance after volume is restored:
    • ≤10 kg: 100 mL/kg per 24 hours
    • 10 to 20 kg: 1000 mL plus 50 mL/kg per 24 hours
    • >20 kg: 1500 mL plus 20 mL/kg per 24 hours
- Moderate shock (25% to 40% of blood volume loss)
  –Initial volume: 20 mL/kg NS or RL; repeat immediately if not improved. If no improvement, alternative therapy includes 20 to 40 mL/kg NS or RL again, or 10 to 20 mL/kg packed red blood cells and surgical intervention.
  –Total volume: If improved, run NS or RL at 5 mL/kg per hour for several hours. If child remains stable, adjust intravenous rate toward maintenance levels. May need transfusion depending on clinical response and hematocrit.
- Severe shock (≥40% of blood volume loss)
  –Initial volume: Push NS or RL until blood available. Push packed red blood cells or whole blood. Surgery.
  –Total volume: Replace with type-specific blood.

Pneumatic Antishock Garment. An adjunct previously used in pediatric shock cases is the pneumatic antishock garment (PASG). The PASG may have some benefit in patients with pelvic and lower extremity fractures in which it may assist in splinting fractures and diminishing venous bleeding; however, the PASG is no longer recommended for the treatment of shock.

Disability

AVPU. A rapid neurologic evaluation is part of the primary survey. This neurologic evaluation should include assessment of only pupillary response, patient's level of consciousness, and any obvious localizing finding such as paralysis or paresis of an extremity. A simple method for evaluating level of consciousness involves the mnemonic **AVPU**:

A – Alert
V – Responds to verbal stimuli
P – Responds to painful stimuli
U – Unresponsive

A more in-depth neurologic assessment should

be performed during the secondary survey (see Chapter 6).

Glasgow Coma Scale. The Glasgow Coma Scale score can be used to assess the verbal and nonverbal child (see Chapter 6).

Exposure and Examination

It is important that the patient's clothing be removed completely to allow full assessment of the extent of injury and a complete examination. However, in an open space, such as the emergency department, a small child may quickly become hypothermic after exposure. A radiant warmer, warming blanket, or air convection unit may be required to maintain the child's temperature at 36° to 37°C.

If not already done, place a nasogastric tube (after excluding evidence of midfacial fracture) and insert a urinary catheter (unless there is suspected urethral injury, such as with a pelvic fracture or when blood is at the urethral meatus).

Secondary Survey

The secondary survey is a timely, directed evaluation of each body area that proceeds from head to toe. It should answer the following questions:

- Is an injury present in the anatomic area under evaluation?
- If so, what type of injury is present, and which organ is injured?
- What is the severity of the injury, including both the anatomic and physiologic severity, to each organ?
- What is the appropriate definitive care for the injury?
- What is the priority of therapy for this injury compared with other injuries identified in the secondary survey?

The components of the secondary survey are:

- History
- Complete examination
- Laboratory studies
- Radiographic studies
- Problem identification

During this phase, complete the history and perform a thorough physical examination. Pay attention to the adequacy of cervical stabilization obtained during the primary survey and continue aggressive resuscitation.

History

The history should include the mechanism of injury, time, status at scene, changes in status, and complaints that the child may have. Obtain a history using the mnemonic **AMPLE**:

A – Allergies
M – Medications
P – Past illnesses
L – Last meal
E – Events preceding the injury

The child's parents may be quite useful not only for the history but also in assessment of the child's interactions with them.

Physical Examination

Head. Begin the secondary survey with an evaluation of the eyes, including conjunctiva, pupillary size and reaction, retinal appearance, and vision, if possible. Examine the face for evidence of maxillofacial trauma by palpating bony prominences. Check the dentition. Examine the scalp carefully for laceration or underlying soft tissue injury. Suspect basilar skull fracture if the **Battle's sign** or **raccoon eyes** are present or if hemotympanum, cerebrospinal fluid, rhinorrhea, or otorrhea occurs. Check for symmetric voluntary movement and neurologic function of the facial muscles.

Neck. Examine the neck for subcutaneous emphysema, abnormal tracheal position, hematoma, or localized pain. Palpate the cervical spine for stepoffs, swelling, or tenderness. Neck vein distention also should be assessed.

Chest. Reevaluate the chest visually for adequacy of respiratory excursion, asymmetry of chest wall motion, or the presence of a flail segment. After observation, carefully palpate the chest and auscultate the lung fields and cardiovascular system.

Abdomen. Examine the abdomen next; it is important to remember that specific diagnoses usually are not possible immediately. Examination of the abdomen includes inspection for ease of movement with respiration, bruises, seatbelt marks, tire marks, and lacerations; auscultation of bowel sounds; and gentle palpation for localized findings. Observe and palpate the flanks. The abdomen may need to be examined several times to make an accurate assessment.

Pelvis. Palpate the bony prominences of the pelvis for tenderness or instability. Carefully examine the perineum for laceration, hematoma, or active bleeding. Check the urethral meatus for blood.

Rectum. A rectal examination is necessary; evaluate the integrity of the wall, displacement or distortion of the prostate, sphincter muscle tone, and occult gastrointestinal hemorrhage.

Extremities. Examine the extremities for signs of fracture, dislocation, abrasion, contusion, or hematoma formation. Note bony instability, and perform a neurovascular evaluation.

Back. Examination of the back should not be neglected. With the neck immobilized, if spinal injury or paralysis has not been excluded, gently roll the patient to examine the entire back and spine.

Skin. Examine thoroughly for evidence of contusions, burns, and petechiae, as in traumatic asphyxia.

Neurologic. Perform an in-depth neurologic examination, including motor, sensory, and cranial nerves and level of consciousness. Reexamine the fundi. Check the nose for rhinorrhea.

Laboratory and Radiographic Studies

The first laboratory study should be typing and cross-matching blood for possible transfusion. A more extensive laboratory database for a significantly injured child will be highly individualized and driven by clinical judgment. At a minimum, in the seriously injured child, hematocrit or hemoglobin, white blood cell count, glucose, and urinalysis are needed; serial determinations may be helpful.

A cervical spine radiographic series is required if a neck injury is suspected or the child has serious multisystem trauma or head injury. A chest radiograph often is needed, and other radiographs are obtained as directed by physical findings and history. More sophisticated studies for severely injured children usually include computed tomography, especially if there is a head injury.

Continuously monitor and frequently reevaluate the patient. A high index of suspicion and constant alertness for signs of deterioration or the development of new problems will allow early diagnosis and management of ongoing pathophysiology.

It is important that those involved with emergency treatment of seriously injured children understand the principles of care and priorities of treatment in multiple trauma. The person who performs the initial evaluation and stabilization should remain the child's responsible practitioner and function as his or her advocate until responsibility for the child's total care is undertaken by another. Appropriate consultations must be requested by the captain of the trauma team.

Document initial assessment and all resuscitation procedures. Such records are essential in monitoring improvement or deterioration. Frequently, in the "heat of battle," important data and observations are lost; this can be avoided by adequate preplanning and assignment of record-keeping to experienced personnel.

Problem Identification

Head and Spinal Cord Injuries. See Chapters 6 and 7.

Chest Injuries. Blunt **thoracic trauma** is encountered commonly in children and may cause injuries that require immediate correction to establish adequate ventilation. A child's chest wall is very compliant and allows energy transfer to the intrathoracic structures, frequently without any evidence of injury on the external chest wall. The elasticity of the chest wall increases the likelihood of pulmonary contusions and direct intrapulmonary hemorrhage, usually without overlying rib fractures. Significant thoracic injuries rarely occur alone and usually are a component of major multisystem injury.

Children with **pulmonary contusion** manifest few physical findings. Early radiographs may show minimal changes. Such patients require careful monitoring and serial evaluations of ventilatory status. Observe for development of tachycardia, rales, hemoptysis, and a falling PaO_2. Early recognition is important. Provide oxygen, elevate the head of the bed, and limit fluids unless the patient is in hypovolemic shock.

Pneumothorax can occur with blunt or penetrating trauma and consists of air in the pleural space from lung or tracheobronchial tree injury or external leakage. Minimal collections of air in the pleural space may be undetected on examination and are seen best on an expiratory chest radiograph, although even then they may be obscured if the film is taken with the patient in the supine position.

Collapse of one lung may produce signs of hypoxia, hyperresonance to percussion, asymmetry of chest wall movement, and decreased breath sounds on the affected side. Treatment involves tube thoracostomy with underwater seal drainage. Bilateral pneumothoraces and tension pneumothorax are life-threatening injuries. With bilateral pneumothoraces, the patient is hypoxic, has minimal or absent breath sounds bilaterally, and is typically hypotensive. A needle or an over-the-needle catheter device placed in the second intercostal space anteriorly or in the fourth to fifth intercostal space (Appendix 5-5) in the axillary line (at the level of the nipple) may be life saving until chest tubes can be placed. Remember to administer oxygen to all patients who sustain significant blunt chest trauma.

An **open pneumothorax** may be sucking or nonsucking, depending on size and other factors. Intrathoracic and atmospheric pressures equilibrate; thus, if the opening is as large or larger than the airway, no effective ventilation occurs. Place an occlusive dressing (gauze impregnated with petroleum jelly) over the wound and tape it on three sides. Insert a chest tube immediately (Appendix 5-6). If the patient exhibits sudden respiratory embarrassment after the closure, suspect tension pneumothorax. Remove the dressing briefly to let any air under pressure escape until the chest tube is placed.

A **tension pneumothorax** is a common lethal chest injury. It frequently develops after the patient's arrival in the hospital and especially may occur in ventilated patients who receive high inspiratory volumes under positive pressure to potentially injured lung parenchyma. The pathophysiology is that of sudden combined cardiorespiratory failure. The pleural pressure rises and the lung collapses. The mediastinum shifts and the opposite lung is compressed. The superior vena cava kinks, and there is decreased venous return. The resulting decreased cardiac output is the immediate threat to life.

The diagnosis must be established by physical examination prompted by a high index of suspicion. The neck veins are distended and the trachea is deviated. These findings may not be present in children with tension pneumothorax,

and a high index of suspicion must be maintained. There are decreased breath sounds with tympany and hypotension.

Immediate treatment is required to improve cardiac output. First, perform needle thoracostomy, and convert the tension pneumothorax to a simple pneumothorax. Needle thoracostomy can be performed within seconds and will provide several minutes of stability while a chest tube is inserted.

Traumatic hemothorax is treated with chest tube insertion and concomitant volume replacement. If massive bleeding is noted, the chest tube should be clamped and the patient prepared for immediate thoracotomy. Continued bleeding (>10 mL/kg per hour) indicates major vascular injury and the need for open thoracotomy.

Traumatic asphyxia occurs with sudden massive compression of the chest. The pressure is transmitted to the heart, lungs, vena cava, neck, and head. Clinical signs include petechiae of the head and neck, subconjunctival hemorrhages, and, occasionally, depressed level of consciousness. Hemoptysis, pulmonary contusion, and great vessel injury may be present. Treatment consists of management of component injuries. Supply oxygen, place chest tubes as needed, limit fluids, and elevate the head of the bed. If PaO_2 falls, the use of positive end-expiratory pressure and mechanical ventilation may be indicated.

Cardiac tamponade more commonly occurs as an iatrogenic injury after cardiac catheterization, postoperative open heart surgery, or placement of a central venous catheter. It also may occur with a penetrating or crush injury. There is an accumulation of blood in the pericardial sac so the heart cannot fill during diastole, causing low cardiac output. The diagnostic triad is shock (look for narrowed pulse pressure), distended neck veins (also massive hepatomegaly), and muffled heart sounds. Treatment consists of a large fluid bolus and pericardiocentesis (Appendix 5-2). The aspiration of a small volume of fluid from the pericardial space may be life saving. If there is time, an echocardiogram can be helpful in securing the diagnosis.

Abdominal Injuries. The onset of symptoms of abdominal injury may be rapid (due to the massive hemorrhage) or slow in evolution (primarily due to bacterial or chemical peritonitis). Children with such injuries may only need to be observed carefully, with judicious fluid and blood replacement. The decision to observe injuries of this type can be made only with the surgeon who will be responsible for emergency laparotomy if such becomes necessary. If the abdominal injury results in significant blood loss that prevents successful reestablishment or maintenance of vital functions after 40-mL/kg volume restoration, immediate surgical intervention may be necessary.

It is important to remember that the abdominal examination initially may fail to show significant abdominal pathology and that sequential reexamination is essential to rule out an evolving abdominal problem. Perform such reexaminations periodically while other organ systems are being evaluated. The abdominal girth should be measured serially.

Computed tomography, serial abdominal examination, and monitoring are used in children more often than diagnostic peritoneal lavage. Even in centers in which radionuclide scanning, computed tomography, and ultrasonography are used to evaluate the intra-abdominal contents, diagnostic peritoneal lavage still can play a helpful role in the child with a depressed level of consciousness whose injuries require immediate surgical intervention on another organ system. This situation may include a child who requires neurosurgical exploration or open fracture irrigation and debridement. A peritoneal tap to determine significant abdominal injury is, however, seldom used in a lucid child who does not require immediate surgery.

Priority of abdominal injury management in a child with multiple trauma depends on the severity of insult and the other systems involved. A child with multiple trauma and a severe cerebral insult, who can be easily stabilized, can have cerebral diagnostic and resuscitative efforts take precedence over a self-limited abdominal injury. The suspected abdominal injury, however, must be evaluated systematically and defined accurately. Capability to intervene surgically in the abdomen requires the presence of a surgeon on the evaluating team in all seriously injured children.

Liver and Spleen Injuries. The liver and spleen are organs commonly injured from blunt trauma in the child. These injuries may be sufficiently extensive to require immediate exploration, but recent experience indicates that in children they are frequently self-limited. This has stimulated the evolution of nonsurgical protocols in which stable children are managed expectantly with intensive care monitoring and surgical supervision because the option of immediate surgical intervention must be available at all times. This decision to treat nonsurgically is solely the responsibility of the surgeon and must be based on personal examination and evaluation.

Pancreatic/Duodenal Injuries. High-speed deceleration or direct blows to the upper abdomen may produce pancreatic or duodenal trauma. The most commonly reported pancreatic lesions are fractures and severe contusions, usually in the midportion of the gland as it overlies the lumbar spine. This may present as relatively acute onset peritonitis, or it may produce a posttraumatic pseudocyst that develops within days to weeks of injury. Duodenal injury may produce retroperitoneal leak as well as frank duodenal disruption. It should be considered in any child subjected to abuse. Intramural duodenal hematoma is a lesion frequently seen in children who sustain blunt abdominal trauma. It commonly causes signs and symptoms of upper intestinal obstruction. As with pancreatic injuries, a high index of suspicion is the key to expedient and accurate recognition.

Intestinal Injuries. The intestine may be perforated by deceleration trauma, but this is relatively uncommon. Intestinal perforation may be present immediately with the development of free air, notable on abdominal radiographs, or it may present with the evolution of bacterial peritonitis over a period of 12 to 24 hours. Mesenteric injuries occur infrequently after trauma from improper seatbelt position. Less frequently, the intestine may be perforated by a deceleration or whiplash injury.

Genitourinary Injuries. Retroperitoneal injuries involving the kidney vary from simple contusion to major renal pedicle disruptions with perinephric hematomas and complete loss of renal function. A high index of suspicion must be present to diagnose serious conditions early in the patient's course so suitable management can be introduced quickly.

The combination of significant flank trauma and hematuria (even microscopic) in a seriously injured child is an indication for a computed tomography scan with intravenous contrast to assess bilateral function and absence of extravasation. If abnormal, surgical consultation should be obtained. In some centers, a sonogram is the initial diagnostic tool used to evaluate for renal abnormalities.

Lower urinary tract disruption occurs primarily in association with severe pelvic trauma, the prototype of which is the straddle (bicycle) injury. A child who has blood at the urethral meatus requires retrograde urethrography to determine whether a lower urinary tract injury is present.

DISPOSITION

After initial assessment, resuscitation, and stabilization, a decision must be made about definitive care. Admission to the local hospital may be indicated if the injuries are not life threatening and appropriate supportive and consultative services are available. In cases in which more comprehensive or specialized care is needed, rapid safe transport must be arranged. For such transfer to be effective, the patient must be stabilized. Practitioner-to-practitioner discussion between transferring and receiving hospitals is mandatory before, during, and after transport (see Chapter 20).

Considerations for interhospital transport include personnel to accompany the child and medication and equipment necessary for safe effective transfer. Clear written instructions to transferring personnel should augment established protocol. All pertinent records and radiographs should be transferred with the patient, as well as identification of family and referring practitioner. Give the child's family support in obtaining parallel transportation to the receiving hospital. Allow them to see and touch the child as soon as possible and keep separation to a minimum.

SUMMARY

The gradual development of more sophisticated and complete emergency medical systems is improving the quality of pediatric trauma care by establishing well-defined primary and definitive care centers and protocols for transfer. Predetermined referral patterns and transfer agreements will facilitate and standardize the optimal regional care provided to an injured child.

ADDITIONAL READING

American Academy of Pediatrics. *Guidelines for Air and Ground Transport of Neonatal Pediatric Patients.* Elk Grove Village, Ill: American Academy of Pediatrics; 1993.

Cooper A, Barlow B, DiScala C, et al. Mortality and truncal injury: the pediatric perspective. *J Pediatr Surg.* 1994;29:33-38

Cooper A. Pediatric trauma (basic principles). In: Ayres SM, ed. *Textbook of Critical Care*, 3rd ed. Philadelphia, Pa: WB Saunders; 1995:1465-1475.

Eichelberger MR, ed. *Pediatric Trauma: Prevention, Acute Care, Rehabilitation.* St Louis, Mo: Mosby–Year Book; 1993.

Fleisher GR, Ludwig S. *Textbook of Pediatric Emergency Medicine*, 3rd ed. Baltimore, Md: Williams & Wilkins; 1993.

Mayer T, Walker ML, Johnson DG, et al. Causes of morbidity and mortality in severe pediatric trauma. *JAMA.* 1981;245:719-721.

Rang M, ed. *Children's Fractures*, 2nd ed. Philadelphia, Pa: JB Lippincott Co; 1983.

Tepas JJ, DiScala C, Ramenofsky ML, et al. Mortality and head injury: the pediatric perspective. *J Pediatr Surg.* 1990;25:92-95.

Tepas JJ. Pediatric trauma. In: Feliciano DV, Moore EE, Mattox KL, eds. *Trauma.* Stamford, Conn: Appleton & Lange; 1996:879-898.

Tepas JJ: Problems and solutions. In: Arensman RM, ed. *Pediatric Trauma: Initial Care of the Injured Child.* New York, NY: Raven Press; 1995:1-5.

Trauma resuscitation. In: Chameides L, Hazinski MF, eds. *Textbook of Pediatric Advanced Life Support.* Dallas, Tex: American Heart Association; 1997:8-1 to 8-9.

Wesson DE, Filler RM, Ein SH, et al. Ruptured spleen—when to operate? *J Pediatr Surg.* 1981;16:324-326.

Appendix 5-1. Cricothyroidotomy.

Cricothyroidotomy (Figure 5-4) rarely is necessary in the pediatric patient and should be attempted only if other airway methods have been unsuccessful. It can be performed with the patient's head in a neutral position, with adequate cervical spine stabilization. After preparation of the neck with antiseptic solution, use one finger to palpate the cricothyroid membrane in the midline, between the thyroid and cricoid cartilages. It is critical to stay precisely in the midline during this procedure to ensure the airway is cannulated appropriately and significant bleeding is avoided. Have an assistant hold the child's head and neck to facilitate this midline position. Once the cricothyroid membrane has been identified clearly, attach a 10-mL syringe to a large (14-gauge) over-the-needle catheter device.

While palpating the cricothyroid cartilage in the midline, insert the needle with catheter just below the midpoint of the cricothyroid membrane, with the needle angled 45 degrees caudally. Rapid aspiration of air into the syringe indicates entry into the tracheal lumen. Withdraw the needle carefully while advancing the plastic catheter caudally into the trachea, taking care not to perforate the posterior tracheal wall. Recheck the position of the catheter through aspiration with the syringe. Attach the hub of the catheter to an adapter and then to a connector between the oxygen and the cannula. Oxygen flow should be ≥15 L/min. Intermittent ventilation can be provided by a jet ventilator or even by occluding the open port of the Y connector with the thumb placed on for 1 second and off for 4 seconds. This technique allows 30 to 40 minutes of oxygenation and is a temporizing measure until more secure airway control can be obtained. It is important to remember that carbon dioxide retention may occur even with adequate oxygenation and may be especially hazardous in the head-injured child.

Open surgical cricothyroidotomy is a useful procedure in older children and adolescents when performed by appropriately trained physicians, but it is a potentially dangerous procedure in young children because the cricoid cartilage is the narrowest level of the pediatric airway. In addition, significant bleeding can be encountered if the cricothyroid artery, which extends horizontally over the upper portion of the cricothyroid membrane, is injured. Reserve surgical cricothyroidotomy for those extremely rare circumstances in which intubation cannot be performed and needle cricothyroidotomy is not satisfactory.

FIGURE 5-4.
Needle cricothyroidotomy. A, Anatomy of cricothyroid area. B, Insertion of angiocatheter. C, Attach Luer-lock to oxygen source. D, Surgical cricothroidotomy (very rarely indicated).

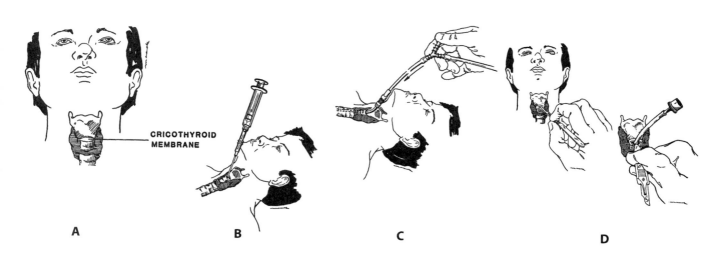

CRICOTHYROID MEMBRANE

A   B   C   D

Appendix 5-2. Pericardiocentesis.

Insert an 18-gauge angiocatheter into the subxiphoid area just to the left of midline. Aim the needle tip for the left scapula, 45 degrees laterally and 45 degrees superiorly (Figure 5-5). Aspirate on the syringe during needle advancement. Blood aspirated from the pericardial sac will not clot; blood aspirated from the heart chambers will clot within 4 to 6 minutes. Remove the needle and leave the catheter in the pericardial space in case further aspiration is required. Careful ECG monitoring is necessary to watch for ST-segment changes.

FIGURE 5-5.
Pericardiocentesis.

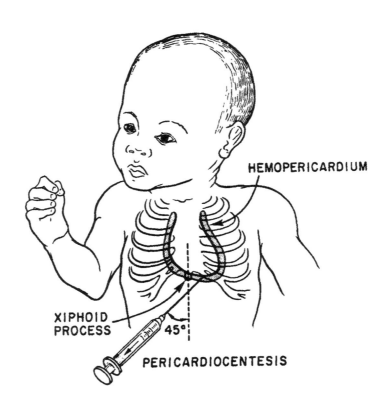

Appendix 5-3. Intraosseous Infusion.

After preparing the skin antiseptically and securing the leg adequately, choose a site on the anteromedial portion of the tibia, 1 to 2 cm distal and medial to the tibial tuberosity. Specially manufactured intraosseous infusion needles are optimal for the procedure, but a Jamshidi bone marrow aspiration needle or any 14- to 18-gauge needle with a stylette can be used in an emergency. Holding the needle at a 60-degree caudal angle, advance firmly using rotary motion until the cortex is penetrated and the marrow cavity entered (Figure 5-6). Evidence that the needle is adequately within the marrow includes:

- A soft pop and lack of resistance to forward motion after the needle has passed through the cortex
- Aspiration of bone marrow into the needle
- Free flow of fluid into the marrow without evidence of subcutaneous infiltration

Consider intraosseous infusion of fluid, blood, and medication during the initial minutes of resuscitation if percutaneous venous cannulation has been unsuccessful. Because the flow rate is limited, the intraosseous route alone seldom will be sufficient for prolonged resuscitation.

FIGURE 5-6.

Intraosseous infusion. A, Standard anterior tibial approach. The insertion point is in the midline on the medial flat surface of the anterior tibia, 1 to 2 cm (two fingers' breadth) below the tibial tuberosity. B, Anterior tibial approach for young infants. The insertion point is at the level of the tibial tuberosity.

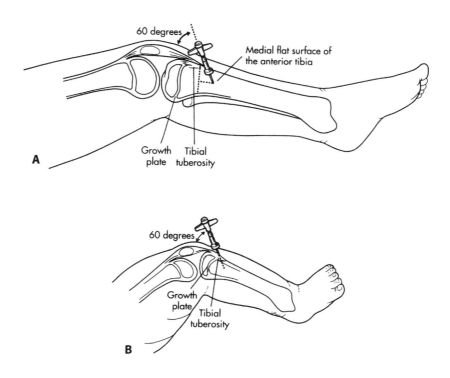

From Dieckmann RA, Fiser DH, Selbst SM, eds. *Illustrated Textbook of Pediatric Emergency & Critical Care Procedures.* St Louis, Mo: Mosby; 1996:222. Adapted with permission.

Appendix 5-4. Venous Cutdown.

Regardless of the site chosen for cannulation, the technique for cutdown should be the same. After preparation of the skin with antiseptic and anesthetic, make a 1- to 2-cm skin incision, taking care to incise only the skin. Ligate or cauterize small vessels in the wound (easily performed with a sterile, hand-held electrocautery device) because even minor bleeding may obscure adequate cannulation. Place a small curved hemostat in the wound to gently probe for the vein.

After placing the hemostat underneath the vein, gently open the instrument to free the vein gradually from the surrounding tissue. Clear surrounding tissue from the vein as much as possible because that tissue may impair cannulation by creating false tracks around the vein. Once the vein has been dissected free for a distance of 1 to 2 cm, place strands of 4-0 absorbable suture under the vein. Place the distal suture around the most distal aspect of the vein at the inferior border of the wound margin. Neither suture is tied at this point but simply provides countertraction while the vein is cannulated. Puncture the vein directly with an over-the-needle catheter device and advance the catheter into the vein (Figure 5-7). Secure the catheter in place by tying the proximal suture around the vein and catheter.

FIGURE 5-7.
Saphenous vein cutdown. A, Anatomy of skin incision. B, Scoop vein off tibial periosteum. C, Puncture the vein directly with an over-the-needle catheter device and insert catheter with stylet removed to avoid marking a false passage.

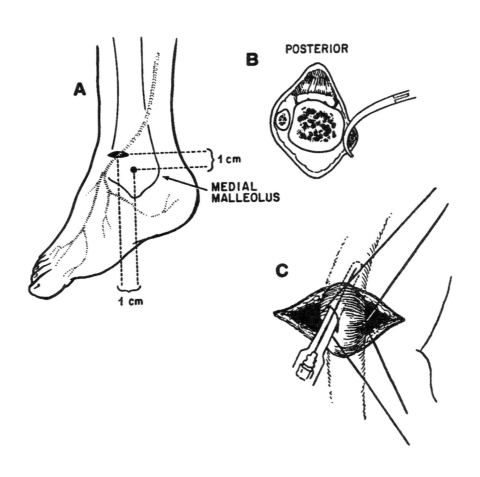

Appendix 5-5. Needle Thoracostomy.

Equipment required for needle thoracostomy includes the following:
- 14- or 16-gauge over-the-needle catheter
- 3-way stopcock
- 60-mL syringe

Attach the needle to the stopcock and syringe. Insert the needle just over the rib in the second interspace at the midclavicular line or the fourth interspace at the anterior axillary line. As the needle is advanced through the chest wall, aspiration suddenly will become very easy as the pleural space is entered and decompressed. Leave the catheter in the pleural space and open to atmospheric pressure (Figure 5-8). After the thoracentesis, perform a tube thoracostomy. Attach the chest tube to a one-way valve for transport; an underwater seal is used in the hospital.

FIGURE 5-8.
Needle thoracostomy.

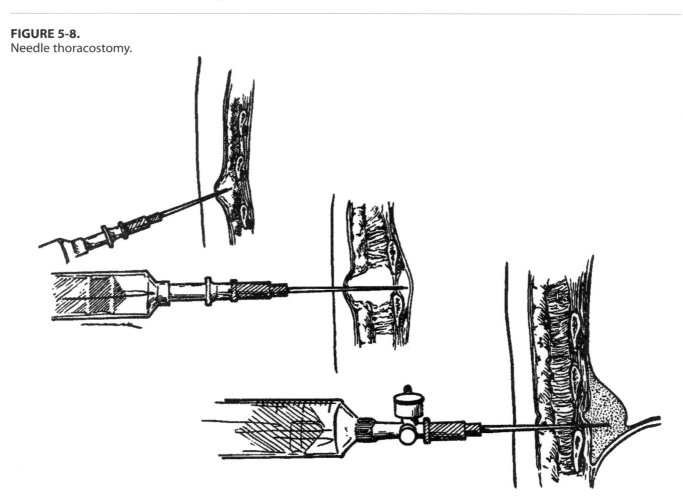

Appendix 5-6. Insertion of a Chest Tube.

Identify the side or sides with the hemothorax or pneumothorax through physical examination and, **if time allows**, a chest radiograph. Initiate treatment of cardiorespiratory disturbances before beginning the procedure (Figure 5-9). If abdominal distention is present, pass a large-bore nasogastric tube to reduce diaphragmatic elevation.

Restrain the child if necessary. Locate the landmarks, and cleanse the site with povidone-iodine solution. Wearing sterile gloves, use a local anesthetic (1% lidocaine) in an awake child to infiltrate the skin, subcutaneous tissue, and periosteum of the upper rib border. Make the skin incision one intercostal space below the rib over which the catheter will pass. That provides an oblique trajectory for the chest tube, which helps maintain a seal when the tube is in position and after its removal.

Using a curved hemostat or Kelly clamp, bluntly dissect through the muscle and fascial layers to the upper surface of the chosen rib. Determine proper location by palpation with the tip of the instrument. Slide the instrument over the superior rib margin, puncturing the intercostal muscles and pleura well below the neurovascular bundle of the adjacent cephalad rib. Open the instrument widely to provide an opening through the intercostal muscles and pleura that is ≥1.5 to 2.0 cm in diameter. At that point, any fluid or air under pressure in the pleural space may surge out.

Grasp the chest tube between the tips of the curved hemostat or clamp. Advance the instrument through the incision and up the previously dissected tract to the pleural space. When the tube tip has entered the cavity, open the hemostat and advance the catheter until all holes of the tube are well within the chest. The tip will most likely be at the apex of the hemithorax. Approximate the incision with several sutures, some of which should encircle the tube to secure it in place. Apply a sterile occlusive dressing to the wound. Further taping will help prevent dislodging. After the tube has been attached to the drainage set and when the patient is stable, obtain an upright or a decubitus chest radiograph.

FIGURE 5-9.
Tube thoracostomy. A, Location of chest tube insertion site. B, Skin incision and thoracic wall entry site. C, Retract skin superiorly to superimpose skin and chest wall entry sites. D, Final position of chest tube and pursestring suture. Attach tube to underwater drainage.

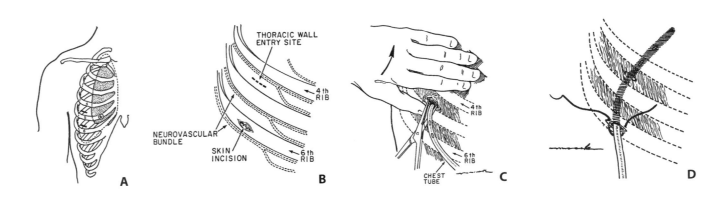

Chapter 6

Head Trauma

OBJECTIVES

1. Identify the primary and secondary causes of brain damage, including increased intracranial pressure, after head trauma.

2. Assess the patient using the AVPU system and Glasgow Coma Scale.

3. Provide optimal initial therapy and appropriate triage for children with head injuries.

4. Identify appropriate diagnostic imaging modalities for head-injured patients.

5. Recognize the various clinical manifestations of head trauma, including epidural and subdural hemorrhage.

6. Describe the indications and guidelines for intubation and hyperventilation in a head-injured patient.

In children, head injury accounts for ≈4% to 8% of visits to pediatric emergency departments. Although most injuries are trivial, ≈80% of traumatic deaths in children result from head injuries. The assessment, treatment, and triage of the head-injured child are anxiety provoking because failure to appreciate the extent of the injury and anticipate and treat sequelae may result in increased morbidity and sometimes mortality.

The type of injury varies with the age of the child. In the neonate, head injuries may be sustained at birth as a result of a traumatic forceps extraction, but neonates with head injuries rarely present to the emergency department. The practitioner, however, will be faced with infants who have sustained nonaccidental head injury as a result of child abuse and who may have no external signs of trauma. It has been determined that child abuse is common in children younger than 2 years who are admitted to tertiary care hospitals because of head trauma. Children who are ambulatory and younger than 5 years are likely to sustain head injuries as a result of falls at home; those older than 5 years are more likely to be involved as pedestrians or cyclists in collisions with motor vehicles. This is the most common cause of traumatic death in children. At any age, head trauma may be sustained by passengers in motor vehicle collisions.

Because of anatomic and physiologic differences, the child's response to trauma is significantly different from that of the adult. An appreciation of these differences is the first step in the proper management of these children. The goal of emergency care should be the prevention of secondary cerebral insults. The practitioner should be able to assess the patient with head injuries, initiate resuscitation and stabilization, request appropriate diagnostic studies, consult with specialists, and appropriately triage these patients. This chapter is intended to provide information to assist in the management of a wide spectrum of insults due to head trauma.

PATHOPHYSIOLOGY

Brain insults may occur at the time of impact and usually are due to damage sustained as a result of direct trauma to the skull and intracranial structures. These injuries include scalp lacerations and skull fractures, as well as traumatic neuronal and vascular injuries. Primary injuries sustained at the time of impact only rarely are influenced by therapeutic interventions; however, secondary brain injury may occur as a result of the ongoing pathophysiologic derangements. In addition, failure to recognize and treat disorders of other organ systems, including the cardiovascular and respiratory systems, may further potentiate brain injury. Iatrogenic factors, such as overzealous hydration, also may contribute to cerebral swelling and secondary brain damage (Figure 6-1). The final common pathway leading to secondary brain injury usually is increased intracranial pressure (ICP) and decreased cerebral perfusion pressure (CPP). Maintenance of adequate CPP relies on maintenance of a normal blood pressure with appropriate volume expansion and inotropic support when necessary, as well as maneuvers to maintain ICP within normal limits.

Determinants of Cerebral Perfusion Pressure

CPP is calculated as the mean arterial pressure (MAP) minus ICP. Increased ICP is the most common cause of decreased CPP in the head-injured child; this occurs because of the unyielding nature of the cranial vault and relative low compliance of the intracranial contents. The intracranial cavity contains cerebrospinal fluid (CSF), brain, and cerebral blood.

Intracranial volume (IC_{vol}) is represented by the following formula:

$$IC_{vol} = CSF_{vol} + Blood_{vol} + Brain_{vol}$$

Under normal circumstances, the intracranial volume is maintained relatively constant because of compensatory adjustments in these three components. As such, ICP is kept relatively constant (<15 mm Hg) and fluctuates minimally with the Valsalva maneuver, respiration, pulse, and position. Once the compliance of the intracranial vault is exceeded, small changes in volume cause

FIGURE 6-1.
Dynamics of traumatic brain damage.

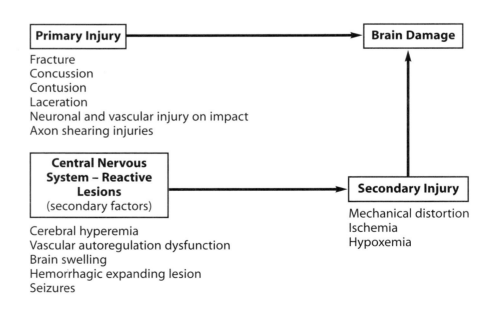

SYSTEMIC INJURY

Pulmonary
Hypercarbia
Hypoxia
Cardiovascular
Decreased cardiac output
Hypotension
Hypertension
Hematologic
Anemia
Coagulopathy
Thrombosis
Skeletal
Fat embolism
Miscellaneous
Electrolyte disturbance
Hyperthermia
Infection

Primary Injury ⟶ **Brain Damage**

Fracture
Concussion
Contusion
Laceration
Neuronal and vascular injury on impact
Axon shearing injuries

Central Nervous System – Reactive Lesions (secondary factors)

Cerebral hyperemia
Vascular autoregulation dysfunction
Brain swelling
Hemorrhagic expanding lesion
Seizures

Secondary Injury

Mechanical distortion
Ischemia
Hypoxemia

massive increases in ICP (Figure 6-2).

Buffering Mechanisms

Cerebrospinal Fluid

The CSF is an important early buffer for the maintenance of ICP. The CSF comprises ≈10% of the intracranial volume, and most is displaced easily into the spinal subarachnoid space when intracranial volume increases. With further increase in brain swelling, the ventricular system is compressed. This causes further displacement of CSF, which again diminishes the intracranial CSF volume. When CSF volume is almost totally displaced, intracranial compliance is diminished, and at this time, pressure-volume relationships are occurring in the steep part of the volume-pressure curve (Figure 6-2). At this point, minimal changes in intracranial volume may produce marked and sustained rises in ICP. In most cases, patients presenting with increased ICP have exhausted the CSF compensatory mechanism, so therapy to decrease ICP relies on other mechanisms, including manipulation of cerebral blood volume.

Cerebral Blood Volume

Blood comprises ≈8% of the intracranial volume. Most of the cerebral blood is in thin-walled venous capacitance vessels. Extrinsic pressure from a mass lesion may displace blood from these vessels. However, cerebral blood flow (CBF) may be increased in response to head trauma in childhood.

This global increase in CBF (cerebral hyperemia) may occur shortly after injury. Although the underlying reasons for this increase in CBF and intracranial blood volume are unknown, it is well established that CBF is responsive to changes in $PaCO_2$ and PaO_2 (Figures 6-3 and 6-4).

Hypocarbia of 25 to 30 mm Hg reduces cerebral blood volume by ≈50% from baseline levels at $PaCO_2$ of 40 mm Hg. This is important because children with severe head injury may hypoventilate and become hypercapnic, with resultant cerebral hyperemia. The CO_2 response is the rationale for hyperventilating the child with severe head injury and increased ICP. However, recent evidence suggests that prolonged hyperventilation to $PaCO_2$ levels of <35 mm Hg offers little benefit and that levels of <25 mm Hg are potentially hazardous as a result of reduction in global CBF achieved mainly by decreasing flow to undamaged brain tissue. The provision of adequate oxygenation (PaO_2 >80 mm Hg) also is important because hypoxemia may be accompanied by an acute rise in cerebral blood volume as well as secondary hypoxic neuronal damage. Seizure activity or hyperthermia increases cerebral metabolic rate and oxygen demand and may potentiate neuronal injury if metabolic demands are not met.

Brain

The brain parenchyma occupies ≈80% of the intracranial volume. It is minimally compressible

FIGURE 6-2.
Relationship of expanding intracranial volume to intracranial pressure.

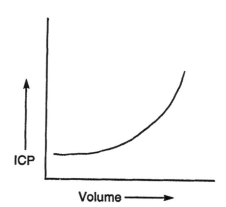

FIGURE 6-3.
Relationship of $PaCO_2$ to cerebral blood flow.

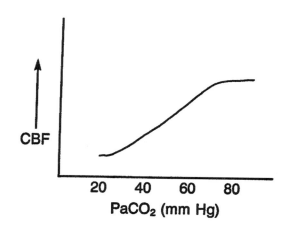

and contributes very little to the intracranial volume-buffering system. In children with no significant underlying brain lesions, rapid recovery will occur if CPP is maintained within normal limits. However, in children with diffuse impact injuries, initial control of hyperemia will maintain a normal ICP, but delayed elevation of ICP may occur due to cellular edema. Control of this edema can be achieved in part through avoidance of overhydration. Water restriction is no longer recommended because its salutary effects on ICP may be countered by untoward effects on MAP, thereby decreasing ICP.

MANIFESTATION OF HEAD TRAUMA IN CHILDREN

The type and extent of head injury in children vary tremendously and depend on the age of the child and nature of the traumatic event. Injuries may vary from relatively minor injuries to the scalp to very severe disruptions of brain tissue.

Extracranial Head Injuries

Lacerations and Hematomas

These are fairly common injuries and, fortunately, usually minor. When scalp lacerations are extensive, local hemostasis is a priority. If direct pressure does not control the hemorrhage, either infiltration of lidocaine with epinephrine ($\leq$7 mg/kg) or hemostat application to the galea with

external reflection will temporarily control most bleeding areas. The wound then should be explored with a gloved finger. Evidence of bone fragments or open or depressed fractures necessitate neurosurgical consultation before closure. Pressure applied directly to the repaired wound also enhances hemostasis.

Subgaleal Hematoma

These injuries occur frequently in children younger than 1 year. The child may have a lump that is not noticed for several days. Children with subgaleal hematomas commonly present with a soft, boggy swelling, occasionally in association with a linear fracture. Because of the fluctuant nature of these lesions, they often are diagnosed as having a CSF collection that has leaked through the fracture. However, these swellings usually are liquified subgaleal blood and can spread circumferentially around the entire skull. These lesions should be left alone because attempts at surgical treatment, including aspiration, predispose to infection. Sufficient blood leakage may occur into the subgaleal space in an infant to produce anemia.

Skull Fractures

Linear Skull Fractures. Skull fractures are not synonymous with significant intracranial injury; often, they are only confirmatory evidence that a force has been applied to the skull. Most skull fractures that occur in children are linear and extend across the cranial vault. Children with such injuries frequently are asymptomatic except for swelling and tenderness over the fracture site. In younger children, even if the external signs are minimal but a skull fracture is suspected, radiographic evaluation should be undertaken for documentation.

Depressed Skull Fractures. Depressed skull fractures usually are more obvious on physical examination. They commonly are associated with a significant traumatic force acting on a small cross-sectional area (eg, a blow from a hammer). Depressed skull fractures may be associated with underlying brain damage and, occasionally, dural tears. Depressed fractures may in some instances be compound or comminuted. Neurosurgical evaluation is mandatory in all cases to decide

FIGURE 6-4.
Relationship of hypoxemia to increase in cerebral blood flow.

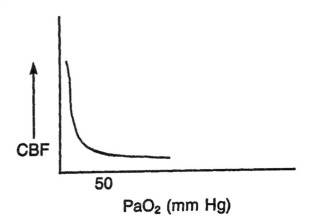

whether surgery is necessary.

Basilar Skull Fractures. Basilar skull fractures are found in the basal portion of the skull and may occur in the anterior, middle, or posterior cranial fossa. These fractures usually are characterized by periorbital subcutaneous hemorrhages (**raccoon eyes**), CSF rhinorrhea, or otorrhea, cranial nerve palsies, hemotympanum, or postauricular ecchymosis (**Battle's sign**). These signs may appear at the initial assessment but also develop during stabilization; hence, serial examinations are important. In the young child, the dura closely adheres to the basilar skull and may lead to meningeal tears in basilar fractures. Children with CSF rhinorrhea should have a neurosurgical consultation and be admitted and cared for in bed in the sitting position. Any child who is suspected of having an anterior fossa basilar skull fracture is at risk for intracranial penetration with nasogastric tubes, so orogastric intubation is preferred for gastric decompression.

Concussions

A concussion is a transient state of neuronal dysfunction as a result of trauma. It may manifest as transient confusion or loss of consciousness. In the infant and young child, there is a characteristic concussion syndrome that is seen minutes to hours after a fall. Consciousness rarely is lost; however, the child becomes very sleepy and pale and may begin to vomit. Examination usually reveals a pale child with tachycardia, clammy skin, normal blood pressure, no evidence of focal neurologic deficit, and a soft fontanel. The level of consciousness varies from spontaneous movements of all extremities to deep stupor with responses to pain only. These symptoms usually subside rapidly. Occasionally, however, hospitalization and judicious administration of intravenous fluids may be necessary for ≥24 hours. An older child may present with irritability and vomiting. Amnesia of the events leading to the accident (retrograde amnesia) or post-traumatic (antegrade) amnesia is fairly common in older children. The length of the post-traumatic amnesia usually correlates with the severity of head injury. Recovery from concussion usually is uneventful.

Diffuse Brain Injury

Diffuse brain injury in children younger than 1 year commonly occurs as a result of child abuse. The shaken baby syndrome is an important example. Pathologically, there is tearing of the anterior bridging veins, petechial hemorrhage in the white matter and deep gray structures with shearing of myelin and axons, contusions of the corpus callosum, subarachnoid hemorrhage, and acute intracranial hypertension. These children often are brought to medical attention after hours of coma and usually have sustained several previous but less major injuries. On examination, there often is no evidence of external trauma but perhaps some bruising or pinch marks on the upper arms. They may present in several ways, including deep coma with decorticate posture or flaccidity, fixed dilated pupils, and apnea or bradycardia. They sometimes are arousable to painful stimulation, move all extremities, and breathe well spontaneously. In severe cases, the fontanel is full and tense. In almost all cases, retinal hemorrhages can be detected on ophthalmoscopic examination.

Diffuse brain injury in the older child may result from primary impact injury to the cerebral cortex. Pathologically, this is due to areas of disruption of the blood-brain barrier and small intracranial hemorrhages, but it also may be due to significant contusions and lacerations as a result of shearing forces. More commonly, a pattern is seen of bilateral diffuse swelling produced by vasodilatation and hyperemia after trauma. This swelling is produced mainly by an increase in intracerebral blood volume; however, redistribution of blood from the subarachnoid and pial vessels into the intraparenchymal regions is a contributory factor. A child with a deteriorating neurologic status after a period of lucency is more likely to have generalized cerebral swelling than intracranial hemorrhage, but significant brain edema may be superimposed on this hyperemia. This is likely to occur in children who present in immediate deep coma, suggesting a significant degree of neuronal injury at impact. This primarily is due to white matter edema caused by disruption of the blood-brain barrier and may cause an increase in ICP that cannot be adequately controlled through hyperventilation.

Intracranial Hemorrhage

Epidural Hematoma

Epidural hematomas are relatively rare (<3%),

even in severe trauma in children. Most epidural hematomas originate from a hemorrhaging middle meningeal artery that quickly separates the meningeal dura layer from the inner table of the skull. In children, however, most epidural hematomas are due to meningeal and diploic vein hemorrhage. These hematomas occasionally occur in the posterior cranial fossa due to a bleeding deep-venous sinus. In contradistinction to the adult, the dura matter in the young child is tightly adherent to the skull. This factor probably is responsible for the varying and occasional subacute presentation of epidural hemorrhages in children.

In the infant and young child, an epidural hematoma usually results from a fall from a height onto a hard surface or a motor vehicle crash. Acute epidural hematoma in infancy may be associated with anemia and shock because a large amount of blood can accumulate in the head due to the greater compressibility of the brain and the expandable nature of the cranial vault. If an associated skull fracture is present, the hematoma can decompress into the subperiosteal galea with an even greater blood loss. This is an exception to the general rule that shock does not result from head injury alone. Children younger than 5 years with epidural hematomas rarely present with the classic pattern of a lucid period followed by rapid neurologic deterioration occurring within hours of injury. The period of lucidity usually is not a totally asymptomatic interval but simply stabilization or an improvement in the level of consciousness. Many children at this age never become deeply unconscious but present within 48 hours of injury with papilledema, bradycardia, continued moderate lethargy, and sometimes recurrent vomiting over several days. These signs usually signify increased ICP and impending transtentorial herniation. Cranial vault fractures occur in only ≈50% of children with epidural hemorrhages. In a child, epidural hemorrhage also can occur in the posterior cranial fossa after occipital trauma, and it commonly causes nuchal rigidity, cerebellar signs, vomiting, and continued impaired consciousness. Improved outcome from epidural hematomas relies on prompt recognition and treatment.

Subdural Hematoma

Post-traumatic subdural hemorrhages are an important source of neurologic morbidity in children. Subdural hematomas occur 5 to 10 times more frequently than bleeding in the epidural space and tend to occur in infants more often than in older children. These hemorrhages are almost exclusively venous in origin, mostly due to cerebral vein disruption at the sagittal sinus. In a young infant, the onset of symptoms may be relatively slow because of the venous rather than arterial source of bleeding and the relative plasticity of the skull due to open sutures. These infants may present with nonspecific symptoms such as vomiting, irritability, and low-grade temperature. Some infants, however, will not present until the subacute or chronic phase of subdural collection. In the subacute phase, the subdural blood organizes into a hemorrhagic cyst over several weeks and expands in size due to the osmotic pressure of red blood cell breakdown products. The usual presentation is that of a child with an enlarged head and no history of trauma. Occasionally, these patients may present with focal or generalized seizures. Physical examination often reveals an irritable, lethargic baby with a bulging fontanel, "sunsetting" eyes, retinal and preretinal hemorrhages, and hypertonic musculature. Older children with subdural bleeding tend to present more acutely with symptoms and signs of increased ICP and impending transtentorial herniation.

Intracranial Hypertension and Herniation

Intracranial hypertension is common in children with severe head injury, even in the absence of a mass lesion. The ICP may be elevated early or become elevated after several days because of persistent or uncontrollable cerebral hyperemia or vasogenic or cytotoxic cerebral edema. Symptoms of increased ICP occurs only after the compensatory mechanisms for maintaining normal ICP have been exhausted. Early symptoms and signs of increased ICP include headache, vomiting, altered mental status, respiratory irregularity, and abnormal posturing. Prompt therapy should be instituted to avoid further increases in ICP, decreased CPP, or brain herniation (Figure 6-5). Hypertension, bradycardia, and pupillary dilatation are late manifestations of raised ICP, so they should not be relied on for establishment of the diagnosis. Herniation of the brain may take place at any of three anatomic sites: transtentorial incisura, inferior edge of the falx cerebri, and foramen magnum. The most common herniation is a central transtentorial herniation of diffusely swollen cerebral hemispheres. When this occurs, the diencephalon and upper brainstem are compressed initially, causing a deterioration in level of consciousness, respiratory irregularity, pupillary dilatation, upward gaze limitation, and progressive hypertonia. With continued caudal progression, decorticate posturing, pupillary dilatation, and hyperventilation develop. Basilar artery compression and brainstem ischemia also will develop and lead to further deterioration (Figure 6-5).

Seizures

Seizures have been reported in some series in as many as 10% of children seen in emergency departments after experiencing head trauma. Post-traumatic seizures may be temporally divided into those of immediate, early, and late onset. An **immediate seizure** occurs within seconds of impact and may represent a traumatic depolarization of the cortex. This seizure can occur with mild trauma, is brief, and has no prognostic significance.

Early seizures account for ≈50% of post-traumatic seizures; they take place within the first week of the traumatic event and usually are due to focal brain injury. Young children are more susceptible to the development of early post-traumatic seizures within the first 24 hours after trauma. Apparently equivalent numbers of patients have generalized or focal seizures, and 10% to 20% develop status epilepticus. Approximately 25% of children with early seizures continue to have seizures after the first week.

Late post-traumatic epilepsy probably reflects cortical scarring. The severity of head injury, dural laceration, and intracranial hemorrhage are factors that determine whether late-onset seizures occur. Approximately 5% of hospitalized patients with head trauma develop late post-traumatic seizures. The long-term prognosis is worse in these patients because as many as 75% will develop a chronic seizure disorder.

ASSESSMENT

A thorough history and physical examination are essential to determine the severity of the intracranial injury, identify those at risk for secondary injuries (ie, assignment of risk categories), and identify injuries to other organ systems that may contribute to morbidity or mortality.

History

Events surrounding the injury should be elicited, such as the mechanism of injury, patient's neurologic status before and after the accident, presence of associated injuries, and prehospital

FIGURE 6-5.
Herniation of the brain due to cerebral edema and mass lesion.

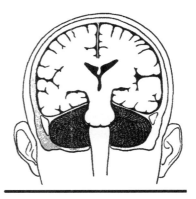

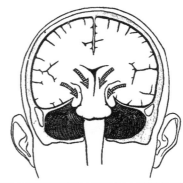

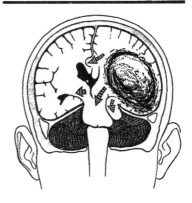

From Plum F, Posner JB. *The Diagnosis of Stupor and Coma*, 3rd ed. Philadelphia, Pa: FA Davis; 1980. Reprinted with permission.

care. The mechanism of the injury may increase the likelihood of specific pathology. For example, a diving accident immediately raises the possibility of a cervical spine injury. The height from which the patient fell, quality of impact surfaces, and shape and velocity of striking objects also may influence the diagnostic plans. Although reports of events may be inconsistent and therefore unreliable, the progression of neurologic signs or symptoms since injury provides valuable data to assist in clinical decision-making. The patient who is verbally responsive should be questioned about head or neck pain, visual changes, paresthesia, paresis, and amnesia.

Parents or prehospital personnel can reliably report any changes in level of consciousness and prehospital care the patient received. The past medical history relating to previous predisposition to seizures, bleeding diathesis, allergies, chronic illness, or current medications, is important for further management. A diagnosis of child abuse may be suggested if the history is incompatible with physical findings.

Physical Examination

The patient with severe head trauma often requires simultaneous physical examination and therapy. Table 6-1 outlines the salient points in physical examination. Abnormalities of airway, breathing, or circulation should be detected and treated before continuation of the physical assessment. The presence of a **Cushing response** (bradycardia and hypertension) indicates increased ICP but is a late response and therefore not helpful in guiding initial management in most cases. A rapid pulse often signifies blood loss and should lead to a search for non-central nervous system injuries.

A neurologic flow sheet facilitates an objective and serial recording of the patient's status. This is best accomplished initially using the AVPU system (see Chapter 5) or the Glasgow Coma Scale (GCS) (Table 6-2). The GCS is an important tool that influences both treatment decisions and outcome. Although modifications of the GCS for preverbal children have not been specifically validated, the GCS may be used in children younger than 2 years with limited verbal skills by assigning a full score if the child cries with stimulation. To be meaningful, the motor, verbal, and eye-opening responses of the

GCS should be elicited in the proper manner. When recording motor response as an indication of the functional state of the brain as a whole, the best or highest response from any limb is recorded. However, any difference between the responsiveness of one limb and that of another may indicate focal brain damage, and for this purpose, the worst (most abnormal) response also should be noted. For motor response, it is best to initially apply pressure to a nail bed with a pencil. This may result in either flexion or extension of the elbow. If flexion is observed, stimulation is applied to the head and neck or trunk to test for localization. Raising the hand above the chin in response to supraorbital pressure is a localizing response. The eye-opening response to speech does not necessarily require a command to open the eyes.

The minineurologic examination should include an extremity examination to determine whether there are focal differences in tone, reflexes, or response. Pupillary reflexes and observation of extraocular movements also are essential. The size and reactivity of the pupils may give the first clue to impending transtentorial herniation. The oculocephalic (**doll's eyes**) reflex should not be done at this stage because of the possibility of cervical spine injury. The minineurologic examination should assist in determination of the presence of focal neurologic signs due to an intracranial mass or of an impending cerebral herniation due to increased ICP. In all cases, scalp hematomas and contusions should be palpated (for

---

TABLE 6-1.
Features of physical and neurologic examination of children who have sustained head trauma.

Physical Examination
  ABCs
  Determination of vital signs
  Investigation for signs of skull fracture
    Hemotympanum
    Periorbital or postauricular ecchymosis
    Cerebrospinal fluid otorrhea and rhinorrhea
    Depressed fracture or penetrating injury
Neurologic Examination
  Glasgow Coma Scale
  Pupillary light reflexes
  Cranial nerve examination
  Movement of extremities
  Plantar responses

underlying depressions for depressed skull fracture). All full-thickness skull lacerations should be explored to ensure that the underlying bone is intact before suturing. The presence of other organ injuries, such as thoracic or abdominal injuries, should be sought because these may contribute to the morbidity and mortality. Data obtained from the history and physical examination should be sufficient for initiation of therapy and determination of risk of intracranial injury.

Classification of Risk of Intracranial Injury

Table 6-3 classifies the severity risk of intracranial injury based on history and physical examination. Triage and referral guidelines should be based on the risk of intracranial injury, need for immediate therapy, and availability of resources at the treating hospital. The correction of cardiorespiratory instability, stabilization of the cervical spine, and initial treatment of increased ICP should precede any triage decisions.

Patients with mild intracranial injury may be discharged home with instructions concerning head injury observation and precautions (Table 6-4). These patients do not require any specific therapy but may pose a diagnostic dilemma when child abuse is suspected.

Patients with a moderate risk of intracranial injury require close observation for ≥6 hours after the injury. If progressive improvement occurs during the observation period, these patients may be discharged home when asymptomatic. In this group of patients, however, other factors may dictate the need for admission, such as the possibility of child abuse, serious facial or spinal trauma, internal organ injury, and preexisting neurologic or hematologic illness. Patients who are discharged should be given appropriate instructions and have a reliable caregiver in charge of neurologic observation. If any of the criteria for neurologic normality are not met, extended observation in the hospital is recommended for 24 to 48 hours or until normality is attained. The role of radiographic

---

TABLE 6-2.
Glasgow Coma Scale.

Eye Opening Response

Spontaneous	4
To speech	3
To pain	2
None	1

Verbal Response*

Oriented	5
Confused conversation	4
Inappropriate words	3
Incomprehensible sounds	2
None	1

Best Upper Limb Motor Response

Obeys commands	6
Vocalizes	5
Withdraws	4
Abnormal flexion	3
Extensor response	2
None	1

*Children younger than 2 years should receive full verbal score for crying after stimulation.

TABLE 6-3.
Classification of severity of intracranial injury.

Mild
Asymptomatic
Mild headache
Three or fewer episodes of vomiting
Glasgow Coma Scale score of 15
Questionable or brief loss of consciousness

Moderate
Loss of consciousness for ≥1 minute
Progressive lethargy
Progressive headache
Vomiting protracted (more than three times) or associated with other symptoms
Post-traumatic amnesia
Post-traumatic seizure
Multiple trauma
Serious facial injury
Signs of basal skull fracture
Possible penetrating injury or depressed skull fracture
Glasgow Coma Scale score of 11 to 14

Severe
Glasgow Coma Scale score of 10 or a decrease of ≥2 points not clearly caused by seizures, drugs, decreased cerebral perfusion, or metabolic factors
Focal neurologic signs
Penetrating skull injury
Palpable depressed skull fracture
Compound skull fracture
Shaken baby impact syndrome

studies, including computed tomography (CT) scan, in this group of patients has not been clearly defined; however, if there is no improvement or deterioration during the observation period, a CT scan should be obtained. A few children who have a GCS score of 15 on presentation but have history of loss of consciousness will have positive findings on the CT scan. Patients who do not improve or deteriorate require neurosurgical or critical care consultation. *In all doubtful cases, a consultation with a neurosurgeon is warranted.* If these children require observation, the decision to provide care in a community hospital may best be made after careful clinical assessment and appreciation of the possible adverse outcomes and on the basis of the availability of treatment resources.

Patients at high risk of cerebral injury should be admitted to a tertiary care facility and seen by a trauma surgeon, neurosurgeon, and critical care specialist with pediatric expertise. However, cardiorespiratory stabilization and treatment of ICP should be instituted immediately and are more important than immediate referral. If the child presents to a non–tertiary care center, consultation with a trauma surgeon, neurosurgeon, and critical care physician at the referral center is advisable before transfer. These patients are best transported by a critical care transport team and should not undergo further radiographic evaluation, even CT scan, before transport unless requested by the referral center specialists. If definitive therapy is not available at the community hospital, transport should not be delayed. Investigations for child abuse should be undertaken, particularly if the patient is an infant with retinal hemorrhage and subarachnoid or intracerebral hemorrhage, regardless of whether external signs of injury are present. These evaluations, however, should not delay transfer because they can be accomplished later.

MANAGEMENT

Airway and Breathing

Children with head injuries may hypoventilate for a variety of reasons, including upper airway obstruction (eg, due to tongue displacement, airway trauma, or aspiration of stomach contents), seizures, or primary neurologic injury. Aggressive airway management is required to control

oxygenation and ventilation and thus avoid secondary brain injury. Suctioning of the oropharynx and the jaw thrust may be all that are necessary to open the airway. An oropharyngeal airway should not be used if it stimulates a gag or cough response because it may aggravate increased ICP. One hundred percent inspired oxygen should be administered in all cases to maintain SaO_2 at 90% to 95%. Head-injured patients may require intubation and ventilation for the following reasons:

- Hypoxemia from a variety of causes
- Hypoventilation from a variety of causes
- GCS score of ≤8
- Need for controlled ventilation to treat increased ICP

Endotracheal intubation always should be conducted in a controlled manner with in-line cervical stabilization (see Chapter 7). In addition, it always should be preceded by bag-valve-mask ventilation to achieve proper oxygenation and hypocarbia. Patients in whom increased ICP is suspected should undergo a rapid sequence induction (see Chapter 2).

Severe facial fractures may mandate an emergency needle cricothyroidotomy (see Chapter 5, Appendix 5-1) with transtracheal catheter ventilation. Patients should be ventilated to maintain SaO_2 at >90% to 95% and $PaCO_2$ of 30 to 35 mm Hg. These patients should be monitored with the use of continuous cardiorespiratory, transcutaneous oxygen saturation, and end-tidal

TABLE 6-4.
Instructions to parents or caregivers for observation at home of children who have sustained head trauma.

Bring child immediately to emergency department if any of the following signs or symptoms appears within the first 72 hours after discharge:
Any unusual behavior
Disorientation as to name and place
Unusual drowsiness and sleepiness
Inability to wake child from sleep
Increasing headache
Seizures, twitching, or convulsions
Unsteadiness on feet
Clear or bloody drainage from ear or nose
Vomiting more than two or three times
Blurred or double vision
Weakness or numbness of face, arms, or legs
Fever
Stiff neck

carbon dioxide monitors. Meticulous attention to proper endotracheal tube placement, fixation, and tracheal toilet is mandatory.

Circulation

The patient's perfusion should be assessed on the basis of parameters such as the quality of the peripheral pulse, capillary perfusion, heart rate, blood pressure, and urine output. If hypotension is present in the patient with head trauma, it is likely that an extracranial source of hemorrhage exists. In infants who have a large subdural or subgaleal hemorrhage and in patients in whom falling blood pressure is a terminal event, hypotension may occur in the absence of extracranial trauma, but this is rare.

Hypotension should be treated aggressively with isotonic saline, colloid solutions, and inotropes in an attempt to maintain normal vascular volume and CPP. However, if there is no evidence of hemodynamic instability, an intravenous solution of 5% dextrose in half normal saline may be infused at a strict maintenance rate because overzealous hydration may increase morbidity and mortality.

Bradycardia in a pediatric patient is a late sign of increased ICP and impending herniation. It is a signal to intensify neuroresuscitative efforts. Occasionally, bradycardia also may occur because of unopposed parasympathetic tone in a cervical spine injury. In this situation, accompanying signs are those of neurogenic shock (hypotension with

---

TABLE 6-5.
Emergency therapy for children who have increased intracranial pressure caused by head trauma.

Establish controlled ventilation ($PaCO_2$ of 30 to 35 mm Hg).
Maintain oxygenation.
Stabilize the cervical spine.
Keep head and neck in midline position.
Minimize stimuli (ie, suctioning and movements).
Institute fluid resuscitation for shock and hypovolemia.
If not in shock, restrict fluids to about three fourths of maintenance.
Monitor heart rate, respirations, blood pressure, cardiac rhythm, and, if indicated, pulse oximetry.
Prescribe mannitol 0.25 to 0.5 g/kg IV in cases of documented deterioration despite above measures.
Use central venous pressure monitoring to assess intravascular volume.

---

warm, flushed skin) and spinal shock (decreased deep-tendon reflexes, decreased sensory level, flaccid sphincters, and hypotonia).

Brain Resuscitative Measures

Close attention to airway, breathing, and circulation represents the most important therapeutic maneuvers in the treatment of severe brain injury. If immobilization of the cervical spine was not accomplished before arrival, it should be done as soon as the patient arrives. Neck immobilization should be continued throughout resuscitation, and a cross-table lateral neck radiograph should be obtained when convenient. However, immobilization should be maintained despite a normal radiograph because the view obtained may not show subtle bony injuries and children may sustain severe spinal cord damage in the absence of radiologic abnormalities. Patients with severe head injuries should be afforded therapy as outlined in Table 6-5. Frequent serial neurologic examinations and close monitoring, including arterial blood pressure and ICP, are necessary.

Diuretic therapy with mannitol (0.25 to 0.5 g/kg) may be used as rescue therapy in patients who, despite all efforts, continue to show signs of markedly increased ICP, including signs of herniation and pupillary dilatation. In general, this therapy is not necessary in the initial resuscitation of most pediatric patients. In addition, patients may become hypotensive when this therapy is instituted because other injuries (abdominal and thoracic) may have been overlooked. Mannitol, therefore, should be used cautiously in acute resuscitation and only when other measures (Table 6-5) have been instituted and failed to control increased ICP. Central venous pressure monitoring is needed when mannitol is used.

Seizures should be treated aggressively with anticonvulsants to prevent increased brain metabolism and CBF. Initial therapy may include a short-acting anticonvulsant (0.1 to 0.3 mg/kg **diazepam**, 0.05 to 0.1 mg/kg **lorazepam**), followed by a long-acting anticonvulsant (10 to 20 mg/kg **phenytoin** or **fosphenytoin**). Phenytoin should be infused at 1 mg/kg per minute or 50 mg/min, whichever is the slower rate. Fosphenytoin can be infused much faster, at rates up to 150 mg of phenytoin equivalents per minute. Prophylactic anticonvulsant therapy also may be indicated if extensive cortical lesions are evident on examination or CT scan.

Systemic factors that can affect cerebral function also must receive careful attention. Struggling due to pain and agitation should be managed with analgesics and neuromuscular blocking agents. Sedation also is important to prevent unnecessary coughing. Strict adherence to suctioning protocols should be maintained to prevent marked increases in ICP. Similarly, hyperthermia, which causes increased CBF and metabolism, must be reduced rapidly with cooling blankets and antipyretics. Anemia and coagulation deficits also may occur in the head-injured patient and require prompt correction.

The definitive treatment of epidural and subdural hematomas is drainage in the operating suite. If, however, life-threatening increases in ICP develop in an infant with an open fontanel before a neurosurgeon is available, **bilateral subdural aspirations** can be performed. These are accomplished under aseptic conditions by perforating the scalp with a 23- or 25-gauge butterfly needle inserted perpendicularly ≥2 cm lateral to the midline at each lateral corner of the fontanel or within the medial coronal sutures. If there is an accumulation of fluid or blood, it will be under pressure and flow freely.

DISPOSITION

After they are stabilized, these patients should be transferred to the appropriate area for further treatment (ie, intensive care unit, surgical suite, or referral center). The transport unit should be equipped to provide care similar to that of a tertiary care intensive care unit, including appropriate monitoring and medications to treat any complications. The mortality and morbidity from severe head injury can be reduced by the application of physiologic principles to cerebral resuscitation, meticulous attention to systemic disorders, and safe patient transport.

ADDITIONAL READING

Bruce DA. Head trauma. In: Fleisher GR, Ludwig S, eds. *Textbook of Pediatric Emergency Medicine*, 3rd ed. Baltimore, Md: Williams & Wilkins; 1993.

Duhaime AC, Alario AJ, Lewander WJ, et al. Head injury in very young children: mechanisms, injury types, and ophthalmologic findings in 100 hospitalized patients younger than 2 years of age. *Pediatrics*. 1992;90:179-185.

Emergency Paediatrics Section, Canadian Paediatric Society. Management of children with head trauma. *Can Med Assoc J*. 1990;142:949-952.

Kissoon N, Dreyer J, Walia M. Pediatric trauma: differences in pathophysiology, injury patterns and treatment compared with adult trauma. *Can Med Assoc J*. 1990;142:27-34.

Luerrsen TG, Klauber MR, Marshall LF. Outcome from head injury related to patient's age: a longitudinal prospective study of adult and pediatric head injury. *J Neurosurg*. 1988;68:409-416.

Masters SJ, McClean PM, Arcarese JS, et al. Skull x-ray examinations after head trauma: recommendations by a multidisciplinary panel and validation study. *N Engl J Med*. 1987;316:84-91.

Pascucci RC. Head trauma in the child. *Intens Care Med*. 1988;14:185-195.

Plum F, Posner JB. *The Diagnosis of Stupor and Coma*, 3rd ed. Philadelphia, Pa: FA Davis; 1980.

Zimmerman RA, Bilaniuk LT. Pediatric head trauma. *Neuroimag Clin North Am*. 1994;4:349-366.

Chapter 7

Cervical Spine Trauma

OBJECTIVES

1. Identify signs and symptoms of cervical spine and cord injury.

2. Discuss goals of initial management, including adequate and correct immobilization with the use of cervical collars, hard spine board, spacing devices, and securing straps.

3. Recognize anatomic and growth differences between the pediatric and adult cervical spine.

4. Describe techniques for airway intervention in a patient with airway compromise and a possible cervical spine injury.

5. Describe radiographic assessment of the cervical spine and the ABCs (alignment, bones, cartilage, soft tissues) method of evaluation.

6. Discuss radiographic findings seen with injuries of the cervical spine, including Jefferson fracture, hangman's fracture, atlantoaxial subluxation (transverse ligament rupture), dens fracture, distraction injury, SCIWORA, torticollis, and rotary subluxation.

Cervical spine injuries are relatively uncommon in children, but it should be assumed that all children who have sustained multiple trauma or head or neck trauma (blunt or penetrating), have been involved in a high-risk mode of injury (eg, motor vehicle crash, sports injury, fall, or dive), or have been shaken vigorously have a cervical spine injury until proved otherwise. In pediatrics, most cervical spine injuries occur in boys and are secondary to blunt trauma, most often motor vehicle crashes. As many as 20%, however, are secondary to penetrating injury, often from knives and bullets.

Signs and symptoms of cervical spine or cord damage include altered level of consciousness, abnormal neuromotor or neurosensory examination or report of neurologic abnormality at any time after injury, neck tenderness, crepitus or pain on palpation or movement, limitation of neck motion, or unexplained hypotension (Table 7-1).

Goals in the care of children with cervical spine trauma include effective stabilization of the primary spinal injury and prevention of progression to a more severe or significant injury. Patient management involves recognition of the possibility of cervical spine injury and taking steps to prevent secondary injury by adherence to the ABC approach of resuscitation, along with steps to prevent further movement or displacement of a potentially unstable cervical spine. The devastating nature of a cervical cord injury makes it imperative that a potentially unstable cervical spine injury not be missed; it has been estimated that 3% to 25% of cervical cord damage with resultant neurologic compromise or death results from inadequate management of patients with unrecognized unstable cervical spine injuries.

Cervical spine and cord injury may present anywhere along the degree of severity continuum. The cervical column may incur a fracture that is stable and not a neurologic threat, whereas at the other end of the spectrum, a patient may have no evidence of bony injury but have a complete cervical cord transection. It is important to realize there is a set of pediatric patients (ie, those with Down's syndrome) whose underlying medical problems make them more susceptible to cervical cord injuries, even as the result of relatively trivial trauma.

PATHOPHYSIOLOGY

It has been estimated that 1% to 2% of pediatric patients with multiple trauma have a cervical spine injury. Many, if not most, patients with spinal column injuries present without overt neurologic deficits. In several studies, most patients with spinal injuries had evidence of concurrent head injury.

Neurologic damage from spinal injuries can be caused by many different anatomic problems. The spinal canal may be impinged on by fracture fragments, blood, or a herniated disc or the cord may be compromised directly by edema, hypoperfusion, contusion, laceration, or transection. The effects of a head injury may make diagnosis of concurrent neck injury difficult if not impossible in the early stages of evaluation. Although spinal injury must always be assumed, it is helpful when possible to distinguish between neurologic deficits that result from brain trauma and those that result from spinal cord trauma. Brain-injured patients often have diffuse or regional deficits (one side of the body), spasticity, and intact bulbocavernosus and anal reflexes, whereas patients with spinal cord injuries often present with neurologic deficits in a myotome distribution, neuromotor disparity between arms and legs, flaccidity and absent reflexes, and loss of sphincter tone (spinal shock).

The pediatric cervical spine is sufficiently flexible that even significant distortions may revert to normal, so the physical or radiographic examination may appear unremarkable even after a significant spine injury.

INITIAL MANAGEMENT

Goals of management for a patient with a suspected cervical spine injury are to ensure airway patency and respiratory sufficiency, control hemorrhage, maintain osseous stability, and identify and prevent progression of all injuries.

If a protective helmet is in place, this should be removed slowly and carefully, with lateral expansion of the helmet, rotation of the helmet to clear the occiput, neck support, and stabilization during the removal process. Evaluation and care of the possibly injured cervical spine begin with proper immobilization in an attempt to avoid further damage to a potentially unstable spine.

Several concepts should be kept in mind concerning cervical immobilization in children. Soft cervical collars offer no protection to an unstable spine, and hard collars (Philadelphia, StiffNeck) alone may still allow flexion, extension, and lateral movement of the cervical spine. **Ideal immobilization** includes a hard cervical collar in conjunction with a full spine board and soft spacing devices between the head and securing straps. The patient should be secured to the spine board by tape or straps that cross the forehead, anterior portion of the cervical collar, and bone prominences of the shoulders and pelvis. Incorrect immobilization may contribute to secondary spine or cord injury as a result of neck hyperextension or malposition or may compromise respiration by obstructing chest rise. The securing straps should be assessed periodically to ensure adequate and safe attachment of the patient to the spine board.

Care should be taken with the type of spacing devices used with spinal immobilization. The traditional sand bag should be replaced with lighter-weight spacers (towel rolls, specialized

TABLE 7-1.
Signs and symptoms of cervical spine injury.

Abnormal motor examination (paresis, paralysis, flaccidity, ataxia, spasticity, rectal tone)
Abnormal sensory examination (pain, sensation, temperature, paresthesias, anal wink)
Altered mental status
Neck pain
Torticollis
Limitation of motion
Neck muscle spasm
Neck ecchymosis or swelling
Abnormal or absent reflexes
Clonus without rigidity
Diaphragmatic breathing without retractions
Neurogenic shock (hypotension with bradycardia)
Priapism
Decreased bladder function
Fecal retention
Unexplained ileus
Autonomic hyperreflexia
Blood pressure variability with flushing and sweating
Poikilothermia
Hypothermia or hyperthermia

From Woodward G. Neck trauma. In: Fleisher GR, Ludwig S, eds. *Textbook of Pediatric Emergency Medicine*, 3rd ed. Baltimore, Md: Williams & Wilkins; 1993. Adapted with permission.

spacing devices) to avoid the inadvertent risk of secondary neck injury with "log rolling" of the spine board. Many specialized spinal immobilization devices are available with soft spacers as part of the immobilization package. Although these are adequate for adults and young children, improvisation must be used for infants and toddlers in whom cervical injury is suspected.

When a hard spine board is used for a pediatric patient, remember that the child's head is disproportionately large compared with the adult head. Fifty percent of the postnatal head circumferential growth occurs by age 18 months, whereas 50% of the postnatal growth of the chest does not occur until age 8 years. The disparate growth of the head and trunk results in the neck being flexed into a position of relative kyphosis when a child is placed on a hard spine board. Suggestions have been made to allow a recess in the head area of the spine board to accommodate a child's large occiput or to place a spacing device such as a blanket under the torso to allow the neck to rest in a neutral position. Cervical spine alignment can be greatly affected and improved by these techniques, with avoidance of inadvertent flexion and anterior displacement of a potentially unstable spine. These amendments to the cervical spine board can be discontinued for patients ≥8 years, in whom cervical spine and body proportions approximate those of the adult.

TRAUMA RESUSCITATION

When administering the basic ABCs of trauma resuscitation, stabilization of the cervical spine should not be neglected. Airway management will have to be modified somewhat in the patient in whom a cervical spine injury is suspected. Gentle use of the jaw thrust will be helpful in treating airway obstruction, although vigorous use may inadvertently hyperextend an unstable cervical spine. Hyperextension of the neck to facilitate intubation clearly should be avoided. Gentle cricoid pressure should not cause excessive movement to the cervical spine, but if used too vigorously, it may result in neck flexion. In-line manual neck immobilization (performed by a caretaker whose sole responsibility is to ensure there is no neck motion) should be used to assist with airway maneuvers. Care should be taken to avoid significant traction to the cervical spine to prevent longitudinal stress and secondary cord injury.

ARTIFICIAL AIRWAY

Indications for an artificial airway with neck trauma include stridor, dyspnea, hypoxia, rapidly expanding hematoma, altered mental status, quadriplegia, hemiparesis, and other signs of vascular, airway, or neurologic insufficiency. Orotracheal intubation with manual in-line stabilization is the preferred method in children. Debate continues regarding the preferred method of airway management in the patient with a proven cervical spine injury or the child who has a suspected injury but in whom time or severity of presentation does not allow prior radiographic evaluation. Orotracheal intubation with manual in-line stabilization is appropriate in this setting. However, a surgical airway or fiberoptic-assisted intubation performed by personnel skilled in its use should be considered in patients with proven unstable spinal injury or in whom a strong suspicion of cervical injury is present before radiographic evaluation. This does not suggest, however, that all trauma patients who require airway intervention also require a surgical airway if normal cervical spine radiographs are not available.

If the patient has signs of neurologic impairment that may be secondary to a cervical cord injury, it is prudent to proceed with a technique of airway management that is unlikely to worsen a preexisting injury. Barring obvious signs or symptoms of cervical spine or cord damage, orotracheal intubation performed by someone experienced in pediatric trauma intubations is an acceptable and expedient method of securing the airway. When intubation is performed, neutral neck positioning should be maintained with stabilization from below and care taken to notify the intubator if there appears to be excessive flexion or extension of the head or neck. The cervical collar may be opened when the intubation is ready to commence to facilitate the intubation by allowing anterior movement of the jaw and tongue. Avoid the temptation to perform nasal intubation in the trauma patient who is <8 years. The anteriorly located glottis may make intubation difficult, and bleeding that can result from adenoid or mucosal damage can greatly hinder subsequent airway status and management.

INTRAVENOUS FLUIDS AND MEDICATIONS

Intravenous access is mandatory, as is precise assessment of fluid status and needs in any severely traumatized patient. The patient with a cervical spine injury may show signs of autonomic dysfunction and present in neurogenic shock (hypotension, bradycardia, peripheral flush) from the loss of vascular sympathetic input, increased venous capacitance, loss of arterial vasoconstriction, and unchecked cardiac vagal tone. Concurrent blood loss may make initial diagnosis and management of neurogenic shock difficult, but neurogenic shock should be suspected if the patient is bradycardic and vasodilated while demonstrating signs of hypovolemia or shock. These patients need moderate fluid resuscitation and may require inotropic support, such as dopamine, ephedrine, or phenylephrine.

A study by Bracken et al suggests that **methylprednisolone** (Solu-Medrol) in a dose of 30 mg/kg over 15 minutes, followed by infusion of 5 to 6 mg/kg per hour for 23 hours begun within 8 hours after cervical trauma, may improve functional outcome in some patients with spinal cord injury. Although this study specifically excluded children younger than 13 years, the poor functional outcome of patients with documented spinal cord injury has led many experts to recommend use of this still controversial protocol in children and adults.

CLINICAL PRESENTATIONS

Evaluation of a child with a potentially injured cervical spine begins with a thorough history and physical examination. There are many clues that can aid in the diagnosis of a cervical cord injury (Table 7-1). The signs and symptoms may be obvious or they may be masked by other abnormalities, such as altered level of

FIGURE 7-1.
Radiographic versus clinical evaluation of the cervical spine in the traumatized patient.

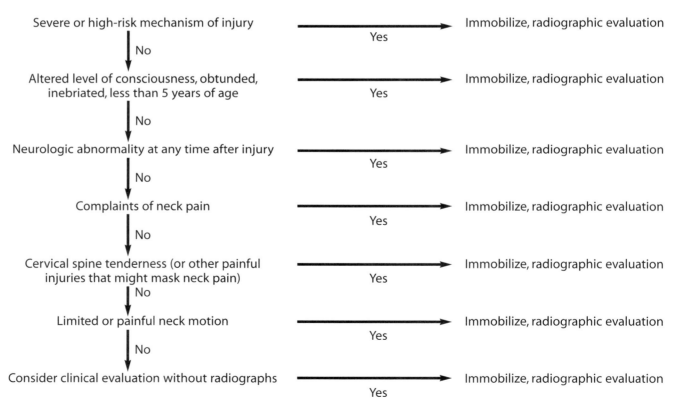

From Woodward G. Neck trauma. In: Fleisher GR, Ludwig S, eds. *Textbook of Pediatric Emergency Medicine*, 3rd ed. Baltimore, Md: Williams & Wilkins; 1993. Reprinted with permission.

consciousness, hypovolemic shock, or a concurrent head injury. Head and neck injuries may present with overlapping abnormal neurologic signs, and differentiation of causation may be difficult. A complete history is imperative to assess whether abnormal neurologic function, such as paresthesias, paralysis, or paresis, was present at any time after injury. These symptoms may have been transient and may not be present at the time of the examination or volunteered by the patient during the history taking but may suggest an underlying cervical cord injury. The physical examination should include assessment of the patient for neck tenderness, pain, limitation of motion, and muscle spasm, as well as for the neurologic signs, particularly those of neurogenic shock (ie, hypotension, bradycardia, peripheral flush) and spinal shock (ie, flaccidity, areflexia, loss of anal sphincter control).

In the patient who has sustained cardiac arrest shortly after trauma, a catastrophic neck injury should be strongly suspected. Resuscitation plans may need to be modified accordingly.

DIAGNOSTIC AIDS

Pediatric Versus Adult Anatomy

The pediatric cervical spine anatomy and its evaluation differ in many ways from those of the adult spine. The fulcrum of the cervical spine of an infant is at approximately C2-3 and at C3-4 by age 5 to 6 years, whereas the adult fulcrum is at C5-6. This is in part due to the relatively large head size of a child compared with that of an adult. At the age of 8 years, the fulcrum and other characteristics of the cervical spine approximate those of an adult. The higher fulcrum of a child's spine, along with relatively weak neck muscles and poor protective reflexes, accounts for young children often having fractures that involve the upper cervical spine, whereas older children and adults have fractures

FIGURE 7-2.
Approach to radiographic evaluation of the patient with a suspected neck injury. If fracture is identified, further emergent radiographic evaluation often is not necessary. Further evaluation with computed tomography may be indicated to evaluate fracture.

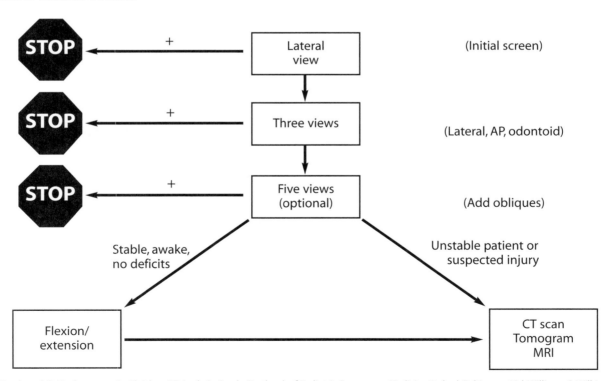

From Woodward G. Neck trauma. In: Fleisher GR, Ludwig S, eds. *Textbook of Pediatric Emergency Medicine*, 3rd ed. Baltimore, Md: Williams & Wilkins; 1993. Adapted with permission.

that more often involve the lower cervical spine.

The large amount of cartilage in the pediatric cervical spine may cushion forces that are distributed to the spine, but it also can make radiographic evaluation challenging. The radiolucent nature of cartilage makes the ability to evaluate and appreciate soft tissue abnormalities on the radiograph extremely important. The pediatric cervical spine appears to have more anterior and posterior movement than its adult counterpart, due not only to the radiolucent cartilage but also to ligamentous laxity and relatively horizontal facet joints. These differences in part account for the anterior pseudosubluxation (physiologic subluxation) that can be seen between C2-3 and C3-4 up to the age of 16 years. These factors also allow the apparent predental space (between the dens and anterior ring of C-1) to be increased to a maximum of 5 mm (adult maximum is 3 mm). The cartilage growth centers (synchondroses) also suggest fractures to the untrained eye.

The pediatric cervical spine also has the ability to revert to a relatively normal appearance after a significant distortion, which can hinder the radiographic search for abnormalities. Neurologic symptoms from compressive problems, including epidural hematomas, may be slower to manifest in a young child than in an adult due to the increased room around the spinal cord within the spinal column in a young child.

Plain Radiography, Computed Tomography, and Magnetic Resonance Imaging

Radiographic evaluation of the cervical spine is

TABLE 7-2.
Radiographic characteristics of the pediatric cervical spine.

Cartilage artifact
    Tapered anterior vertebrae
    Apparently absent anterior ring of C-1
    Atlas (C-1) body not ossified at birth and may fail to close
    Axis (C-2) four ossification centers
    Apex of odontoid ossifies between ages of 12 and 15 years
    Spinous process ossification centers
Increased mobility
    Pseudosubluxation
    C-1 override on dens
    Increased predental space (5 mm maximum)
    Ligament laxity
    Facet joints shallow
Growth plates (synchondrosis)
    Dens ossifies between ages of 3 and 8 years (may persist into adulthood)
    Posterior arch of C-1 ossifies at age 3 years
    Anterior arch of C-1 ossifies at age 6 to 9 years
C-1 internal diameter reaches adult size at age 3 to 4 years
C-2 through C-7 internal diameter reaches adult size at age 5 to 6 years
Lack of cervical lordosis
Fulcrum varies with age (see text)
Soft tissue variability with respiration
Congenital clefts or other bony abnormalities (os odontoideum), spondylolisthesis, spina bifida, ossiculum terminale
Rare compression fractures
Approaches adult characteristics by age 8 years

FIGURE 7-3.
Lordotic curves seen with normal cervical spine alignment. 1, Anterior spinal line. 2, Posterior spinal line (anterior spinal canal). 3, Spinolaminal line (posterior spinal canal). 4, Spinous process tips.

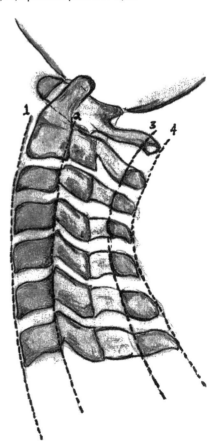

an essential step in the assessment. Options include radiography, computed tomography (CT), and magnetic resonance imaging (MRI).

MRI scans are more appropriate for evaluation of the subacute or chronic stages of injury or an acute problem with cord impingement by blood or soft tissues. The MRI does not image cortical bone as well as other modalities and should not be used to evaluate the cervical spine for fractures. The CT scan, however, demonstrates fractures quite clearly. A CT scan often is used as a secondary screen when adequate plain radiographs cannot be obtained or to confirm suspected fractures. The CT scan will give good soft tissue detail and allows for the possibility of reconstruction images but does not provide the intrathecal, ligamentous, disc, or vascular detail that can be obtained with an MRI scan.

The plain radiograph remains the initial test of choice in the acutely traumatized patient. Several authors have attempted to devise criteria to limit the number of patients who should receive cervical spine radiographs. The perception of unnecessary tests must be balanced against the severity of consequences that may occur with a missed cervical spine injury. The literature suggests that if the patient does not have a high-risk mechanism of injury (eg, motor vehicle crash, sports injury, fall, dive, or penetrating neck injury), is awake and alert, can have an interactive conversation (eg, not inebriated, no altered level of consciousness, older than 4 to 5 years), does not complain of cervical spine pain, has no tenderness or muscle spasm on palpation (especially in the midline), has normal neck mobility without limitation of motion, has a completely normal neurologic examination without history of abnormal neurologic signs or symptoms at any time after the injury, and has no other painful injuries that may mask neck pain, then the patient probably does not need radiographic evaluation of the cervical spine. There are published case reports, however, of cervical fractures in patients (mainly adults) who apparently did meet the criteria to forego a radiographic evaluation.

When radiographs are obtained, remember, *a normal lateral radiograph does not "clear" the cervical spine* but does allow assessment of gross malalignment or distraction. The sensitivity of a lateral cervical spine radiograph varies between 82% and 98% in the literature.

In evaluation of a lateral cervical spine radiograph, C1-7 as well as the C-7/T-1 junction should be included. Additional films, including an anteroposterior (AP) view of C3-7 and an open-mouth view (AP) of C1-2, will increase the sensitivity of the initial radiographic evaluation to >95%. If at any point during the radiographic evaluation a fracture is identified, further plain radiographs often are not necessary. CT at that point may be more useful in delineating the extent of the injury. An algorithm for considering radiographic evaluation is presented in Figure 7-1. An approach to ordering cervical spine imaging studies is shown in Figure 7-2.

The cervical spine has anterior (vertebral bodies, intervertebral discs, ligaments) and posterior (lamina, pedicles, neural foramen, facet joints,

FIGURE 7-4.
Jefferson fracture. A, Offset of lateral mass of C-1 >1 mm indicates possible fracture. B, Cross-section from A demonstrating multiple fracture sites (see arrows).

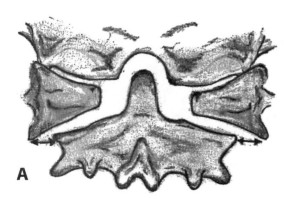

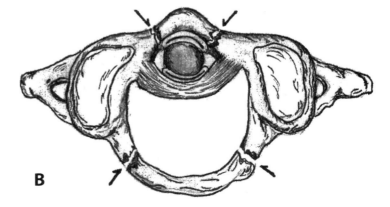

spinous processes, ligaments) components. The initial three-view series can provide a good evaluation of the anterior cervical spine, but it is not ideal for evaluation of the posterior cervical spine. Oblique (pillar) views will be helpful in evaluation of the posterior elements. Flexion and extension films for assessment of ligamentous stability can be obtained in an awake patient by having the patient flex and extend the neck as able without discomfort. These films often will be inadequate because the neck muscles have splinted the cervical column in a position of comfort or stability and subsequent alignment will not change with flexion or extension. If questions remain concerning the integrity of the cervical spine after obtaining these radiographs, CT should be considered. Radiographic tomograms also can be performed but require patient movement, are time consuming, and are not easily performed with an acutely ill patient.

Evaluation of Radiographs

When evaluating radiographs of the cervical spine, use a systematic approach. The ABCs (alignment, bones, cartilage, soft tissues) method of evaluating the lateral cervical radiograph is a useful system. Alignment is assessed, as demonstrated in Figure 7-3, keeping in mind that the spinal cord lies between the posterior spinal line and the spinolaminal line. The usual lordotic curve of these lines may not be present in children younger than 6 years, in those on hard spine boards (the large occiput forces the neck in a flexed direction), in those with cervical collars, or in those with cervical neck muscle spasm. As mentioned, pseudo- or physiologic subluxation may be seen in the upper cervical spine until the age of 16. Gross abnormalities should be detectable through assessment of alignment.

In evaluation of the bones, look for typical abnormalities that may be quite subtle. In assessment of vertebral body sizes, look for compression fractures as suggested by differences in the heights of adjacent vertebral bodies. Be aware that structures including the skull and teeth, which overlay the spine, may simulate fractures, as can the cartilage growth centers (Table 7-2).

Assess cartilage after the bones. Cartilage is radiolucent on plain radiographs. Pediatric spinal columns contain a large amount of cartilage that

can make radiographic evaluation challenging. The cartilaginous areas include the synchondroses or growth plates and intervertebral disc spaces. The growth plates may mimic fractures and be confusing to those who are unaware of their presence. Growth plates can be differentiated from fractures by their location and regular, smooth, sharp borders compared with the irregular appearance and often different locations of fractures. Growth centers in the anterior-superior vertebral bodies cause a sloped appearance that may look like anterior compression fractures to the untrained eye. The vertebral disc space also should be evaluated because abnormalities may suggest specific mechanisms of injury. A vertebral disc space that is narrowed anteriorly may indicate disc extrusion from compression, whereas a widened space suggests a hyperextension injury with posterior ligamentous disruption.

Evaluation of the soft tissue is extremely important. Abnormal soft tissue spaces may be the only clue to the underlying ligament, cartilage, or subtle bone injury that may not be overt on the radiograph. Soft tissue thickening may represent blood or edema, which suggests an underlying injury. A rule of thumb is that the prevertebral

FIGURE 7-5.
Hangman's fracture (traumatic spondylolisthesis of C-2). Note abnormal posterior cervical line.

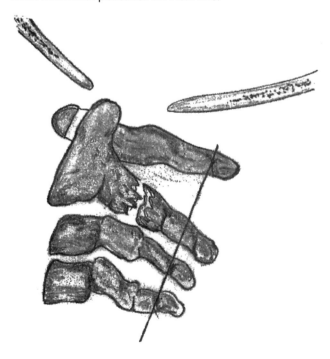

(retropharyngeal) space at C-3 should be less than two thirds the anteroposterior width of the adjacent vertebral body. This space will approximately double below C-4 (the level of the glottis) because the usually non–air-filled esophagus is included in this area. Crying, neck flexion, or the expiratory phase of respiration may produce a pseudothickening in the prevertebral space. Soft tissue abnormality should be reproducible on repeated radiographs if there is an underlying injury.

Multiple types of neck injuries can be seen in the pediatric patient, ranging from minor muscular strains with torticollis to stable bony injuries to unstable cervical injuries with and without neurologic damage. Five percent or more of patients with a cervical spine injury will have an additional spinal injury at another level, and these injuries should be actively sought.

SPECIFIC INJURIES

The **Jefferson fracture** is a bursting fracture of the ring of C-1 secondary to an axial load (Figure 7-4). Although the fracture may be unstable, neurologic impairment often is not present initially since the fracture fragments splay outward and do not physically impinge on the spinal cord. The fracture usually is seen best on the open-mouth odontoid view; the radiographic criterion for diagnosis of a Jefferson fracture is lateral offset of the lateral mass of C-1 of >1 mm from the vertebral

body of C-2. Neck rotation may give a false-positive radiograph. Approximately one third of Jefferson fractures are associated with other fractures, most often involving C-2. The pseudo-Jefferson fracture of childhood is present in 90% of children at the age of 2 and usually normalizes by 4 to 6 years. The pseudo-Jefferson fracture has the radiographic appearance of a Jefferson fracture due to increased growth of the atlas (C-1) compared with the axis (C-2) and radiolucent cartilage artifact. If a Jefferson fracture is suspected in a child younger than 4 years, a CT scan may be necessary to further elucidate the suspected injury. The CT scan is quite helpful in the evaluation of suspected injuries in the C1-2 area.

The **Hangman's fracture** is a traumatic spondylolisthesis of C-2 (Figure 7-5). This injury occurs as a result of hyperextension that fractures the posterior elements of C-2. Hyperflexion after the hyperextensions leads to anterior subluxation of C-2 on C-3 and subsequent cervical cord damage. The subluxation seen with a hangman's fracture can sometimes be mistaken for the pseudo- or physiologic subluxation seen in the C2-3 or C3-4 region in ≈25% of children younger than 8 years, and which may occur up to the age of 16. Distinguishing between a subtle hangman's fracture and pseudosubluxation can be accomplished using the **posterior cervical line of Swischuk**, as described in Figure 7-6. A value of >1.5 to 2 mm indicates an occult hangman's fracture as the source

FIGURE 7-6.
Posterior cervical line. Use only to assess anterior displacement of C-2 and C-3. A line is drawn from the cortex of the spinous process of C-1 to the cortex of the spinous process of C-3, and the relationship to the cortex of spinous process of C-2 is noted. A, Normal line passing through cortex of C-2. B, Normal line passing within 1.5 mm of cortex of C-2. C, Abnormal line passing >2 mm anterior to cortex of C-2, suggesting underlying fracture of posterior elements of C-2.

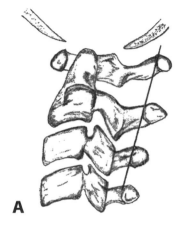
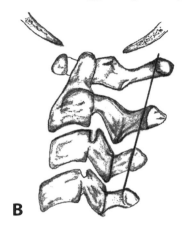
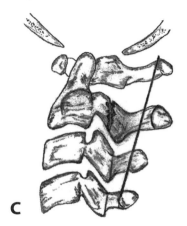

A   B   C

of the anterior subluxation of C-2 on C-3. This line should be used only for evaluation of anterior subluxation of C-2 on C-3.

Atlantoaxial subluxation is the result of movement between C-1 and C-2 secondary to transverse ligament rupture or a fractured dens (Figure 7-7). Ligament instability precipitated by tonsillitis, cervical adenitis, pharyngitis, arthritis, connective tissue disorders, or Down's syndrome may allow minor trauma to result in ligamentous damage. Subluxation due to transverse ligament disruption will be evidenced by a widened predental (preodontoid) space on a lateral radiograph. Normal predental measurement in children is <5 mm compared with <3 mm in adults. Steel's **rule of three** states that the area within the ring of C-1 is composed of one third odontoid, one third spinal cord, and one third connective tissue. Space therefore is available for limited dens movement or predental space widening without neurologic compromise. Neurologic symptoms often are not seen until the predental space exceeds 7 to 10 mm. Dens fractures cause atlantoaxial subluxation more often than ligamentous disruption in a young child because the weakest part of the child's musculoskeletal system is the osseous component. These fractures often are seen in young infants secondary to a rapid deceleration while in improperly positioned forward-facing car seats.

Distraction injuries result from a longitudinal stress to the cervical column. These injuries actually may contribute to a significant percentage of deaths in pediatric acute trauma. Although severe distraction injuries may be incompatible with long-term survival, initial cardiopulmonary resuscitation may be possible. These injuries may be obvious or subtle on the lateral radiograph. Increased space between the occiput and C-1 or widening of an intervertebral disc space without an obvious adjacent compression fracture indicates the possibility of a distraction injury. Distraction injuries also may be seen with difficult newborn deliveries. They may not be visible on a plain radiograph because the pediatric cervical spine can distract 2 inches before there is radiographic evidence of spinal column distraction. The spinal cord, however, can distract only one fourth of an inch before there is permanent neurologic damage. An MRI scan will be useful in assessing an infant or other stable patient with diminished motor activity who is suspected of having a distraction injury.

Rotary subluxation is a cervical spine injury that often is missed or undiagnosed due to difficulty in interpreting the radiographs of patients with these injuries. Rotary subluxation or displacement may follow minor or major trauma or apparently may be spontaneous. These patients rarely present with abnormal neurologic findings. They present in the typical (cockrobin) position, with the muscle spasm of the sternocleidomastoid on the same side to which the chin points. In contrast, in patients with muscular torticollis, the chin points to the side opposite that involved. This is logical considering that the action of the sternocleidomastoid is an attempt to reestablish normal neck position.

FIGURE 7-7.
A, Dens fracture. B, Widened predental space secondary to transverse ligament rupture. C, Cross-section of C1-2 with transverse ligament rupture.

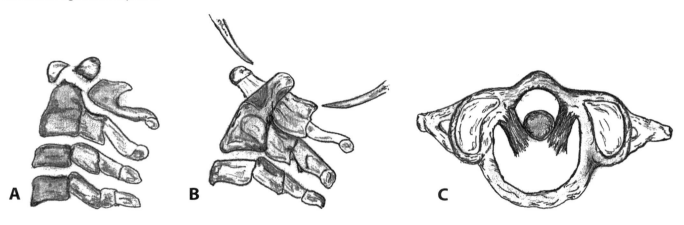

Radiographs may help distinguish between muscular torticollis and rotary subluxation, although the radiographs may be normal in both cases. Suspect rotary subluxation if on an open-mouth radiograph one of the lateral masses of C-1 appears forward and closer to the midline while the opposite lateral mass appears narrow and away from the midline (lateral offset). Caution should be used in interpreting these films because simple neck rotation can give the appearance of subluxation. Cineradiography can demonstrate that C1-2 will move as a unit, although the CT scan appears to be the most useful diagnostic tool in rotary subluxation. Patients with mild rotary subluxation should be treated with a cervical collar and analgesia for comfort; those with moderate rotary displacement need immobilization and occasionally traction. If there is anterior displacement of C-2 on C-1, there may be a need for longer immobilization to allow injured ligaments to heal.

Spinal epidural hematomas also are seen in the pediatric population. These are venous bleeds that compress the adjacent spinal cord and present with ascending neurologic symptoms hours or days after often apparently minor trauma. An MRI scan can be quite helpful in the evaluation of these patients. Rapid evaluation and surgical decompression are mandatory to prevent further neurologic compromise.

SCIWORA (Spinal Cord Injury Without Radiographic Abnormality) is a syndrome that has been described in as many as 67% of children with cervical cord injuries, but most studies report a prevalence of 25% to 50%. These injuries occur mainly in children younger than 8 years who present with or develop symptoms consistent with cervical cord injuries without radiographic or tomographic evidence of bone abnormality. The etiologies are unclear, but many include vascular injury (occlusion, spasm, infarction), ligamentous injury, disc impingement, or incomplete neuronal destruction. There is a subset of patients who have initial transient neurologic symptoms, as described earlier, who apparently recover and then return an average of 1 day later with significant neurologic abnormalities. For this reason, many recommend hospitalization and immobilization for young patients who have experienced transient neurologic symptoms.

MANAGEMENT SUMMARY

Treatment of patients with suspected cervical spine injuries involves basic and advanced life support measures, immobilization, neurosurgical consultation, and consideration of pharmacologic treatment. Consider airway support for a patient with an upper cervical cord injury because respiratory embarrassment will occur as they tire. Patients may present in neurogenic shock and require fluid and inotropic medication support. The use of steroids may offer some promise for the patient with a spinal cord injury. The need for immediate surgical stabilization is unusual in children, whereas other forms of immobilization are more common. Patients with proven or suspected cervical spine injuries should remain immobilized with permanent or semipermanent immobilization decisions made in conjunction with a neurosurgical consultant. Patients with altered levels of consciousness from other injuries should have immobilization continued until neurologic function can be assessed completely.

ACKNOWLEDGMENT

Figures 7-3 through 7-7 were prepared by Stephen Ostergaard, PNP.

ADDITIONAL READING

Bonadio WA. Cervical spine trauma in children: Part I. General concepts, normal anatomy, radiographic evaluation. *Am J Emerg Med.* 1993;11:158-165.

Bonadio WA. Cervical spine trauma in children: Part II. Mechanisms and manifestations of injury, therapeutic considerations. *Am J Emerg Med.* 1993;11:256-278.

Bracken MB, Shepard MJ, Collins WF, et al. A randomized, controlled trial of methylprednisolone or naloxone in the treatment of acute spinal-cord injury: results of the Second National Acute Spinal-Cord Injury Study. *N Engl J Med.* 1990;322:1405-1411.

Curran C, Dietrich AM, Bowman MJ, et al. Pediatric cervical-spine immobilization: achieving neutral position? *J Trauma.* 1995;39:729-732.

Davis JW, Parks SN, Detlefs CL, et al. Clearing the cervical spine in obtunded patients: the use of dynamic fluoroscopy. *J Trauma.* 1995;39:435-438.

Laham JL, Cotcamp DH, Gibbons PA, et al. Isolated head injuries versus multiple trauma in pediatric patients: do the same indications for cervical spine evaluation apply? *Pediatr Neurosurg.* 1994;21:221-226.

Nypaver M, Treloar D. Neutral cervical spine positioning in children. *Ann Emerg Med.* 1994;23:208-211.

Pang D, Pollack IF. Spinal cord injury without radiographic abnormality in children—the SCIWORA syndrome. *J Trauma.* 1989;29:654-664.

Woodward GA. Neck trauma. In: Fleisher GR, Ludwig S, eds. *Textbook of Pediatric Emergency Medicine,* 3rd ed. Baltimore, Md: Williams & Wilkins; 1993.

Chapter 8

Burns: Thermal and Electrical Trauma

OBJECTIVES

1. Explain the pathophysiology of thermal injury and burn classification.

2. Quantify the size of the burn.

3. Explain the initial assessment and stabilization.

4. Explain outpatient treatment of burns.

5. Define high- versus low-voltage electrical injury.

6. Describe special problems of the pediatric burn.

7. Explain pure thermal and electrical injury, renal insult, underestimation of extent of injury, and occult nature of deep injury.

Thermal injury is the second most common cause of traumatic pediatric death in the United States. It is estimated that there are ≈3000 pediatric deaths from burns annually and probably three times as many disabling injuries. Most burn accidents occur in the home. Scalding injuries are most commonly seen in children younger than 3 years; a significant minority of scalds occur as a result of intentional injury. Flame-related injuries most often occur in children older than 3 years. The latter group represents most major burns and fatalities.

Electrical injuries account for ≈5% of burn unit admissions in the United States. About 1300 fatalities are reported each year, as well as approximately four times as many nonfatal injuries. Most electrical injury victims (93%) are male. Pediatric patients account for approximately one third of all victims, including toddlers injured while playing with electrical appliances and adventurous adolescent boys climbing trees or poles near high-tension lines.

THERMAL TRAUMA

Pathophysiology

Thermal burns are classified according to the extent of surface area involved and the depth of injury created. **First-degree** burns, which are characterized by erythema, involve only the epidermis and have little or no physiologic significance. Deeper **partial-thickness (second-degree)** burns involve the dermis and may be characterized by blisters and extreme sensitivity and pain. Deep partial-thickness burns may be difficult to distinguish from full-thickness burns. **Full-thickness (third-degree)** burns usually are pain free because they involve destruction of the full thickness of the dermis, including hair follicles and nerve endings. Third-degree burns are characterized by anesthesia and a brawny or tallow-like feel and appearance. **Fourth-degree** burns are rare; they extend through the subcutaneous tissue and involve muscle and other deep structures. These commonly occur with high-voltage electrical injuries.

Partial-thickness burns heal through spontaneous regeneration of the epidermis because the epidermal appendages (eg, hair follicles, sweat glands) are spared; therefore, partial-thickness burns usually do not require grafting. Full-thickness injury destroys those appendages, and grafting almost always is required.

The interaction of two major factors, temperature and duration of contact, determines the depth of tissue injury. For example, at 44°C (111°F), cellular destruction will not occur for ≈6 hours of contact in adults and older children. For each degree of temperature elevation above that level, the time needed for cellular destruction is reduced by half. Epidermal injury will occur within ≈1 minute at 51°C (125°F) and 1 second at 70°C (158°F). Children have thin skin compared with adults, so they are more prone to sustain deep burn injury.

Different types of thermal exposure have different effects. Flash injuries dissipate a large amount of heat, but the duration of exposure usually is short; the usual result is a nearly uniform partial-thickness burn. Scalding injuries generally involve skin contact for <4 seconds at temperatures of <100°C. These burns are in general partial thickness, except for hot oil scalds and burns in young infants or burns resulting from hot fluid being held close to the body by the clothes. The presence of full-thickness burns in a child with a history of brief scald injury may suggest the possibility of nonaccidental trauma.

Flame burns can produce high temperature with prolonged contact, so they are associated with the highest risk of serious full-thickness injury. Full-thickness injury is associated with the highest risk of physiologically significant injury. The presence of full-thickness injuries from flame injury also is suspicious for nonaccidental trauma.

Hot metal, such as radiators, floor heating grates, or oven racks, often produces full-thickness burns. More fire-related deaths are secondary to smoke inhalation than to the thermal injury (see Chapter 9). The most common cause of death during the first hour after burn injury is respiratory failure, either from smoke inhalation with its attendant hypoxia or carbon monoxide poisoning or from mechanical effects, such as airway edema and respiratory compromise from circumferential burns of the chest or abdomen that inhibit chest wall expansion. If the patient's airway is stabilized, the next few hours provide a relatively stable period during which it is optimal to transfer appropriate patients to a burn unit before burn shock sets in.

After the first few hours, the most common cause of death is **burn shock**. The capillary permeability of burned tissue in patients who have sustained partial- or full-thickness burns is increased markedly. Although fluid losses usually are proportional to the depth and size of the burn, if burns involve >30% of the body surface, generalized systemic capillary permeability occurs. This results in the extravasation of large amounts of fluid from the intravascular to the extravascular space with a dramatic decrease in intravascular volume, hypoperfusion, and edema of both the burned area and other tissues.

Hypoperfusion can produce hypovolemic shock and lactic acidosis. Thermal effects may destroy red blood cells, and particularly in electrical accidents, muscle tissue may be destroyed. The resultant hemoglobinuria and myoglobinuria along with hypovolemia can interact to precipitate renal injury, which used to be a major cause of death a few days after the injury. With proper early fluid resuscitation and alkalinization to blood pH 7.35 to 7.40 in cases involving myoglobinuria, there should never be renal failure from burn shock and myoglobinuria.

Late causes of death include infection, tetanus, and iatrogenic effects. Other complications may include vascular compromise as edema from circumferential full-thickness burns constricts the blood flow to the distal extremity or if the vessels are thrombosed from severe burns. Gastrointestinal ileus also is common with more severe burns.

Initial Survey and Management

Airway

Direct initial attention toward the airway regardless of how dramatic the child's other injuries may appear. The most common airway problem is progressive upper airway edema. Significant inhalation injuries initially may present subtle signs, and carboxyhemoglobin levels should be obtained early. The following signs are indicative of inhalation injury:

- Cyanosis
- Carbonaceous sputum
- Oropharyngeal carbon deposits, blistering, and

inflammatory changes of the tongue and palate
- Voice change, hoarseness, and persistent coughing
- Facial burns, singeing of the eyebrows and nasal hairs
- History of closed space confinement
- Altered level of consciousness related to hypoxemia or increased carboxyhemoglobin

Within a short time, these signs can progress; with fluid resuscitation, the supraglottic and glottic airway may obstruct. The patient must be evaluated carefully for endotracheal intubation and maintenance of patent airway. Oxygen should be administered via nonrebreather mask for any suspected inhalation injury and to treat carbon monoxide inhalation.

In general, intubation should be done earlier rather than later; by the time it is necessary, the swelling may have progressed to the point at which it is impossible.

Estimating Severity

The depth of a burn injury is classified as erythema, superficial or deep partial thickness, or full thickness. A **first-degree** burn damages only the epidermis. The surface is erythematous, and there is local pain but no blister formation. First-degree burns should not be included when estimating the total extent of a burn injury.

Second-degree burns result in partial-thickness skin loss. The skin appears pink or mottled red. Blisters are commonly seen (superficial second degree), and the surface of the skin is moist. These burns are very painful when touched. A deep partial-thickness burn has an even more mottled appearance, and the skin assumes a waxy character.

Full-thickness burns involving the epidermis, dermis, and subcutaneous tissues appear to be pale white or black and do not contain blisters. The skin has a dry, hard, and leathery appearance and a loss of normal elasticity. Thrombosed vessels may be seen. These areas are painless when touched because the nerve endings have been destroyed.

Deep partial-thickness burns often are difficult to distinguish from full-thickness (third-degree) burns. That is not of immediate concern, however, because the initial treatment for the two injuries is the same.

The total skin surface involved with full- and partial-thickness burns (except for areas of first-degree burn) is included in the estimation of the total body surface area involved (Figure 8-1). Fluid resuscitation is guided by this estimation, and prognosis is related closely to the extent of the burn.

FIGURE 8-1.
Lund and Browder chart. "Rule of nines" divides the body surface into areas of approximately 9% or multiples of 9%; the head and neck and an upper extremity each represents 9%; a lower extremity and the front and back of the torso each represents 18%; the perineum 1%. This method of estimation is sufficiently accurate for emergency situations. It is modified in children from birth to 1 year of age to allow 19% for the head and neck and 13% for each lower extremity. One percent is subtracted from the head and neck and added to the lower extremities for each year from ages 1 to 10.

Area	Age (Years)					% 2°	% 3°	% Total
	0–1	1–4	5–9	10–15	Adults			
Head	19	17	13	10	7			
Neck	2	2	2	2	2			
Ant. Trunk	13	17	13	13	13			
Post. Trunk	13	13	13	13	13			
R. Buttock	2½	2½	2½	2½	2½			
L. Buttock	2½	2½	2½	2½	2½			
Genitalia	1	1	1	1	1			
R. U. Arm	4	4	4	4	4			
L. U. Arm	4	4	4	4	4			
R. L. Arm	3	3	3	3	3			
L. L. Arm	3	3	3	3	3			
R. Hand	2½	2½	2½	2½	2½			
L. Hand	2½	2½	2½	2½	2½			
R. Thigh	5½	6½	8½	8½	9½			
L. Thigh	5½	6½	8½	8½	9½			
R. Leg	5	5	5½	6	7			
L. Leg	5	5	5½	6	7			
R. Foot	3½	3½	3½	3½	3½			
L. Foot	3½	3½	3½	3½	3½			
					Total			

Weight _____
Height _____

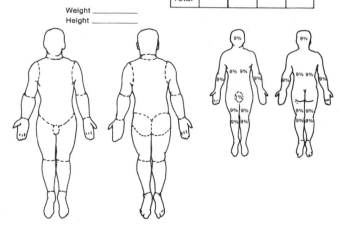

From Callaham ML, ed. *Current Practice in Emergency Medicine*, 2nd ed. Philadelphia, Pa: B.C. Decker; 1991: 879. Reprinted with permission.

Vascular Access and Fluid Therapy

Management of the burn patient must begin from the moment of arrival. Initial measures include establishment of a flow sheet, insertion of a Foley catheter, and consideration of the need for a central venous line. Stringent adherence to aseptic technique is required because sepsis is a major cause of death in hospitalized burn patients.

Initial laboratory studies for major or moderate thermal injury involving >10% of body surface area should include CBC, electrolytes, carboxyhemoglobin level, typing and cross-matching, urinalysis, and arterial blood gas determinations. A chest radiograph also should be obtained.

Although it is preferable to cannulate a peripheral vein in an unburned region of the body, if the injuries are extensive, access may be obtained through the burned surface. Unlike the adult, in whom the incidence of thrombophlebitis is greatly increased when cannulating lower extremity veins, the pediatric patient will better tolerate short-term use of an intravenous catheter in these sites. In some patients, vascular access represents a significant challenge. When faced with a small infant with a significant burn wound who requires urgent resuscitation, an intraosseous technique can be used for initial access and fluid administration. When adequate perfusion has been established, appropriate peripheral access may be obtained more easily.

It is necessary to use intravenous resuscitation for any child with a burn of >15% of body surface. At times, small children with even less burned surface will be resistant to oral hydration and require parenteral fluids. If shock is present, lactated Ringer's solution or normal saline should be given rapidly in 20-mL/kg boluses.

Fluid resuscitation may proceed with normal saline without dextrose at 3 to 4 mL/kg body weight per percent body surface area burned (Table 8-1). One half of the fluid should be administered within the first 4 to 6 hours after burn injury, and the remainder should be administered during the ensuing 18 hours. Pediatric patients, especially infants and toddlers with small burns, will require maintenance fluids in addition to the calculated burn wound resuscitation volume. This also may be given as lactated Ringer's solution with careful monitoring of urinary output to maintain urine volume of ≥1 mL/kg per hour. It is essential to monitor serum electrolytes and pulmonary function to avoid excess sodium and volume resuscitation. Blood glucose levels must be monitored frequently because small infants may require dextrose-containing solutions during the first 24 hours of resuscitation. After the first 24 hours, decreasing amounts of sodium and increasing amounts of potassium are administered as indicated. The urine also should be analyzed for myoglobinuria.

Burn Wound Care

While intravenous access and fluid resuscitation are attended to, attention can also be directed to burn wound care and management of the other problems frequently associated with thermal injury, including gastric ileus and pain.

Initially, the child must be completely undressed to facilitate a complete examination. However, care must be taken to prevent hypothermia. External heating devices should be used judiciously. Although the application of cool water compresses

---

TABLE 8-1.
Initial fluid therapy.

Burns of <35% of Body Surface Area (BSA)
 First 24 Hours
  Correct hypovolemia with boluses of normal saline or lactated Ringer's at 20 mL/kg as needed
  3 to 4 mL/kg per percent of BSA (plus maintenance in children with burns of <20% BSA)
  One half to be given within the first 4 to 6 hours after burn event
  One fourth to be given within the subsequent 6 hours
  One fourth to be given within the remaining 12 hours
 Second 24 Hours
  One half to three fourths of the first 24 hours' requirement
Burns of ≥35% of BSA
 Regimen as above, except that 4 mL/kg per percent of BSA is used as the guideline for estimating fluid requirements. Maintenance requirements must be added to the fluid calculation for children younger than 5 years.
Guidelines for Adequacy of Fluid Replacement
 Urine output of ≥1 mL/kg per hour
 Adequate estimated cardiac output
 Monitor glucose levels

may soothe the first- and second-degree burn wound, the patient may rapidly develop a falling core temperature. Use these compresses only in burns of <10% total body surface area.

The burns can be washed with either warm water or saline. Blisters should be left intact, especially on the palmar surface of the hands and soles of the feet, unless they are large and prone to rupture with the dressing application. Dead skin can be debrided with a wiping motion of a moist gauze sponge or with instruments.

Analgesics must be administered with careful monitoring. Full-thickness burns usually are insensate and require only minimal analgesia. Partial-thickness burns may be exquisitely sensitive. Narcotics should be given intravenously in small, frequent doses. Morphine sulfate may be used at a rate of 0.1 mg/kg per dose, given intravenously over 10 to 15 minutes and repeated as needed. Respiration, pulse, and blood pressure should be monitored carefully.

After debridement and initial cleansing, the wound may be managed with open or closed technique. Small superficial partial-thickness burns may be left open, or petrolatum gauze may be used and a bulky dressing applied. Deep partial- and full-thickness wounds require a topical antimicrobial agent; **silver sulfadiazine** is the preparation of choice. The wounds then may be left open or covered with a thin dressing.

Escharotomy should be considered in the presence of circumferential full-thickness burns of the trunk or limb that cause difficulty in breathing or compromise of circulation. This may be limb or even life saving.

Facial burns should be treated with an antibiotic ointment that is safe to use around the eyes. An ophthalmic preparation is a good choice. Debridement of the face, especially the ears, eyelids, and nose, should be minimal to preserve as much viable tissue as possible. The use of systemic antibiotics rarely is indicated in the initial management of the burn wound.

Because burns often are associated with gastric ileus, placement of a nasogastric tube should be considered in patients with extensive burns.

Tetanus immunization should be brought up to date.

If a decision is made to proceed with extensive wound care, the following steps must be taken:

1. Place the patient on a sterile sheet.
2. Outfit members of the resuscitation team with surgical caps, masks, and gloves.
3. Gently scrub the wound with warm water or saline.
4. Limit debridement to necrotic tissue or blisters that rupture during cleansing. Do not open intact blisters.
5. Apply silver sulfadiazine cream and dress wounds with a limited-thickness dressing of gauze or leave it open if the patient is admitted.
6. Escharotomy may be necessary for constricting full-thickness burns of the trunk or extremities if there is ventilatory or neurovascular compromise.
7. Check tetanus immunization status and determine whether there is any preexisting disease, the patient is on any medication, or there are medication allergies.

Pitfalls in Burn Care

Failure to recognize a respiratory or inhalation component of a burn that occurred in an enclosed space or associated multiple trauma can result in a major catastrophe. Avoid underestimation of burn size and depth by approaching the assessment in a disciplined fashion. The extent of the burn depth or the possibility of later grafting is not predictable at the time of initial assessment. It is best to be cautious about prognosis.

Nonrecognition of myoglobinuria or hemoglobinuria and of the attendant need for alkalinizatoin of the urine can lead to kidney failure.

Failure to perform escharotomy and fasciotomy when appropriate can lead to respiratory compromise or loss of an extremity.

Guidelines for Triage and Disposition

The guidelines in Table 8-2 can be used in determining disposition. If there is any doubt, admit a burned child to the hospital. Apply these guidelines based on the circumstances of each patient, including age, preexisting medical conditions, extent and nature of thermal injury, and social circumstances involved.

Transfer to a major burn center can be facilitated through direct telephone communication between the referring and receiving physicians. Preexisting transfer plans are very helpful.

Maintain adequate records to provide continuity in observation and care. Before a patient leaves the primary facility, prepare him or her for transport with a secure airway, working intravenous line, nasogastric tube, urinary catheter, proper burn dressing, and adequate analgesia.

ELECTRICAL TRAUMA

Pathophysiology

A number of factors determine the effect of electrical current on the body.

Resistance. Wet skin or water immersion decreases resistance precipitously, thereby increasing current delivered to tissue but resulting in few surface burns. In contrast, in and around tissue with high resistance such as callouses, more heat will evolve, resulting in cellular necrosis and worse surface burns.

Current Type. Alternating current (AC) is much more dangerous at lower voltage than direct current (DC) and may provide ventricular fibrillation at very low voltage. AC also causes tetanic muscle contractions that make many electrical injury victims unable to "let go" after contact with a circuit.

TABLE 8-2.
Guidelines for burn triage and disposition.

Outpatient Management
  Partial-thickness burn <10% body surface area (BSA)
  Full-thickness burn <2% BSA
Inpatient General Hospital Management
  Partial-thickness burn <25% BSA
  Full-thickness burn <15% BSA
  Partial-thickness burn of face, hands, feet, and
    perineum
  Questionable burn depth, extent
  Chemical burn, minor
  Significant coexisting illness or trauma
  Inadequate family support
  Suspected abuse
  Fire in an enclosed space
Burn Center
  Partial-thickness burn >25% BSA
  Full-thickness burn >15% BSA
  Full-thickness burn of the face, hands, feet, and
    perineum
  Respiratory tract injury
  Associated major trauma
  Major chemical and electrial burns

Current Pathway. Current follows the pathway of least resistance from contact point to the ground. Current that crosses the heart or brain is most dangerous.

The most frequent and serious problems involved in electrical injury include burns, cardiopulmonary arrest or injury, associated physical trauma, infection of burned tissue, myoglobinuria and third-space loss with renal injury, neurologic injury, tympanic membrane rupture, cataracts, and peripheral vessel occlusion.

Four types of electrical burn injury can occur, as follows:
- Direct injury from contact with the electrical source
- Flash burn (similar to a gas flame flash burn)
- Arc burn (measured at 2500°C)
- Flame injury from ignition of clothing

In addition, blunt injury can occur if a person is thrown by the intense muscle spasm that may be triggered by the electrical current or from falls.

Prolonged hypotension and massive muscle necrosis predispose the burn patient to severe infections, the most common cause of death among those who initially are resuscitated. It is critically important to remember that although victims of electrical injury may have minimal external manifestations, extensive underlying tissue damage and occult trauma often exist.

Lightning injuries, which follow the same laws of physics as other electrical injuries, usually present somewhat differently. Victims of lightning strike rarely have external or deep internal burn injuries. Cardiac arrest is the main cause of death, although permanent neurologic sequelae often occur in those who survive the initial incident.

Assessment

Life support protocols may be used for treating patients in cardiopulmonary arrest. If the victim of electrical injury is in hypovolemic shock, fluid resuscitation, as with thermal burns, is appropriate, including alkalinization of the urine if there is myoglobinuria. The deep injuries may produce massive muscle necrosis and myoglobinuria.

Lightning injuries rarely have myoglobinuria, and fluid resuscitation may be contraindicated unless there are massive burns. In patients injured by generated electrical power sources, care must be taken by rescuers to avoid injury to themselves.

Management

Maintain ventilation with high-flow oxygen and endotracheal intubation if necessary because many patients will exhibit persistent apnea. Hypotension usually is secondary to hypovolemia; treat it initially with a crystalloid fluid challenge of 20 mL/kg, which may be repeated as necessary. If a pressor agent is needed to achieve adequate perfusion, low-dose dopamine is the agent of choice because of the beneficial effect on renal perfusion.

Perform a thorough physical assessment after the primary survey, paying special attention to potential intracranial injury; entrance and exit burn wounds; signs of intra-abdominal hemorrhage, peritonitis, or ileus; evidence of fractures or dislocations; and diminished or absent pulses. Assess the patient for signs of blunt injury that may occur as a result of a fall or being thrown by intense muscle spasm.

Traditional burn formulas frequently underestimate crystalloid requirements in patients with electrical injury because of the massive third-space shift that may occur. In addition, fasciotomies, not just escharotomies, may be necessary because of deep muscle injury.

An indwelling urinary catheter to monitor urine output and a central venous line may be useful. Blood transfusion usually is not required within the first 24 hours of care unless there is ongoing occult hemorrhage.

Cardiac dysrhythmias, acidosis secondary to muscle necrosis, renal injury, and gastric dilation may be encountered. If myoglobinuria is present, the goal of fluid resuscitation should be a urine output of 1.0 to 1.5 mL/kg per hour while the urine is pigmented and 0.5 to 1.0 mL/kg per hour after the urine clears. Sodium bicarbonate may be added to one-half normal saline (or more-dilute crystalloid solutions) to promote alkalinization of the blood to pH ≥ 7.35 to 7.40, which will enhance urinary excretion of myoglobin. **Mannitol** (0.25 to 0.5 g/kg IV bolus followed by continuous infusion at 0.25 to 0.5 g/kg per hour) may be indicated to enhance renal perfusion and avoid myoglobinuric renal failure, one of the main causes of death in the past.

Because lightning injuries seldom involve deep injuries or myoglobinuria, fluid loading, osmotic diuresis, and fasciotomies rarely are needed.

Cranial computed tomography scanning is indicated for unexplained coma, deterioration of mental status, or development of lateralizing neurologic signs. Emergent fasciotomy or escharotomy may be required if vascular or respiratory compromise is present. Administer tetanus prophylaxis if indicated.

Disposition

Electrical burns are considered major burns according to the American Burn Association classification system. Transfer to a burn center is appropriate for all seriously injured patients.

Admission to the hospital is recommended for severe electrical burns. However, for the stable patient with relatively isolated burns, including lip burns, studies have shown that the patient may be safely released after 4 hours of observation in the emergency department, provided caretakers are instructed regarding proper methods of controlling late hemorrhage, which can occur from the labial artery.

Cardiac monitoring is controversial. Those with low-voltage electrical injuries probably can be safely discharged if they display no mental status changes or cardiac dysrhythmias. Creatine phosphokinase level has no relationship to the amount of burn or to the overall prognosis of the electrically injured patient.

Surgical consultation or follow-up is necessary for victims of electrical injury. Close follow-up is necessary for all patients with burn injuries. For cases of arc burns to the lip, consultation or follow-up with an experienced oral or plastic surgeon is necessary because severe bleeding may occur when the burn eschar separates from the underlying labial artery (usually 5 to 9 days after the injury) and because long-term splinting, particularly when the burn involves the commissure, may be necessary to avoid microstomia. Growth retardation of the mandible, maxilla, or dentition may occur.

Lightning victims may present more as cardiac or neurologic emergencies than as burn or trauma patients. A baseline ECG is indicated. Changes include nonspecific ST-T wave changes, T-wave changes, axis shift, QT prolongation, and ST-segment elevation. Admission usually is indicated, but children with completely normal examinations, laboratory tests, and ECGs may be discharged if there is adequate home observation and close follow-up.

OTHER BURNS

Abuse

An alarming number of children are subjected to maltreatment (see Chapter 12). Nonaccidental injury should be suspected and thoroughly investigated if there is evidence of any unusual pattern of the burn wound or the history given does not explain the nature of the injury. A clenched fist and "gloved" forearm burn distribution or bilateral lower extremity and buttocks injuries suggest involuntary submersion. Cigarette and steam iron-pattern burns are suspicious findings that warrant a social services investigation.

Chemical Burns

Early management of most chemical burns, particularly strong acid and alkali burns, must include irrigation with copious amounts of water or saline to dilute any chemical substance. Alkali burns usually are more significant than acid injuries because they penetrate deep into the tissue. After removal of all the chemical substance, the burn wound can be managed with debridement, applications of topical antibiotic creams, and dressings.

Circumferential Full-Thickness Burns

Extremities may be burned circumferentially. With fluid resuscitation, there is increasing edema beneath the unyielding burn eschar, which may lead to decreasing or absent distal vascular perfusion within the first 12 to 24 hours after the injury. This usually is a problem only with full-thickness burns.

It is important to evaluate the overall status of perfusion serially with Doppler ultrasound. When signs of decreasing flow are present, longitudinal incisions (escharotomies) should be made on the medial and lateral aspects of the extremity. This often will decrease the elevated compartment pressure and enhance peripheral circulation.

The thorax and abdomen also may sustain extensive full-thickness injury, resulting in respiratory embarrassment. Escharotomies on the chest, back, and abdomen may facilitate more adequate ventilation.

Fasciotomy may be necessary with electrical burns to salvage an extremity because of the incidence of deep muscle damage and edema within a fascial compartment.

ADDITIONAL READING

Andrews CJ, Cooper MA, ten Duis HJ, et al. The pathology of electrical and lightning injuries. In: Wecht CJ, ed. *Forensic Sciences.* New York, NY: Matthew Bender & Co; 1995.

Baker MD, Chiaviello C. Household electrical injuries in children. Epidemiology and identification of avoidable hazards. *Am J Dis Child.* 1989;143:59-62.

Capelli-Schellpfeffer M, Toner M, Lee RC, et al. Advances in the evaluation and treatment of electrical and thermal injury emergencies. *IEEE.* 1995;31:1147-1152.

Cherington M, Martorano FJ, Siebuhr LV, et al. Childhood lightning injuries on the playing field. *J Emerg Med.* 1994;12:39-41.

Cooper MA. Lightning injuries: prognostic signs for death. *Ann Emerg Med.* 1980;9:134-138.

Cooper MA, Andrews CJ. Lightning injuries. In: Auerbach P, ed. *Wilderness Medicine: Management of Wilderness and Environmental Emergencies,* 3rd ed. St Louis, Mo: Mosby–Year Book; 1995:261-289.

Del Vecchio DA, Whitaker LA. Facial trauma and plastic surgical emergencies. In: Fleisher GR, Ludwig S, eds. *Textbook of Pediatric Emergency Medicine,* 3rd ed. Baltimore, Md: Williams & Wilkins; 1993.

Hammond J, Ward CG. Myocardial damage and electrical injuries: significance of early elevation of CPK-MB isoenzymes. *South Med J.* 1986;79:414-416.

Harmel RP Jr, Vane DW, King DR. Burn care in children: special considerations. *Clin Plast Surg.* 1986;13:95-105.

McLoughlin E, Joseph MP, Crawford JD. Epidemiology of high-tension electrical injuries in children. *J Pediatr.* 1976;89:62-65.

Nichter LS, Morgan RF, Bryant CA, et al. Electrical burns of the oral cavity. *Compr Ther* 1985;11:65-71.

O'Neill JA. Burns in children. In: Artz CP, Moncrief JA, Pruitt BA Jr, eds. *Burns: A Team Approach.* Philadelphia, Pa: WB Saunders; 1979.

O'Neill JA. Fluid resuscitation in the burned child—a reappraisal. *J Pediatr Surg.* 1982;17:604-607.

O'Neill JA, Meacham WF, Griffin JP, et al. Patterns of injury in the battered child syndrome. *J Trauma.* 1973;13:332-339.

Purdue GF, Hunt JL. Electrocardiographic monitoring after electrical injury: necessity or luxury. *J Trauma.* 1986;26:166-167.

Robinson M, Seward PN. Electrical and lightning injuries in children. *Pediatr Emerg Care.* 1986;2:186-190.

Schwartz LR. Thermal burns. In: Tintinalli JE, Ruiz E, Krome RL, eds. *Emergency Medicine: A Comprehensive Study Guide,* 4th ed. New York, NY: McGraw-Hill; 1996:893-898.

Silverglade D, Ruberg RL. Nonsurgical management of burns to the lips and commissures. *Clin Plast Surg.* 1986;13:87-94.

Thompson JC, Ashwal S. Electrical injuries in children. *Am J Dis Child.* 1983;137:231-235.

Wallace BH, Cone JB, Vanderpool RD, et al. Retrospective evaluation of admission criteria for paediatric electrical injuries. *Burns.* 1995;21:590-593.

Environmental Emergencies

Chapter 9

Toxicology: Ingestions, Inhalation Injuries, Envenomations

OBJECTIVES

1. Explain the general management principles for ingestions and toxic exposures.

2. Identify methods used to minimize drug absorption.

3. Describe the specific therapies for common poisonings, including antidotes.

4. Identify the resources available for consultation for managing the child with poisoning or toxin exposure.

PART 1: INGESTIONS

Since the early 1960s, there has been a 95% decline in the number of pediatric poisoning deaths. Child-resistant product packaging, heightened parental awareness of potential household toxins, and a more sophisticated medical intervention at the poison control, emergency, and intensive care levels have all helped to reduce morbidity and mortality. Nevertheless, poisoning continues to be a preventable cause of pathology in children and adolescents. It is imperative that pediatricians, family physicians, and pediatric emergency physicians be familiar with the general approach to the poisoned child as well as the latest treatment methods available.

More than 60% of calls received by regional poison control centers in the United States involve children younger than 17 years. Most exposures in this group are accidental and result in minimal toxicity. The highest morbidity and mortality rates occur in adolescent and adult patients, but younger children also can be severely affected. Because of the potential for death or severe disability, prompt and effective management is crucial if the outcome is to be optimal. Toxins can cause a myriad of symptoms and conditions. Poisoning can occur from ingestion, dermal absorption, or inhalation of toxins. Although many pediatric patients present with a history of a specific toxic exposure, others may present with unexplained signs or symptoms and no history of poisoning.

PATHOPHYSIOLOGY

The mechanisms by which toxic substances act vary. Toxins may act on a cellular level (eg, cyanide) or affect a specific organ system, such as the brain (eg, narcotics, hypnotic sedatives, major tranquilizers), autonomic nervous system (eg, organophosphates), lung (eg, hydrocarbons, paraquat), gastrointestinal tract (eg, caustics, corrosives), liver (eg, acetaminophen), or blood (eg, heavy metals). The range of pathologic processes that may be caused by a noxious agent is great.

INITIAL ASSESSMENT

In the initial assessment, the physician must determine rapidly whether a child is in a life-threatening situation.

Treat the patient, not the poison. Attention to the standard ABCs of resuscitation always is the first priority. Evaluate the presence and adequacy of respirations, and follow with measurement of pulse, capillary refill, and blood pressure. Addressing airway patency is of the utmost importance. Institute airway support when indicated. Administer supplemental oxygen if there are signs of respiratory distress or shock. If indicated, start a large-bore intravenous line with normal saline. Assess the glucose level using a bedside glucose oxidase reagent strip and administer **glucose** (0.25 to 0.5 g/kg of 25% dextrose in water) by intravenous push if indicated. **Naloxone** may be used for any child in a coma at a dose of 0.1 mg/kg; it is also acceptable to start at 2 mg for a child older than 5 years.

Next, attempt to identify the specific poison but do not focus on finding an antidote. Obtain a detailed history from the patient, family members, friends, rescuers, or bystanders. Important points are the identification of ingested substance or substances, amount and time of ingestion, presence of allergies or underlying diseases, and first aid treatment that has been administered. Family, friends, or police may need to search the home for the toxin. Examine clothing and personal effects for ingestants and Medic-Alert identification.

Perform a brief physical examination, concentrating on neurologic and cardiopulmonary status. Identify distinct toxic syndromes if present (Table 9-1).

With an assessment of mental status based on the Glasgow Coma Scale or AVPU system, quantify the level of consciousness (see Chapter 6). Always consider other causes of altered mental status, such as metabolic imbalance or trauma, and rule them out through appropriate evaluation.

Patients with central nervous system (CNS) or cardiopulmonary compromise require cardiac monitoring. If cardiac rhythm disturbances are present or the patient is known to have ingested a cardiotoxic poison (eg, tricyclic antidepressant or digitalis), obtain a 12-lead ECG and closely monitor the blood pressure.

If the level of consciousness is altered or respiratory problems are present, obtain a chest radiograph. Aspiration pneumonitis or noncardiogenic pulmonary edema may be present. Certain medications, such as iron, other heavy metals, and enteric-coated capsules, may be seen on abdominal radiographs.

Serum electrolyte and arterial blood gas

TABLE 9-1.
Toxic syndromes.

Toxin	Syndrome
Opioids	Respiratory failure Coma Miosis
Cyclic antidepressants	Coma Seizures Dysrhythmias QRS >100 sec
Organophosphates, cholinergics	Diarrhea, diaphoresis Urination Miosis Bronchorrhea, bronchospasm, bradycardia Emesis Lacrimation Salivation Vomiting Fasciculations
Anticholinergic	Flushing ("red as a beet") Dry skin and oral mucosa ("dry as a bone") Hyperthermia ("hot as a hare") Delirium ("mad as a hatter") Mydriasis Tachycardia Urinary retention
Sympathomimetic	Mydriasis Anxiousness Tachycardia Hypertension Hyperthermia Diaphoresis

determinations can provide valuable information about possible toxic or metabolic processes. In a patient with a metabolic acidosis, the **anion gap** ($Na^+ - [Cl^- + CO_2]$) will be ≥ 12 if there are unmeasured anions present from a toxic or metabolic source. An **osmolar gap** (measured osmoles – calculated osmoles) of >10 will be present in patients who have ingested ethanol, methanol, isopropanol, or ethylene glycol. Calculated osmoles are derived from the formula $2Na^+ + glucose/18 + blood\ urea\ nitrogen/2.8 + ethanol/4.6$.

Toxicologic screening of blood and urine rarely contributes to the acute management. There may be academic or forensic indications for obtaining these studies, in which case they can be ordered on a routine turnaround time. A negative toxicology screen does not rule out the possibility of a toxin. If a particular drug or class of drugs is suspected, communicate this to the laboratory. Serum levels of specific drugs may be available to guide management or predict prognosis.

The **physical examination** and vital signs may be helpful in identifying particular groups of toxins. **Hypertension** suggests cocaine, amphetamines, phencyclidine, sympathomimetic overdose, or sedative or narcotic withdrawal; **hypotension** suggests β-blocker, sedative-hypnotic, or narcotic drugs. **Tachycardia** can be present in ingestions of the same drugs that cause hypertension; **bradycardia** can be associated with digitalis, β-blockers, calcium channel antagonists, clonidine, or hypothermia. Fever can be produced by salicylates, anticholinergics, or withdrawal from alcohol or narcotics.

Respirations are depressed with sedative-hypnotics and narcotics but increased in cases of pulmonary aspiration (hydrocarbons), pulmonary edema (smoke inhalation, narcotics, salicylates), and metabolic acidosis (ethylene glycol, methanol, salicylates). Pupil size (Table 9-2) and skin signs (Table 9-3) also may be helpful in identifying the class of ingested agent.

MANAGEMENT

Management is based on the following four general principles:

- Provision of supportive care (ABCs)
- Prevention or minimization of absorption
- Enhancement of excretion
- Administration of antidotes

Prevention or Minimization of Absorption

Syrup of ipecac-induced emesis is no longer advocated in the health care setting for the treatment of the acutely poisoned patient. Gastric lavage is indicated only if the patient arrives <1 hour after ingestion, in cases of massive ingestion, or for those substances that do not bind to charcoal.

First-line treatment for significant ingestions consists of a single dose of **activated charcoal** in water. The dose is 1 to 2 g/kg in children younger than 6 years and 50 to 100 g in adolescents or adults. A nasogastric tube often is required for complete administration. There are no contraindications for its use; however, it is ineffective for a small group of substances (Table 9-4). Hyperosmolar adjunctive cathartics (eg, sorbitol, magnesium citrate) are contraindicated in children younger than 6 years because of the potential risk for fluid and electrolyte imbalance.

Whole bowel irrigation may be accomplished

TABLE 9-2.
Toxic pupillary findings.

Miosis (COPS)

C — Cholinergics, clonidine
O — Opiates, organophosphates
P — Phenothiazines, pilocarpine, pontine bleed
S — Sedative-hypnotics

Mydriasis (AAAS)

A — Antihistamines
A — Antidepressants
A — Anticholinergics, atropine
S — Sympathomimetics (cocaine, amphetamines)

TABLE 9-3.
Toxic skin signs.

Diaphoretic skin (SOAP)

S — Sympathomimetics
O — Organophosphates
A — ASA (salicylates)
P — PCP (phencyclidine)

Red skin	Carbon monoxide, boric acid
Blue skin	Cyanosis, methemoglobinemia

through the rapid administration of polyethylene glycol electrolyte lavage solution (Colyte, GoLYTELY) via nasogastric tube. It irrigates out the contents of the gastrointestinal tract and is indicated for the ingestion of significant amounts of iron or delayed-release pharmaceuticals. The rate of administration is 500 mL/hr for preschoolers and 1 to 2 L/hr for teenagers and adults. The end point is a clear rectal effluent that takes several hours. This procedure is contraindicated in patients with ileus, obstruction, perforation, or significant gastrointestinal hemorrhage.

Enhancement of Excretion

There are several techniques aimed at enhancing excretion, and each is indicated in only a few situations.

Ion Trapping

In theory, acidification and alkalinization of the urine enhance the excretion of weak bases and weak acids. The former should be avoided altogether because of the risks of acidemia and exacerbation of rhabdomyolysis. Urinary alkalinization should be considered for significant salicylate and phenobarbital poisonings.

Neutral Diuresis

Urine flow can be increased through the administration of excess intravenous crystalloid and should be considered for significant lithium or bromide poisonings. Pulmonary edema, cerebral edema, and renal failure are contraindications.

Multiple Dose Charcoal

Multiple dose charcoal may be indicated with drugs that undergo enterohepatic or enteroenteric recirculation (eg, phenobarbital, theophylline, carbamazepine). In theory, this technique enhances the excretion of toxins by using the gastrointestinal epithelium as a dialysis membrane (gastrointestinal dialysis). In smaller children, overzealous administration should be avoided to prevent iatrogenic complications such as charcoal aspiration and bowel obstruction.

Hemodialysis

This technique is indicated for methanol, ethylene glycol, significant salicylate, phenobarbital, theophylline, and lithium poisonings.

Charcoal Hemoperfusion

This technique is rarely indicated. It is used most commonly in significant theophylline poisoning.

Administration of Antidotes

Antidotes and antagonists are available for only a minority of poisonings and are not intended for indiscriminate use. Use antidotes carefully, particularly in the pediatric patient with an unknown overdose, because overuse may complicate an initial presentation by producing other forms of poisoning. In weighing the benefits and risks of administering a specific antidote, consider the patient's clinical status, appropriate laboratory values, expected pharmaceutical action

TABLE 9-4.
Substances not absorbed by activated charcoal.

PHAILS
P — Pesticides
H — Hydrocarbons
A — Acids, alkali, alcohols
I — Iron
L — Lithium
S — Solvents

TABLE 9-5.
Antidotes.

Poison	Antidote
Acetaminophen	N-Acetylcysteine (United States, oral; elsewhere, intravenous)
Anticholinergics	Physostigmine
Anticholinesterase insecticides	Atropine, 2-PAM
Benzodiazepines	Flumazenil
β-Blockers	Glucagon
Carbon monoxide	Oxygen
Cyanide	Cyanide antidote kit
Cyclic antidepressants	Sodium bicarbonate
Digoxin	Digibind
Ethylene glycol	Ethanol
Iron	Deferoxamine
Isoniazid	Pyridoxine
Lead	Succimer, BAL, calcium EDTA
Mercury	BAL, DMSA
Methanol	Ethanol
Methemoglobinemia	Methylene blue
Opioids	Naloxone

of the toxin, and possible adverse reactions associated with the antidote. Specific antidotes are listed in Table 9-5.

COMMON INGESTIONS

Several substances are commonly ingested by young children, and their management deserves discussion.

Acetaminophen

Acetaminophen is the most commonly used drug for analgesia and antipyresis in children. Ingestions most often are seen in children younger than 6 years, but overdose also may be associated with suicide attempts in adolescents. Toxicity is unlikely in children younger than 6 years, chiefly because they usually ingest nontoxic amounts. Ingestions in older children are potentially serious, and careful assessment and management are necessary to ensure a good outcome.

Acetaminophen is absorbed rapidly after ingestion, with peak plasma levels at ≈1 hour. The drug is metabolized in the liver, with 2% excreted unchanged in the urine. In older children, 94% is metabolized to the glucuronide and sulfate conjugates, and 4% is metabolized through the cytochrome oxidase P-450 system (which produces a reactive metabolite). When the glutathione stores are ≈30% of normal, the highly reactive metabolite binds to hepatic macromolecules, and hepatic damage ensues.

The clinical course has been divided into four stages:

- Stage 1. This stage consists of the first 24 hours after ingestion. Young children may vomit; older children may have nausea, vomiting, generalized malaise, and diaphoresis. The mean onset of symptoms is 6 hours after the ingestion, with 60% of patients symptomatic by 14 hours. Liver enzymes and prothrombin times are normal.
- Stage 2. Patients are asymptomatic during the second 24 hours (quiescent phase). Liver enzymes may become elevated.
- Stage 3. In serious overdoses, the peak of symptoms and abnormalities is seen 48 to 96 hours after the ingestion. Serum aspartase transaminase (AST) concentrations may be as high as 20,000 to 30,000 IU/L. An elevated prothrombin time is considered to be the best

laboratory guide to the severity of hepatic encephalopathy. Death may occur in this stage from hepatic failure or coagulopathy.
- Stage 4. Approximately 7 to 8 days after ingestion, hepatic abnormalities are almost resolved in survivors. Recovery is complete, and hepatic sequelae are not expected.

Acetaminophen poisoning usually does not present with altered mental status within the first 24 hours after ingestion. Consider the possibility that patients presenting with CNS depression have a multiple-drug overdose. Interpret histories with caution, particularly in the adolescent. It often is difficult to distinguish between toxic and nontoxic overdoses by history alone. Draw blood to determine acetaminophen levels from patients with potentially serious overdoses.

FIGURE 9-1.
Rumack-Matthew nomogram for estimating severity of acute acetaminophen poisoning. The time coordinators refer to time of ingestion. Serum levels drawn before 4 hours may not represent peak levels.

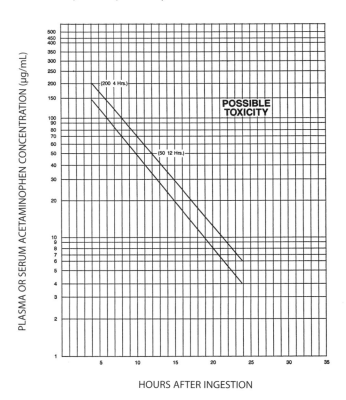

From Rumack BH, Matthew H. Acetaminophen poisoning and toxicity. *Pediatrics.* 1975;55: 871-876. Adapted with permission.

After a brief assessment, administer activated charcoal in water (or mixed with a cathartic if age >6) if <4 hours have elapsed since the ingestion. Activated charcoal binds well to acetaminophen and may lessen a potentially hepatotoxic ingestion. In the older child, a relatively large dose, such as 100 g, may be required because of the large amount of acetaminophen that is typically ingested. In practice, the concern of charcoal adsorbing orally administered N-acetylcysteine (NAC) and diminishing its bioavailability has been overstated. Routine doses of both agents can be administered, but some toxicologists still recommend increasing the dose of NAC by 1.5 times when charcoal has preceded its use.

After a single acute ingestion, blood to determine acetaminophen level is drawn 4 hours after the ingestion. If >4 hours has passed, blood is drawn immediately. Once the plasma level has been determined, plot it on the Rumack-Matthew nomogram to determine whether the level is toxic in relation to time (Figure 9-1). If the level cannot be determined within a time frame of up to 8 hours after ingestion, initiate treatment with NAC after consultation with the poison control center. If the time and amount of ingestion are unknown, determination of acetaminophen level is still recommended with subsequent blood drawn at 4-hour intervals to determine the half-life of the drug. A prolonged elimination half-life of >3 hours is indicative of hepatic damage or delayed absorption.

Oral NAC is available as a 20% concentrate. It has a strong smell of sulfur, which is generally unacceptable to patients. Dilute the concentrate to a 5% concentration (ie, if starting with a 20% concentrate, dilute 3:1). The taste may be improved by mixing it with orange juice or carbonated beverages. Use a cup with a cap and hole for a straw to avoid the smell. The initial dose of NAC is 140 mg/kg with subsequent doses of 70 mg/kg at 4-hour intervals for 17 doses.

Intravenous NAC is licensed in Europe and Canada and available for investigational use in the United States. It is given as three separate infusions: 150 mg/kg over the first 60 minutes, 50 mg/kg over the next 4 hours, and 100 mg/kg over the next 16 hours. Administration of the first infusion over 60 instead of 15 minutes decreases the risk for adverse reactions such as flushing, itching, and hives. The advantages of intravenous therapy are a shorter protocol, no concern that vomiting or charcoal may decrease the bioavailability of the antidote, and ease of administration. It is not unusual for patients receiving intravenous NAC to develop hives, requiring treatment with antihistamines. The efficacy of each protocol is essentially the same.

It is important to follow laboratory parameters in a case of serious poisoning; these include prothrombin time, AST, serum alanine transaminase, and bilirubin, as well as electrolytes, blood urea nitrogen, and creatinine. Most patients (99%) recover within 1 week. Patients requiring careful monitoring may be managed best in a pediatric tertiary care center.

Alcohols

Ethanol

Ethanol poisoning is more likely to occur in an older child, but it can also occur in a toddler. In addition to alcohol-containing beverages such as beer, wine, and hard liquor, children have access to mouthwashes (containing up to 75% ethanol), colognes and perfumes (40% to 60% ethanol), and >700 medicinal preparations containing ethanol. Characteristic breath odor and serum levels make the diagnosis. Mixed drug/ethanol toxicity frequently confounds the clinical picture. A blood ethanol level of 100 mg/dL is considered sufficient to cause intoxication. Levels approaching 500 mg/dL may be lethal. In general, treatment is supportive and may include assisted ventilation. Due to low hepatic glycogen stores, small children are extremely prone to hypoglycemia when intoxicated with ethanol. Intoxication in combination with hypoglycemia can markedly impair mental status.

Methanol and Ethylene Glycol

Very small volumes of methanol or ethylene glycol are life threatening. These toxic alcohols are commonly found in windshield washer fluid and antifreeze products, respectively. They both produce osmolar gap and anion gap metabolic acidosis. Methanol can cause blindness, and ethylene glycol can cause acute renal failure. Both act through the production of toxic metabolites, which can be blocked by ethanol through a competitive inhibition of the alcohol dehydrogenase enzyme.

Treatment consists of the administration of sufficient ethanol to produce a serum concentration of 100 mg/dL. The usual dose is 0.6 g/kg infused over 30 to 40 minutes. Oral ethanol can be used if intravenous ethanol is not readily available. During the infusion of an ethanol drip, the child's glucose levels should be monitored to avoid hypoglycemia. In children with peak serum methanol and ethylene glycol levels of >50 mg/dL, extracorporeal intervention with hemodialysis is indicated. **Folate** (up to 50 mg q4h) is a therapeutic cofactor for methanol, and **thiamine** (up to 100 mg) serves a similar function for ethylene glycol.

Anticholinergic Agents

The symptom complexes associated with anticholinergic overdoses are "red as a beet" (flushing), "dry as a bone" (dry skin, decreased oral secretions), "hot as a hare" (febrile), and "mad as a hatter" (delirium). This complex may be caused by jimsonweed, deadly nightshade, potato leaves, and a number of medications, including antihistamines, benztropine, and tricyclic antidepressants. Most overdoses involving drugs with anticholinergic actions do not result in a pure anticholinergic syndrome; this is especially so for cyclic antidepressants, whose life-threatening toxicity is due to direct myocardial depression. Treatment is mainly supportive. With the exception of tricyclic antidepressants, in severe pure anticholinergic poisoning, consider using the antidote **physostigmine**. Indications include severe agitation, profound hyperthermia, hallucinations, or uncontrollable seizures. Administer in a dose of 0.5 mg IV to a young child and 1 to 2 mg IV to an adolescent over 2 to 3 minutes.

Caustics

Agents such as drain cleaners, Clinitest tablets, oven cleaners, and automatic dishwasher detergents often are ingested by children. Initial treatment may include immediate dilution with water or milk. Children with oral burns or a definite history of significant ingestion should be considered for esophagoscopy within 12 hours of the injury. After ingestion of liquid drain cleaners, esophageal burns can occur without the presence of oropharyngeal burns. Gastric evacuation is contraindicated, and charcoal provides no benefit.

Clonidine

Clonidine is a centrally acting antihypertensive agent. It stimulates α_2-adrenergic receptors in the brain, which makes it effective in lowering blood pressure. It primarily is prescribed for patients with chronic hypertension and narcotic patients in detoxification programs. It is packaged in very small tablets (0.1, 0.2, and 0.3 mg) that can be hard for the elderly to see and easy for a child to swallow. Clonidine also is available in patch form, which can still contain the drug after use. A child can obtain a toxic dose simply by sucking on the patch.

Symptoms of ingestion are low blood pressure, altered mental status, miosis, and respiratory depression. Children present with respiratory rates, blood pressure, and pulse rates that are <50% of normal for their age group. The child who ingests massive quantities of clonidine may present with initial hypertension, usually lasting ≤1 hour. As the brain perceives the hypertension, the central sympatholytic downregulating effects begin to dominate, and the patient becomes hypotensive. This is an accentuation of the mode of action of clonidine. Antihypertensive drugs should not be used because of the transiency of the hypertension.

Treatment is straightforward and supportive. Stimulation of a child with altered mental status often will increase heart and respiratory rate. Apply oxygen. Place the child in a Trendelenburg position. Obtain intravenous access, and be prepared to administer a 20 mL/kg bolus of lactated Ringer's or normal saline. Inotropic drugs seldom are required but are effective. If the respiratory rate does not improve, begin bag-valve-mask ventilation. A few children will require intubation and mechanical ventilation until the drug effects wear off, usually within 24 hours.

Because children with clonidine overdose resemble those with narcotic poisoning, including small pupils, naloxone has been used. In the patient with known clonidine ingestion, however, naloxone is of little use because it is not necessary in the milder cases, it will not correct the severe cases but may sufficiently lighten them so the hypertension may be aggravated, and it is of no help in the hypotensive stage. The symptomatic child will have to be observed in the hospital for 12 to 36 hours because the half-life of clonidine is 12 to 16 hours.

Pediatric fatalities from clonidine toxicity have not been described.

Cyanide

Poisoning with cyanide can occur through dermal exposures or ingestion of silver polish, Laetrile, certain insecticides, specific masticated fruit seeds, and acetonitrile-containing nail cosmetics (nail glue removers). Pulmonary exposure appears frequently in home fires (cyanide gas released from burning synthetic materials); suspect this in smoke inhalation victims. Death can occur within 1 to 15 minutes. Survivors who reach the emergency department may manifest seizures, shock, or coma. Flushing often is a unique sign. *Do not administer mouth-to-mouth resuscitation*; the rescuer may become poisoned. Rapid treatment with 100% oxygen, amyl nitrite, sodium nitrite, and then thiosulfate (cyanide antidote kit) is required for survival. Keep in mind that *the ampule of sodium nitrite in the commercially available cyanide therapeutic kits is an adult dose* and if that dose is given to a child, it could cause profound hypotension, severe methemoglobinemia, and death. The dose of sodium nitrite for a child is 10 mg/kg, or 0.33 mL of 3% solution of sodium nitrite per kilogram of body weight.

Cyclic Antidepressants

Mechanisms of cyclic antidepressant toxicity include direct myocardial (quinidine-like) depression, inhibition of norepinephrine uptake, and anticholinergic activity. Ingestion can produce significant CNS and life-threatening cardiovascular toxicity. Findings include combativeness, delirium, coma, seizures, hypotension, and dysrhythmia. A QRS interval duration of >100 milliseconds is a risk factor for dysrhythmia.

Treat hypotension with a crystalloid challenge; if unsuccessful, proceed to the use of pressors. The drug of choice for the patient with a dysrhythmia is intravenous sodium bicarbonate. A wide QRS interval is an early indication for its use. Alkalinization via hyperventilation also is efficacious. The goal is blood pH 7.45 to 7.55. Physostigmine has no role in cyclic antidepressant overdose, despite the anticholinergic properties; the potent cardiotoxic properties of cyclic antidepressants prevent its use.

Symptomatic patients require an intensive care unit setting; however, long periods of monitoring of asymptomatic patients are not required. For patients with a normal level of consciousness, vital signs, and normal ECG from the outset, a 6-hour period of continuing normality of these parameters is sufficient. Those with an abnormality in any of these three require at least a 24-hour observation period in a monitored setting.

Hydrocarbons

Hydrocarbons are found as solvents, fuels, and additives in household cleaners and polishes. The major toxicity of such compounds stems from their low surface tension and vapor pressure, which allow them to spread over large surface areas, such as in the lungs, leading to a chemical pneumonitis. Patients who ingest hydrocarbons may choke, cough, and gag as the product is swallowed, and they may vomit soon afterward. Aspiration of the product at the time of the initial swallowing may cause aspiration pneumonitis. It originally was believed that the aspiration of those substances into the lungs after the vomiting that accompanies ingestion was responsible for the major pulmonary toxicity. It has been shown, however, that the mere presence of the substance in the hypopharynx can cause chemical pneumonitis by spreading to contiguous surfaces in the airway. In addition to the pulmonary findings, there may be transient associated CNS symptoms, secondary to systemic absorption of some of the hydrocarbons. Rarely, liver, kidney, or myocardial injury occurs.

The amount of a hydrocarbon that has been ingested by a child often is difficult to quantify. Less than 1 mL of some compounds, such as mineral seal oil, when aspirated directly into the trachea, can produce severe pneumonitis and eventual death. Other compounds are difficult to aspirate and are not well absorbed from the gastrointestinal tract. Generally, compounds such as asphalt or tar, lubricants (eg, motor oil, household oil, heavy greases), and liquid petrolatum are not toxic when ingested.

Pulse oximetry and chest radiographs are indicated in patients with respiratory signs or symptoms. Asymptomatic children with a normal physical examination should be observed for 4 to 6 hours in the emergency department. If they remain well, they may be discharged with appropriate instructions for return if fever, tachypnea, or cough develops.

Treatment of hydrocarbon pneumonitis basically is that of supportive care. Antibiotics should not be used prophylactically. The use of corticosteroids in the treatment of aspiration from hydrocarbons has been associated with increased morbidity and is not recommended.

Inducement of emesis with syrup of ipecac or decontamination with gastric lavage is contraindicated. Charcoal administration is not indicated unless the ingested compound contains a dangerous additive that has the potential for systemic toxicity. Other hydrocarbon compounds, including gasoline, kerosene, charcoal lighter fluid, and mineral spirits, are unlikely to produce systemic symptoms after ingestion.

Iron

The lethal dose of elemental iron is 200 to 250 mg/kg, although gastrointestinal symptoms can be seen at doses of 15 to 30 mg/kg. When calculating the ingested dose, remember that the elemental iron per unit dose is only a fraction of the total milligram weight of the tablet. Ferrous sulfate, the most commonly ingested product, is 20% elemental iron; ferrous fumarate has 32% elemental iron, and ferrous gluconate has only 10%. The toxic dose is not absolute, and fatal reactions have been reported with ingestions of only 75 mg/kg. Therefore, all ingestions should be considered potentially dangerous. Significant toxicity, however, is uncommon at amounts <60 mg/kg. All patients who have ingested significant amounts of iron develop gastrointestinal symptoms within 6 hours.

For iron-poisoned patients, the acute pathophysiology and clinical picture have been classified into four stages, as follows:

- Gastrointestinal Stage. The first signs of iron toxicity are gastrointestinal; early symptoms include vomiting, rapid onset of diarrhea, colicky abdominal pain, and gastrointestinal hemorrhage. Iron directly damages the gastrointestinal mucosa and can lead to massive fluid loss and hemorrhage. The gastrointestinal effects may contribute to systemic hypovolemia by the third spacing of the fluid in the small bowel.
- Relative Stability Stage. The gastrointestinal signs and symptoms may ameliorate before the onset of overt shock. In such instances, there is a stage of relative stability. This does not last

longer than 6 to 12 hours, and patients are not really symptom free during this time. Careful assessment will yield evidence of decreased perfusion and acidosis.
- Shock Stage. The third stage is characterized by circulatory failure, profound shock, and acidosis. Shock, the most common cause of fatality in iron poisoning, has a complex etiology that includes hypovolemic, distributive, and cardiac depressant factors. The chief causes of the acidosis are the hydrated unbound circulating iron and lactic acidosis secondary to shock.
- Hepatotoxicity Stage. Hepatotoxicity occurs within the first 48 hours. Earlier onsets correlate with increased severity. This is the second most common cause of mortality.

Gastrointestinal scarring is a late manifestation of iron poisoning, occurring 2 to 6 weeks after ingestion. Typically, it presents as gastric outlet obstruction, but any portion of the small intestine may be involved.

Management of Iron Toxicity

The amount of iron ingested often is hard to quantify, and minimal "safe" levels are not well established. Serum iron levels, if obtained promptly, often correlate with the likelihood of developing symptoms. Usually, iron levels of <350 µg/dL, when drawn 2 to 6 hours after ingestion, predict a benign course. Patients with levels in the range of 350 to 500 µg/dL often show mild phase I symptoms but rarely develop serious complications. Levels of >500 µg/dL suggest significant risk for phase III manifestations. However, serum iron determination is not always available on a "stat" basis.

Prompt clinical assessment coupled with early abdominal radiographs and timely serum iron levels is the mainstay of the management of the iron-poisoned patient (Table 9-6). A radiograph may be used to confirm an ingestion or diagnose concretions. A negative radiograph in a symptomatic patient does not exclude iron ingestion; reasons for a negative radiograph are: iron was not ingested; the ingested iron has dissolved or was absorbed; a liquid iron preparation was ingested; a pediatric multivitamin-plus-iron pharmaceutical with a very small amount of iron per tablet was ingested. The latter pharmaceutical is associated with only mild symptoms.

Although controversial, syrup of ipecac may still play a role in large iron ingestions witnessed in the home setting; however, its use in the emergency department is not recommended. Gastric lavage has little benefit >1 hour after ingestion. In addition, the diameter of the gastric evacuation tube used in a child often is too small to allow removal of significant pill fragments and concretions. Iron is not adsorbed to charcoal. Whole bowel irrigation is considered the technique of choice with large ingestions. Gastrotomies have been performed with massive overdoses. **Intragastric** complexing with bicarbonate, phosphate, or deferoxamine should be avoided because these approaches are ineffective and can be dangerous.

Patients arriving with **severe early symptoms** of iron toxicity, including vomiting, diarrhea, gastrointestinal bleeding, depressed sensorium, or circulatory compromise require urgent, intensive treatment. The first priority is obtaining venous access. Simultaneously, blood should be drawn for complete blood cell count, blood glucose, electrolytes, blood urea nitrogen, liver function tests, serum iron, and typing and cross-matching. The total iron binding capacity (TIBC) level often is inaccurate in the setting of iron poisoning and not useful in the management of an acute overdose. Patients in shock should be supported with normal saline or lactated Ringer's solution and blood transfusions if indicated. These patients often are very acidotic and require large amounts of sodium bicarbonate. Specific chelation therapy with intravenous deferoxamine should be begun immediately in all severely poisoned patients. However, ensure expansion of the intravascular space because fluid-depleted patients treated with deferoxamine are at risk for hypotension, anaphylaxis, and acute renal failure.

Chelation therapy with parenteral deferoxamine enhances the excretion of iron. Indications for chelation are the presence of symptoms or a serum iron concentration of >350 µg/dL. The intravenous dose of deferoxamine is 15 mg/kg per hour up to a maximum of 6 g/day. Indications for cessation of chelation are the absence of symptoms and resolution of acidosis or when the total daily dose has been given. The classic "vin rose" urine color change will result if iron-binding stores are saturated and free iron is complexed with deferoxamine. Although this finding may be helpful in diagnosing toxicity, its results often are subtle; therefore, an absent color change does not rule out significant iron poisoning.

Further problems may include hypotension, profound metabolic acidosis, hypoglycemia or hyperglycemia, anemia and colloid loss due to gastrointestinal hemorrhage (after equilibration), renal shutdown due to shock, and hepatic failure with an associated bleeding diathesis. The maintenance of an adequate urine output is critical to prevent renal failure and promote excretion of the iron/deferoxamine complex. If renal failure occurs, chelation may be continued with concurrent extracorporeal removal, with charcoal hemoperfusion favored over hemodialysis for removal of the iron/deferoxamine complex.

Opioids

Any patient with altered mental status of unknown etiology should receive a trial of an intravenous bolus of **naloxone** (0.1 mg/kg or 2 to 4 mg for age >5). The classic triad of opioid overdose is decreased level of consciousness, depressed

TABLE 9-6.
Management of the iron-poisoned patient.

Assess stability of patient's condition, and stabilize if required.

History: How much? When? Type of iron salt? Enteric coated? Symptoms?

Determine serum iron level.

Obtain abdominal radiograph to corroborate ingestion. Three planes are required to rule out drug concretions or adherence to gastric wall. Consider gastrotomy for presence of concretions, gastric wall adherence, or a potentially fatal amount of iron in the stomach.

If radiograph suggests >30 mg/kg elemental iron in a child or >1.0 g in an adolescent, begin whole bowel irrigation with polyethylene glycol electrolyte lavage solution. Patients with negative radiographs do not require gastrointestinal decontamination. If asymptomatic, they will remain so; if symptomatic, it is too late for it to be of benefit.

Chelate the symptomatic patient with deferoxamine.

Admit to intensive care unit for shock or decreased level of consciousness.

respirations, and pinpoint pupils. If needed, naloxone can be continued intravenously via continuous infusion. Diphenoxylate, propoxyphene, and methadone overdoses may require very large doses of naloxone and prolonged therapy.

Organophosphates

The classic findings of massive cholinergic overdrive are represented by the symptom complex of **DUMBELS**:

D – Diarrhea
U – Urination
M – Miosis
B – Bradycardia, bronchosecretions
E – Emesis
L – Lacrimation
S – Salivation

Vomiting usually is the initial symptom. Other associated symptoms, such as pinpoint pupils, muscle fasciculations, and wheezing, also may be present. Toxicity may mimic gastroenteritis, asthma, seizures, or heat exhaustion. These symptoms usually are seen clinically as a result of toxic exposures of organophosphate and carbamate insecticides.

The most serious symptoms for these patients are overwhelming bronchorrhea and even respiratory failure. The treatment priority is maintenance of the airway, accomplished through intubation. Large doses of atropine (0.5 to 10 mg) may be injected intravenously until the airway has become sufficiently dry that ventilation is no longer a problem. Although those atropine doses are considerably larger than would be given for other situations (bradycardia), they may be required for satisfactory clinical response. With organophosphate insecticide poisoning, a cholinesterase regenerator such as 2-PAM (Protopam) may be required to maintain this satisfactory clinical response. This drug is not indicated in carbamate insecticide poisoning. When managing these patients, skin decontamination is essential, as is protection of the staff from dermal absorption (gloves and protective clothing must be worn).

Salicylates

The usual signs and symptoms of acute salicylate ingestion are nausea, vomiting, hyperventilation, hyperpyrexia, tinnitus, oliguria, disorientation,

coma, convulsions, and hyperglycemia (hypoglycemia in the young child). Less common manifestations include respiratory depression, pulmonary edema, acute tubular necrosis, hepatotoxicity, and syndrome of inappropriate secretion of antidiuretic hormone . In acute ingestions, salicylate levels are prognostic. They have less use in chronic salicylism. The Done nomogram (Figure 9-2) may be useful in determining toxicity if the ingestion is severe. This nomogram should be used only in patients with single acute overdose. Serum levels in patients with chronic toxicity or ingestions of enteric-coated preparations should not be plotted. Because of the potential for delayed salicylate toxicity and

FIGURE 9-2.
Done nomogram for salicylate poisoning. The Done nomogram should be used with the following cautions: (1) The patient has taken a single actue ingestion and is not suffering from chronic toxicity and has not ingested a delayed-release aspirin preparatoin. (2) The blood level to be plotted on the nomogram was drawn ≥6 hours after ingestion. A level of <20 mg/dL at 2 hours indicates a nontoxic ingestion, and additional blood levels are not required.

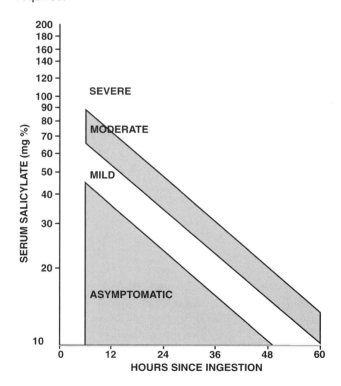

From Done AK. Salicylate intoxication: significance of measurements of salicylate in blood in cases of acute ingestion. *Pediatrics*. 1960;26:800. Adapted with permission.

formation of gastric concretions, more than one salicylate level is recommended to ensure a declining trend. Generally, ingestions of <150 mg/kg are mild; 150 to 300 mg/kg, moderate; 300 to 500 mg/kg, serious; and >500 mg/kg, severe.

Management includes the general principles for all ingestions. Monitor potassium levels carefully because they are usually low. For moderate and severe ingestions, an intravenous line should be established, and 5% dextrose in water with 50 mEq of sodium bicarbonate per liter given at a rate of 10 to 15 mL/kg over 1 to 2 hours. The goal of alkalinization is to maintain urine pH >7; however, this will not be accomplished without aggressive potassium supplementation. Arterial blood gas analysis helps determine the degree of acidosis. If the pH is <7.15, an additional 1 to 2 mEq/kg bicarbonate may be given over 1 to 2 hours. Avoid rapid bicarbonate administration because it may lead to relative CNS acidosis and seizures. Severe, persistent acidosis may require 1 to 2 mEq/kg bicarbonate every 2 hours. Hemodialysis or hemoperfusion may be necessary in unresponsive acidosis (pH <7.1), renal failure, noncardiogenic pulmonary edema, seizures, or progressive deterioration after trials of standard therapy.

DISPOSITION

After being observed for 4 to 6 hours, some patients who have ingested potentially toxic substances and are asymptomatic or marginally affected can be discharged with appropriate instructions for return if necessary. Because repeat ingestions occur in 10% to 50% of children, all discharged patients and their families should be given instructions about poison prevention techniques.

Children with significant toxic ingestions or potential intoxication with substances that have delayed effects (sustained-release products) require admission to the hospital. The specific ingestion and degree of physiologic alteration determine whether treatment in a pediatric intensive care unit is warranted. All patients with intentional overdoses should have a psychiatric assessment.

HAZARDOUS CHEMICAL EXPOSURE

Hazardous chemical exposure includes direct contact with the skin or eye or inhalation of noxious gases. The risk of skin exposure is chiefly from acid or alkali burns due to direct contact. However, systemic toxicity is possible in situations involving lipophilic substances. The concern with eye exposures is for local injury and not systemic toxicity. Inhalation exposures are discussed in detail in the next section.

Ophthalmic and Cutaneous Exposure

Assessment consists of direct inspection of the body part for evidence of caustic or corrosive damage. Copious irrigation of exposed areas with water or saline solution should be initiated immediately, preferably at the scene. Chemical burns are managed as thermal burns. Irrigation of caustic eye injuries should be copious and started as early as possible. Adequacy of irrigation can be judged by checking pH of the tears when acidic or basic compounds have resulted in eye injury. Follow-up management of eye exposures is dependent on the results of the fluorescein examination after irrigation. A negative result requires no interventions; ophthalmologic consultation should be considered for any positive finding.

Health care workers must be careful to avoid personal exposure to toxic chemicals. Appropriate protective clothing is indicated.

ADDITIONAL READING

Albertson TE, Derlet RW, Foulke GE, et al. Superiority of activated charcoal alone compared with ipecac and activated charcoal in the treatment of acute toxic ingestions. *Ann Emerg Med.* 1989;18:56-59.

American Academy of Pediatrics, Committee on Injury and Poison Prevention. *Handbook of Common Poisonings in Children*, 3rd ed. Elk Grove Village, Ill: American Academy of Pediatrics; 1994.

Anderson KD, Rouse TM, Randolph JG. A controlled trial of corticosteriods in children with corrosive injury of the esophagus. *N Engl J Med.* 1990;323:637-640.

Berlin CM. The treatment of cyanide poisoning in children. *Pediatrics.* 1970;46:793-796.

Boehnert MT, Lovejoy FH. Value of the QRS duration versus the serum drug level in predicting seizures and ventricular arrhythmias after an acute overdose of tricyclic antidepressants. *N Engl J Med.* 1985;313:474-479.

Erickson T. General principles of poisoning: diagnosis and management. In: Strange GR, Ahrens WR, Lelyveld S, et al, eds. *Pediatric Emergency Medicine: A Comprehensive Study Guide.* New York, NY: McGraw-Hill; 1996:487-492.

Erickson T. Toxic alcohols. In: Strange GR, Ahrens WR, Lelyveld S, et al, eds. *Pediatric Emergency Medicine: A Comprehensive Study Guide.* New York, NY: McGraw-Hill; 1996:496-500.

Fine JS, Goldfrank LR. Update in medical toxicology. *Pediatr Clin North Am.* 1992;39:1031-1051.

Greensher J, Mofenson HC, Caraccio TR. Ascendency of the black bottle (activated charcoal). *Pediatrics*. 1987;80:949-951.

Henretig FM. Special considerations in the poisoned pediatric patient. *Emerg Med Clin North Am*. 1994;12:549-567.

Henretig FM, Selbst SM, Forrest C, et al. Repeated acetaminophen overdosing. Causing hepatotoxicity in children. Clinical reports and literature review. *Clin Pediatr*. 1989;28:525-528.

Kirk MA, Cisek J, Rose SR. Emergency department response to hazardous materials incidents. *Emerg Med Clin North Am*. 1994;12:461-481.

Koren G. Medications which can kill a toddler with one tablet or teaspoonful. *J Toxicol Clin Toxicol*. 1993;31:407-413.

Kulig K. Initial management of ingestions of toxic substances. *N Engl J Med*. 1992;326:1677-1681.

Kulig K, Bar-Or D, Cantrill SV, et al. Management of acutely poisoned patients without gastric emptying. *Ann Emerg Med*. 1985;14:562-567.

Liebelt EL, Shannon MW. Small doses, big problems: a selected review of highly toxic common medications. *Pediatr Emerg Care*. 1993;9:292-297.

Litovitz T, Manoguerra A. Comparison of pediatric poisoning hazards: an analysis of 3.8 million exposure incidents. A report from the AAPCC. *Pediatrics*. 1992;89:999-1006.

Merigian KS, Woodard M, Hedges JR, et al. Prospective evaluation of gastric emptying in the self-poisoned patient. *Am J Emerg Med*. 1990;8:479-483

Mofenson HC, Greensher J. Physostigmine as an antidote: use with caution. *J Pediatr*. 1975;87:1011-1012. Letter.

Moore RA, Rumack BH, Conner CS, et al. Naloxone: underdosage after narcotic poisoning. *Am J Dis Child*. 1980;134:156-158.

Morelli J. Pediatric poisonings: the 10 most toxic prescription drugs. *Am J Nurs*. 1993;93:26-29.

Notarianni L. A reassessment of the treatment of salicylate poisoning. *Drug Saf*. 1992;7:292-303.

Osterloh JD. Utility and reliability of emergency toxicologic testing. *Emerg Med Clin North Am*. 1990;8:693-723.

Pearn J, Nixon J, Ansford A, et al. Accidental poisoning in childhood: five year urban population study with 15 year analysis of fatality. *Br Med J*. 1984;288:44-46.

Pediatric toxicology. *Pediatric Clin North Am*. 1986;33:245-450.

Rumack BH. Acetaminophen overdose in young children. Treatment and effects of alcohol and other additional ingestants in 417 cases. *Am J Dis Child*. 1984;138:428-433.

Schnell LR, Tanz RR. The effect of providing ipecac to families seeking poison-related services. *Pediatr Emerg Care*. 1993;9:36-39.

Sofer S, Tal A, Shahak E. Carbamate and organophosphate poisoning in early childhood. *Pediatr Emerg Care*. 1989;5:222-225.

Tenenbein M. Whole bowel irrigation as a gastrointestinal decontamination procedure after acute poisoning. *Med Toxicol Adverse Drug Exp*. 1988;3:77-84.

Tenenbein M. Whole bowel irrigation in iron poisoning. *J Pediatr*. 1987;111:142-145.

Tenenbein M. General management principles for poisoning. In: Barkin RM, ed. *Pediatric Emergency Medicine: Concepts and Clinical Practice*. St Louis, Mo: Mosby-Year Book; 1992:463-470.

Victoria MS, Nangia BS. Hydrocarbon poisoning: a review. *Pediatr Emerg Care*. 1987;3:184-186.

PART 2: INHALATION INJURIES

OBJECTIVES

1. Describe the ways in which smoke can be toxic.

2. Discuss the clinical progression of inhalation toxicity.

3. Describe the steps in evaluation and management of the patient exposed to smoke and who may have carbon monoxide poisoning.

Smoke inhalation is a leading cause of morbidity and mortality in the burn victim. Exposure to noxious substances in the atmosphere may directly injure the respiratory apparatus or may indirectly produce systemic intoxication. The nature of the resulting illness depends on the source, intensity, and duration of exposure. Offending agents range from single, well-defined chemicals such as hydrogen cyanide, which produces severe systemic toxicity when inhaled, to the airborne products of a residential fire, a complex matrix of organic and inorganic chemicals, heated atmospheric gases, and the gaseous products of incomplete combustion.

PATHOPHYSIOLOGY

Smoke contains four categories of environmental threat: heat, asphyxiants (chiefly carbon monoxide and hydrogen cyanide), particulate matter, and pulmonary irritants.

Heat

Burns of the upper airway often are encountered in victims of closed-space fire and can occur whenever the temperature of inhaled gas exceeds 150°C. However, thermal injury distal to the vocal cords is quite unusual because the temperature of inhaled smoke decreases rapidly as it passes down the respiratory tree; thus, direct thermal injury to the lung is uncommon. However, significant burns of the supraglottic region or vocal cords frequently produce edema sufficiently severe to result in upper airway obstruction. In contrast, the latent heat of steam is sufficiently high that burns of the distal airway and lung do occur with this toxic inhalation.

Asphyxiants

Asphyxiants include carbon monoxide (CO), which is produced by the incomplete combustion of hydrocarbons such as wood and paper, and hydrogen cyanide (HCN), a byproduct of combustion of nitrogen-containing polymers such as wool or silk. Hydrogen sulfide (H_2S) is a physical asphyxiant that produces hypoxemia through displacement of oxygen from the atmosphere. The characteristic odor of cyanide is that of burned almonds, whereas that of the sulfides is rotten eggs.

CO is the most frequently encountered asphyxiant. This colorless, odorless compound has an affinity for hemoglobin (Hb) that is ≈250 times greater than that of oxygen. Binding of CO to Hb diminishes the oxygen-carrying capacity of blood by a proportion equal to the percentage of carboxyhemoglobin (COHb) and shifts the oxyhemoglobin dissociation curve to the left. In addition, there is evidence that CO interferes with cellular oxygen metabolism at the mitochondrial level. Dissolved oxygen is not affected by CO; therefore, the measured PaO_2 may be normal even when the oxygen saturation (percentage of Hb bound to oxygen) is profoundly depressed.

Venous CO concentrations up to 5% are found in normal individuals. Concentrations of 20% often produce significant neurologic symptoms, but a single level may not correlate with clinical manifestations. Concentrations of >60% frequently are associated with death or neurologic morbidity. In a particular patient, however, specific COHb levels are less important in management than the history of exposure and condition of the patient.

In addition to household fires, children may be exposed to many other sources of CO, including poorly repaired motor vehicles and those left running while parked and malfunctioning or inappropriate household heaters. In rare instances, children are exposed to other asphyxiants such as HCN or H_2S after environmental catastrophes or while playing in an industrial area.

Particulate Matter

Particulate matter consists mainly of carbon. Large particles (ie, >5 μm) are deposited in the trachea or bronchi, and those <1 μm reach the pulmonary alveoli. Although carbon per se is physiologically inert, it may be coated with toxic chemical products of combustion such as acrolein, hydrochloric acid, or aromatic hydrocarbons. In addition, inhalation of carbon dust has been shown to produce airway hyperreactivity.

Pulmonary Irritants

Pulmonary irritants include a heterogeneous

group of compounds that includes ammonia, sulfur oxides, nitrogen oxides, halogen acids (eg, HCl), chlorine gas, aldehydes (eg, acrolein), ketones, and phosgene. These chemicals present both as gases or bound to the surface of small particles and can incite pulmonary edema and mucosal injury.

CLINICAL PRESENTATION

Inhalation injury should be considered in any child who is exposed to fire or presents with a burn injury (other than scald). History of exposure in an enclosed space or physical features such as facial burns, singed nasal hairs, carbonaceous deposits in the pharynx, stridor, or hoarseness suggest the possibility of upper airway injury. Although respirations may be unlabored initially, laryngeal edema is progressive in the smoke inhalation patient and is not maximal until 2 to 8 hours after injury.

The presentation of pulmonary injury ranges in severity from mild wheezing, rales, and rhonchi to frank respiratory failure with cyanosis. After a patient's exposure to fire, an altered sensorium, particularly with loss of consciousness, should be assumed to indicate CO poisoning and central nervous system hypoxia. Concurrent traumatic closed-head injury should remain in the differential diagnosis until excluded.

Non–fire-related toxic inhalation also chiefly involves CO. CO poisoning should be considered in any child with nausea, vomiting, or headache, with or without altered sensorium, when there is no other obvious etiology. Typical presentations include a child who is found unconscious in a home in which a charcoal grill is used for heating, a child who begins to vomit and becomes somnolent while riding in the back seat of an automobile in poor repair, or a child living in a kerosene-heated home. Not infrequently, the child with occult CO toxicity presents with a nonfebrile flu-like illness and improves considerably while under care. The symptoms subside after removal of the child from exposure to a faulty car exhaust or a toxic home environment. A high index of suspicion for CO toxicity must be maintained to prevent recurrent toxicity or even death.

FIGURE 9-3.
General guide for management of children exposed to smoke.

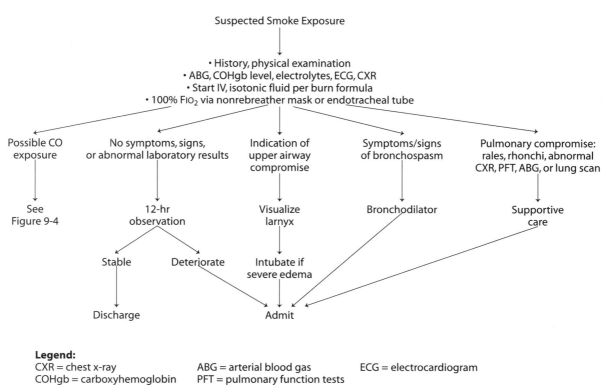

From Thom SR. Smoke inhalation. *Emerg Med Clin North Am.* 1989;7:371-387. Adapted with permission.

DIAGNOSTIC EVALUATION

The diagnostic evaluation of the child after inhalation injury focuses on assessment of airway patency and baseline pulmonary function and determination of whether CO poisoning is present. Children who present with a history consistent with exposure to a fire or CO intoxication require determination of CO level (usually expressed as percent COHb). In most hospitals, this determination is performed with cooximetry, which also indicates the percentage of methemoglobin. Although pulse oximetry is very useful in the evaluation of SaO_2, this technique does not detect the presence of COHb or other abnormal hemoglobins and should never be depended on for this purpose. The arterial blood gas is of value in detecting hypoxemia due to lung injury and metabolic acidosis due to tissue hypoxia produced by severe CO intoxication but cannot be used to evaluate the level of CO.

In room air, the half-life of COHb is ≈4 hours. It decreases to 36 to 80 minutes when the child receives an FIO_2 of 1.0 and 15 to 23 minutes under hyperbaric conditions (3 atmospheres). Because burn victims are generally treated with oxygen ($FIO_2 = 1$) at the scene of the fire and en route to the hospital, significant toxicity may be manifest even when COHb levels are low at the time of presentation. A normal COHb level at the time of admission does not exclude CO poisoning if the history or physical findings suggest that condition to be present.

The chest radiograph is an essential baseline diagnostic study, particularly when exposure occurs in a fire. It initially may be normal but eventually will reveal bilateral patchy and confluent areas of opacification. Other appropriate laboratory studies include a complete blood cell count, urinalysis, and serum electrolytes, blood urea nitrogen, creatinine, and liver function tests. An ECG should be performed to establish a baseline and to detect the presence of myocardial ischemia or infarction.

MANAGEMENT

Care of the child with inhalation injury follows the usual emergency sequence of airway, breathing, and circulation. In addition to administration of oxygen ($FIO_2 = 1$) and routine measures to assess and secure the airway, after stabilization, children at

FIGURE 9-4.

Guide for known or suspected CO poisoning.

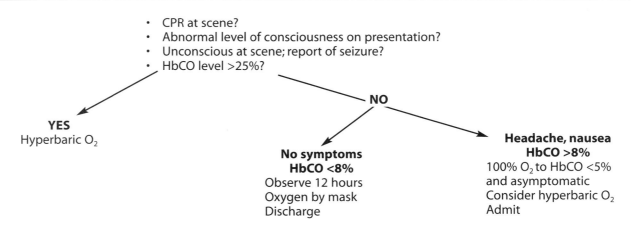

Possible CO Exposure

- ABCs (CPR if needed)
- 100% oxygen
- Cooximetry (HbCO)
- Arterial blood gases, chest radiographs, monitor

- CPR at scene?
- Abnormal level of consciousness on presentation?
- Unconscious at scene; report of seizure?
- HbCO level >25%?

NO

YES
Hyperbaric O_2

No symptoms HbCO <8%
Observe 12 hours
Oxygen by mask
Discharge

Headache, nausea HbCO >8%
100% O_2 to HbCO <5% and asymptomatic
Consider hyperbaric O_2
Admit

From Thom SR. Smoke inhalation. *Emerg Med Clin North Am.* 1989;7:371-387. Adapted with permission.

risk of upper airway thermal injury (facial, oral, or pharyngeal burns; hoarseness; stridor) require urgent bronchoscopy to evaluate for life-threatening airway obstruction. Of course, when airway edema appears to be evolving or signs of obstruction are severe, immediate intubation is required and may prevent catastrophic loss of airway patency.

Aggressive fluid administration, consistent with appropriate burn resuscitation parameters, does not increase the risk of pulmonary edema in the patient with combined burn and inhalation injury. Fluids should not be restricted in an effort to limit the progression of airway and pulmonary compromise.

Diagnostic and management algorithms are presented in Figures 9-3 and 9-4. Oxygen is the initial treatment of choice for most other sequelae of toxic inhalation. As noted previously, oxygen reduces the half-life of COHb, thereby accelerating the rate at which levels decease. Oxygen ($FIO_2 = 1$) is administered until the COHb concentration is <5% and the patient has fully regained normal neurologic function.

In cases of CO poisoning, there is a significant residual tissue burden of CO that remains bound to cellular cytochrome systems and myoglobin even when the blood COHb concentration has returned to normal. Treatment with 100% oxygen under *hyperbaric conditions* (eg, 2 to 3 atmospheres) may accelerate the rate of tissue decontamination. Therefore, when the history suggests exposure to CO, children who are found unconscious at the scene of the exposure, and those with neurologic dysfunction at the time of presentation should be referred to a hyperbaric facility even if the blood COHb concentration has returned to normal. When profound neurologic dysfunction exists at the fire scene, there is a strong probability that CO intoxication is implicated (perhaps in concert with hypoxemia). In this context, direct referral to a cooperating hyperbaric facility from the fire scene may be appropriate before determination of COHb concentration. There are studies suggesting that early application of hyperbaric oxygen may be life saving or reduce the possibility of severe neurologic injury. In addition, all children, even if neurologicly intact, with a measured COHb level of >25% and all pregnant women should be referred.

The decision to refer to a hyperbaric facility will depend on locally available facilities and the stability of the patient. In many communities, hyperbaric chambers are available that are capable of permitting critical care during hyperbaric conditions. After the initial resuscitation and stabilization, assisted ventilation and hemodynamic support need not prevent hyperbaric treatment. Every emergency department should develop referral agreements and protocols with local and regional hyperbaric centers.

Suspected exposure to HCN is treated as described above for cyanide. The treatment for H_2S is the same except that thiosulfate is not needed. Management of other sequelae of inhalation injury follows standard principles of care. Respiratory failure is treated with assisted ventilation, including positive end-expiratory pressure, as indicated. A bronchodilator may be of value, but empiric use of antibiotics or a corticosteroid is discouraged. The management of other aspects of significant fire injury is detailed in Chapter 8.

ADDITIONAL READING

Bresnitz EA. Simple asphyxiants and pulmonary irritants. In: Goldfrank LR, Flomenbaum NE, Lewin NA, et al, eds. *Goldfrank's Toxicologic Emergencies*, 5th ed. East Norwalk, Conn: Appleton & Lange; 1994:1181-1186.

Carvajal HF, Griffith JA. Burns and inhalation injuries. In: Fuhrman BP, Zimmerman JJ, eds. *Pediatric Critical Care*. St Louis, Mo: Mosby–Year Book; 1992:1209-1220.

Clark WR, Neiman GF. Smoke inhalation. *Burns Incl Therm Inj*. 1988;14:473-494.

Goldfrank LR. Hyperbaric oxygen. In: Goldfrank LR, Flomenbaum NE, Lewin NA, et al, eds. *Goldfrank's Toxicologic Emergencies*, 5th ed. East Norwalk, Conn: Appleton & Lange; 1994:1211-1214.

Hampson NB, Dunford RG, Kramer CC, et al. Selection criteria utilized for hyperbaric oxygen treatment of carbon monoxide poisoning. *J Emerg Med*. 1995;13:227-231.

Kirk MA. Smoke inhalation. In: Goldfrank LR, Flomenbaum NE, Lewin NA, et al, eds. *Goldfrank's Toxicologic Emergencies*, 5th ed. East Norwalk, Conn: Appleton & Lange; 1994:1187-1197.

Mosley S. Inhalation injury: a review of the literature. *Heart Lung*. 1988;17:3-9.

Myers RAM. Carbon monoxide poisoning. In: Haddad LM, Winchester JF, eds. *Clinical Management of Poisoning and Drug Overdose*, 2nd ed. Philadelphia, Pa: WB Saunders; 1990:1139-1152.

Nguyen TT, Gilpin DA, Meyer NA, et al. Current treatment of severely burned patients. *Ann Surg*. 1996;223:14-25.

Thom SR. Smoke inhalation. *Emerg Med Clin North Am*. 1989;7:371-387.

Tibbles PM, Edelsberg JS. Hyperbaric-oxygen therapy. *N Engl J Med*. 1996;334:1642-1648.

Tomaszewski C. Carbon monoxide. In: Goldfrank LR, Flomenbaum NE, Lewin NA, et al, eds. *Goldfrank's Toxicologic Emergencies*, 5th ed. East Norwalk, Conn: Appleton & Lange; 1994:1199-1210.

Traber DL, Linares HA, Herndon DN, et al. The pathophysiology of inhalation injury—a review. *Burns Incl Therm Inj*. 1988;14:357-364.

PART 3: ENVENOMATIONS

OBJECTIVES

1. Identify the early manifestations of a serious pit viper envenomation.

2. Initiate the appropriate supportive care for pit viper envenomation.

3. Describe the appropriate use of antivenin for pit viper envenomation.

4. Describe coral snake envenomation and how to evaluate.

5. Describe black widow and brown recluse spider bite recognition and management.

PIT VIPER

Pit viper (*Crotalidae*) envenomation is a rare but important cause of morbidity and mortality in the United States. Although the severity of envenomation varies widely with the species, any member of the family found in North America is capable of inflicting significant damage requiring treatment. The pit viper family includes **rattlesnakes**, **water moccasins**, and **copperheads**.

Pathophysiology

Pit viper venoms may vary widely in the relative amounts of their component parts, including myonecrotic enzymes, cardiotoxins, nephrotoxins, hemotoxins, and neurotoxins. Because of this variation, the clinical presentation also may vary.

After envenomation, the venom produces capillary leak and local tissue necrosis.

After a major envenomation, the release of vasodilatory compounds, hypovolemia from the loss of the integrity of the capillary endothelium, and bleeding may all contribute to the rapid development of circulatory shock.

Assessment

As in all emergencies, first consider the adequacy of the circulatory and respiratory systems. Demographic variables and physical findings should be considered, in the absence of immediate life-threatening symptoms, to assess the severity of the bite. Information regarding the size and species of the snake (if possible), circumstances related to the bite, number of bites inflicted, first aid methods used, time of the bite, and transport time required should be obtained. The severity of the bite should be staged (Table 9-7).

Management

First aid should include reassurance for the child. If the child can be kept quiet, dissemination of the toxins can be lessened. Transportation for medical care should be accomplished as soon as possible. Venom extraction kits that use suction are not harmful and may remove a small amount of the venom if used immediately. Incision of the wound, local ice, electric shock therapy, and venous or arterial tourniquets are not recommended. The

---

TABLE 9-7.
Envenomation staging.

No envenomation
Occurs in ≈25% of strikes; no venom has been released, and only fang marks are present.

Mild envenomation
Fang mark or marks are present, with edema and tissue necrosis confined to the surrounding area. No clinical or laboratory evidence of systemic effects is present.

Moderate envenomation
Edema, bullae, or ecchymoses extending beyond the immediate area of the bite to include a large part of the extremity. Tender adenopathy may be present, depending on the site of the bite. Clinical or laboratory evidence of systemic venom effects may be present, depending on the species.

Severe envenomation
Rapid extension of edema, bullae, or ecchymoses to involve entire extremity; shock as demonstrated by tachycardia, hypotension, poor perfusion, or change in level of consciousness; elevation of hematocrit, prothrombin time, or creatine kinase; depression of platelet count or fibrinogen; bites on the thorax, and especially the head and neck, should be assumed to be severe.

caretakers will be anxious even if the child has no envenomation. For most snakebites in children, reassurance, careful observation, serial measurements, and supportive care are all that are necessary.

Initiate correction of **hypovolemia** with 20 mL/kg crystalloid. A second bolus of 20 mL/kg may be used if needed. The persistence of hypotension mandates invasive monitoring and inotropic support in addition to administration of polyvalent **antivenin**.

Obtain appropriate laboratory studies, including a complete blood count, prothrombin time, fibrinogen degradation products, platelet count, blood urea nitrogen, creatine kinase, and urinalysis. Institute basic and advanced life support, as indicated. Maintain the extremity at heart level. Obtain blood for laboratory studies, and place two intravenous lines. For moderate to severe bites, obtain blood for transfusion and cross-match before starting infusion of antivenin.

In nonenvenomations and mild envenomations, cleanse the wound area. Follow tetanus prophylaxis guidelines for all bites. Prevent secondary infection by administering the appropriate broad-spectrum antibiotics, especially if nonsterile first aid measures were used. Predominantly, Gram-negative bacteria are present in the mouth of a snake. Administer acetaminophen as needed for pain. Do not use sedatives, ice, tourniquets, or aspirin.

Measure the extremity for circumference at a marked location and recheck every 15 to 30 minutes for 6 hours and then at least every 4 hours for a total of 24 hours. Progression of edema beyond the site of the bite may warrant the use of antivenin even after 12 hours. Repeat the laboratory studies every 6 hours; if significant changes occur, treat the patient with polyvalent antivenin.

Use of *Crotalidae* Antivenin

In moderate to severe envenomations, administer polyvalent antivenin. Copperhead bites are often treated without antivenin, but diamondback rattlesnake envenomations are very dangerous. As many as 75 vials of antivenin have been used in a child. In general, children require a greater total quantity of antivenin than do adults. If there are multiple bites, increase antivenin dose by 50%.

When the decision has been made to initiate antivenin therapy, the patient should be skin tested using horse serum material intradermally. In the event of a positive skin test, initiate treatment with antivenin only in an intensive care setting with pretreatment with antihistamines, epinephrine, and adrenocorticosteroids and only for severe envenomations. Be aware that a negative skin test does not always rule out the possibility of an allergic reaction with the actual administration of antivenin.

The initial dose of antivenin is based on the envenomation ranking:

- No envenomation: No skin testing, no antivenin
- Mild envenomation: Skin testing followed by 5 vials
- Moderate envenomation: Skin testing followed by 10 vials
- Severe envenomation: Skin testing followed by 15 vials

Each vial is mixed with 10 mL of saline, and then the total amount (ie, 5 vials [50 mL]) is diluted 1:4 with normal saline or lactated Ringer's solution. Begin to administer the material at the rate of 1 to 2 mL/hr and observe for severe reaction. If none occurs, increase the rate over a 30-minute period to a maximum of 150 mL/hr. In small infants (<10 kg), use a total volume of 100 mL, containing 5 vials, at a maximal rate of 60 mL/hr.

After administration of the amount of antivenin based on the degree of envenomation (5-vial minimum), reassess the patient, including laboratory studies. Continued progression of local or systemic findings suggests the need for additional antivenin therapy. Usually, the initial dose is repeated every 2 hours with reassessment after each step. There is no maximum dose. The total dose is that amount needed to neutralize the poison, as measured by the clinical response. In smaller patients (<45 kg), the antivenin dose required may be ≈50% higher.

Treat mild symptoms of urticaria, itching, and flushing with a decrease in antivenin rate and with **diphenhydramine**. Serious anaphylactic reactions require discontinuation of antivenin, followed by airway control, as needed, and treatment with epinephrine.

Disposition

Asymptomatic patients should be observed and followed with careful measurements for ≥12 hours.

Patients receiving antivenin need careful, continuous monitoring. It is reasonable to initiate antivenin therapy in a monitored setting such as an emergency department. In patients requiring further antivenin for continued progression of symptoms or those with severe envenomations with systemic manifestations, consider transfer to a pediatric intensive care unit or tertiary facility. Arrange follow-up at 5 to 14 days for the possible development of serum sickness from horse serum. These symptoms typically are responsive to diphenhydramine and corticosteroids.

CORAL SNAKE

There are only two species of coral snake (*Elapidae*) in the United States — the Eastern (found in the southeast) and the Sonoran (found in Arizona and New Mexico). Together, they account for only ≈1% of the snake bites in the United States. They are 2 feet long and have a black snout. In North America, wide red and black circumferential bands alternate with a thin yellow band, resulting in the mnemonic verse: "Red on yellow, kill a fellow; red on black, venom lack."

Assessment

The snake has two fangs, which leave two punctures <1 cm apart. There is only mild pain and minimal edema. Paresthesia and weakness are followed by diplopia and bulbar signs, such as dysphagia and dysphoria. Respiratory failure may develop.

Management

Local measures are of no help. Supportive care should be provided as indicated. There is a specific antivenin for the Eastern variety, which tends to be more toxic, but none for the Sonoran. Unlike pit viper bites, the antivenin (3 to 5 vials in 250 mL of normal saline) is recommended for any patient with a documented bite because it is more difficult to monitor the progression of symptoms. Patients should be followed up closely after treatment for serum sickness symptomatology.

BLACK WIDOW SPIDER

The female of the genus *Latrodectus* is noted for her red hour-glass configuration on the ventral side of the abdomen and her ability to envenomate human contacts. The venom of these spiders consists of peptides capable of causing release of acetylcholine at the myoneural junction, thus producing excessive muscle contraction. Norepinephrine also is released by the venom.

Assessment

Black widow spider bites may present as known exposures in the pediatric patient or, more commonly, as an unknown problem with an unusual constellation of symptoms. Consider a child with a sudden onset of irritability and muscle rigidity, particularly of the abdominal musculature, and with perspiration and mild elevation of vital signs, especially hypertension, as possibly having black widow spider envenomation. Other supportive findings include muscle rigidity in one or more extremities, respiratory distress from diaphragmatic muscle paralysis, and periorbital swelling not associated with other signs of angioedema. Rarely, convulsions may occur. Because of the extreme irritability of these children and the rigidity of their abdominal musculature, the possibility of central nervous system infection or an acute intra-abdominal process must be considered. Differentiation of these diagnoses may require a complete blood cell count, abdominal radiographs, and lumbar puncture. If a history of contact with a black widow spider is obtained, those tests may not be necessary. Arterial blood gas analysis may be indicated in children with severe muscle rigidity and suboptimal respirations.

Management

Patients requiring advanced life support or the administration of antivenin should be admitted to a tertiary care facility. Antivenin typically is reserved for younger patients with severe symptoms, such as intractable pain, marked hypertension, or seizures. Administration of benzodiazepines, opiates, or calcium may ease muscle rigidity and spasms. Most patients have a relatively benign course and can be managed with inpatient observation in a monitored setting.

BROWN RECLUSE SPIDER

The brown recluse spider (*Loxosceles reclusa*) is a brown spider 1 to 5 cm long that has a characteristic violin- or fiddle-shaped area on the dorsal cephalothorax. The venom contains calcium-dependent enzyme sphingomyelinase D, which has a direct lytic effect on red blood cells. After cell wall damage, an intravascular coagulation process causes a cascade of clotting abnormalities and local polymorphonuclear leukocyte infiltration, culminating in a necrotic ulcer.

Assessment

The clinical response to loxoscelism ranges from a cutaneous irritation or necrotic arachnidism to a disseminated intravascular coagulation-like life-threatening systemic reaction. Baseline coagulation studies may be predictive of the systemic reaction. There have been no proven fatalities in North America. Signs and symptoms of envenomation most often are localized to the bite area. Typically, there is little pain at the time of the bite. Within a few hours, the patient will experience itching, swelling, erythema, and tenderness over the bite. Classically, erythema surrounds a dull blue-gray macule circumscribed by a ring or halo of pallor. Within 3 to 4 days, the wound forms a necrotic base with a black eschar. Within 7 to 14 days, the wound develops a full necrotic ulceration.

Management

The wound should be cleaned, and tetanus immunization should be updated. The involved extremity should be immobilized to reduce pain and swelling. The early application of ice lessens the local wound reaction; heat will exacerbate the symptoms. Antibiotic treatment is indicated for secondary wound infections. Antihistamines may prove beneficial in children. Some experts advocate the use of a leukocyte inhibitor, dapsone, to diminish the amount of scarring and subsequent surgical complications. However, because of limited studies in humans and the potential for dapsone to induce methemoglobinemia, cautious administration is recommended in pediatric patients. Early excisional treatment can cause complications such as recurrent wound breakdown and hand dysfunction. Delayed closure and skin grafting may be necessary once the necrotic process has subsided several weeks later.

ADDITIONAL READING

Banner W. Bites and stings in the pediatric patient. *Curr Probl Pediatr.* 1988;18:1-69.

Clark RF, Wethern-Kestner S, Vance MV, et al. Clinical presentation and treatment of black widow spider envenomation: a review of 163 cases. *Ann Emerg Med.* 1992;21:782-787.

Cruz NS, Alvarez RG. Rattlesnake bite complications in 19 children. *Pediatr Emerg Care.* 1994;10:30-33.

Erickson T, Herman BE, Bowman MJ. Snake envenomations. In: Strange GR, Ahrens WR, Lelyveld S, et al, eds. *Pediatric Emergency Medicine: A Comprehensive Study Guide.* New York, NY: McGraw-Hill; 1996:590-592.

Erickson T, Herman BE, Bowman MJ. Spider bites. In: Strange GR, Ahrens WR, Lelyveld S, et al, eds. *Pediatric Emergency Medicine: A Comprehensive Study Guide.* New York, NY: McGraw-Hill; 1996:593-598.

Erickson T, Hryhorczuk DO, Lipscomb J, et al. Brown recluse spider bites in an urban wilderness. *J Wilderness Med.* 1990;1:258-264.

Sullivan JB, Wingert WA, Norris RL. North American venomous reptile bites. In: Auerbach PS, ed. *Wilderness Medicine: Management of Wilderness and Environmental Emergencies*, 3rd ed. St Louis, Mo: Mosby; 1995:680-709.

Russell FE, ed. *Snake Venom Poisoning.* Philadelphia, Pa: JB Lippincott; 1980.

Wingert WA, Chan L. Rattlesnake bites in southern California and rationale for recommended treatment. *West J Med.* 1988;148:37-44.

Chapter 10

Submersion Injury

OBJECTIVES

1. Identify the factors responsible for most submersion injuries.

2. Describe the primary and secondary pathophysiologic changes that occur after submersion injuries.

3. Discuss the major management principles of submersion injuries in the prehospital and hospital settings.

Drowning is the third major cause of nonintentional death in children aged 1 to 14 years. In addition, a larger number of children are hospitalized for near-drowning (ie, submersion injury followed by at least temporary survival), but survive. The incidence of submersion injuries is highest in boys younger than 5 years; the next highest incidence is in those between 14 and 19 years old.

The relative availability of different types of bodies of water and the climate, geography, and socioeconomic setting of a community determine the most likely site of submersion for each community. However, unfenced swimming pools represent a major water risk to the unsupervised child younger than 5 years. Although absent adult supervision is a factor in most pediatric submersions, the victim may have predisposing medical conditions such as seizures, alcohol or drug ingestion (especially in preadolescents and adolescents), and trauma, both accidental and nonaccidental (eg, suicide, child abuse, homicide). The possibility of child abuse must be considered in home submersion injuries, such as in bathtubs or water pails. In the absence of child abuse, a history of diving, or trauma, associated injuries are rare.

PATHOPHYSIOLOGY

Prolonged submersion results in global hypoxic injury. The responses of vital end organs to hypoxia and the resulting acidosis follow specific time lines (Table 10-1). Loss of consciousness occurs rapidly. Aspiration of water, which occurs in 90% of drowning victims, causes surfactant washout with subsequent atelectasis. Aspiration and the pulmonary response to hypoxia (reflex-mediated pulmonary hypertension with intrapulmonary shunting) increase the ventilation/perfusion mismatch and oxygen requirement. Myocardial hypoxia results in cardiac arrest within minutes of the submersion. Laryngospasm prevents aspiration in 10% of cases and results in "dry" drowning.

In the child who has been severely asphyxiated, vital organs begin to fail, and cerebral edema, gastrointestinal bleeding, acute respiratory distress syndrome, and myocardial failure develop. Central nervous system hypoxia is the most common cause of death after a successful cardiac resuscitation. Acute respiratory distress syndrome occurs in 5% to 15% of submersion victims in intensive care units. The **delayed immersion syndrome** is an uncommon, delayed acute respiratory distress syndrome-like response to hypoxia occurring up to 24 hours after submersion in victims who initially appear to have minimal injury.

Although uncommon, coagulopathies or renal failure may develop after hypoxia. Myoglobinuria or hemoglobinuria also may precipitate renal failure. Fluid absorption leading to fluid shifts and electrolyte changes are not significant problems for the submersion victim.

The outcome for submersion victims generally is either intact survival or death, and outcome usually can be predicted in the field. Most victims who resume spontaneous ventilations in the field, become responsive, have a sinus rhythm, and have been submerged for ≤5 minutes survive without neurologic sequelae. For victims submerged in waters 5°C or warmer who present in cardiac arrest, aggressive prehospital care may result in return of spontaneous circulation within 10 minutes and intact survival. For victims submerged in nonicy waters (>5°C), the most reliable predictors for death or severe neurologic sequelae include:

- Unresponsiveness on arrival at the hospital
- Elevated blood glucose level
- Fixed pupils in the emergency department
- Cardiac arrest requiring >25 minutes of advanced life support
- Hypothermia

Less reliable outcome predictors in the emergency department are absence of spontaneous respirations and pH <7.1.

On occasion, children submerged in icy waters (≤5°C) have survived neurologically intact despite prolonged (≥60 minutes) submersions and resuscitations. Such rapidly induced hypothermia may provide cerebral protection. These anecdotal survivals and the death-like state induced by severe hypothermia led to the belief that all hypothermic victims should be warmed before cessation of resuscitation. However, data suggest that hypothermia after nonicy but "cold" water (≥5°C) immersion does not provide a protective benefit. Almost all case reports of miraculous survival have followed submersion in icy waters. Knowing the temperature of the immersion water may prove helpful to the practitioner faced with the dilemma of determining whether the victim's hypothermia is due to rapid cooling or prolonged circulatory arrest.

ASSESSMENT

Direct assessment of the ABCs and initiation of critical support are primary. Initial signs and symptoms usually reflect cardiopulmonary and cerebral hypoxic injury. Hypothermia may not be recognized unless a rectal temperature is obtained along with other vital signs. A thermometer capable of measuring temperatures significantly below the normal range is needed to assess the hypothermic patient accurately. Because occult injury to the head, cervical spine, or other areas may be present, all submersion victims are assessed thoroughly for evidence of other trauma. Evaluate all submersion victims for possible abuse or nonaccidental trauma with a social/family evaluation. Evaluate for other

TABLE 10-1.
Timeline of common organ system response to severe submersion.

System	Symptoms and Signs at Scene	Symptoms and Signs Hours Later
Cardiac	Cardiac arrest	Myocardial failure
Central nervous	Loss of consciousness	Cerebral edema (6-12 hr)
Pulmonary	Hypoxia, pulmonary edema	ARDS (may develop at 24 hr)
Gastrointestinal	None	Mucosal sloughing, diarrhea, third spacing of fluids resulting in hypovolemia (6-12 hr)
Renal	None	Renal failure, oliguria/anuria, electrolyte imbalance (6-12 hr)

precipitating causes of submersion injury.

Altered mental status may be due to a combination of cerebral hypoxia and underlying disease processes. Consider drug ingestion, intracranial injury, or a postictal state. Obtain a blood alcohol level and drug screen on all preadolescents and adolescents and blood pH and oxygen saturation on all victims. Further assessment of respiratory status is dictated by the patient's condition. Hematocrit and electrolytes usually are normal.

TABLE 10-2.
Managing the unresponsive patient.

Prehospital

Assess ABCs; ensure cervical spine control; bag-valve-mask ventilate with 100% oxygen; intubate; insert orogastric tube.

Initiate rhythm-appropriate electrical interventions and medication; CPR.

Obtain vascular access; use normal saline to keep open.

Remove wet clothing.

Reassess airway and breathing.

Transport to facility that can provide emergency pediatric care.

Emergency Department

Continue CPR until return of spontaneous circulation or physician decides that resuscitation cannot be accomplished.

Stabilize and evaluate cervical spine.

Assess ABCs; endotracheal tube placement; obtain chest radiograph and arterial blood gases; pass nasogastric tube; monitor oxygen saturation and ECG; assess rectal temperature with a thermometer capable of detecting hypothermia.

Place patient requiring ventilatory support on a respirator; use positive end-expiratory pressure; repeat arterial blood gas determination as indicated.

Ensure vascular access; check glucose using glucose oxidase reagent strip; monitor blood pressure; run fluid to keep open unless treating shock.

Electrical intervention for ventricular dysrhythmias.

Initiate rewarming for hypothermic patients.

Evaluate neurologic status; obtain serum glucose and treat if indicated; assess and treat hypothermia.

Admit to a pediatric intensive care unit.

Repeated assessment of the victim's pulmonary status for evolving sequelae is key. Aggressive, expectant care is the rule. Never underestimate how much near-drowning patients may deteriorate regardless of how "golden" they may appear.

MANAGEMENT

The goal of therapy is reversal of hypoxia. Appropriate aggressive airway management in the field is essential for submersion victims. The usual basic and advanced cardiac life support measures should be applied. Management interventions are described in Tables 10-2 and 10-3.

Positive pressure ventilation and 100% oxygen are key to outcome. Many apneic, unresponsive victims will respond to basic life support efforts to ventilate and will breathe and awaken at the scene. Considerable amounts of water usually are swallowed, and vomiting is likely. Nasogastric intubation and gastric evacuation should be accomplished early in the resuscitation.

Recent studies support the use of standard basic and advanced cardiac life support guidelines. However, many submersion victims are also hypothermic. At temperatures of <30°C, the myocardium is resistant to defibrillation and

TABLE 10-3.
Managing the responsive patient.

Prehospital

Assess ABCs; provide oxygen if any signs of respiratory distress.

Stabilize cervical spine if diving or significant fall.

Remove wet clothing; provide blankets.

Monitor for developing respiratory distress.

Transport.

Emergency Department

Assess ABCs and oxygen saturation; monitor ECG.

Clear cervical spine.

Rule out underlying comorbidity, especially drugs and alcohol.

Monitor glucose level.

Assess rectal temperature.

Admit for any oxygen requirement; observe for delayed oxygen requirement.

pharmacologic agents. If the patient has a nonperfusing rhythm along with monitor evidence of ventricular fibrillation or ventricular tachycardia, defibrillation should be attempted only once. If unsuccessful, CPR should be continued until the patient's temperature is above >30°C, when repeat defibrillation should be performed.

Consideration should be given to warming the hypothermic victim to ≥34°C before the decision to cease efforts is made. Rewarming definitely should be attempted if the victim was submerged in icy, ≤5°C water. When there is no return of spontaneous circulation, the decision to cease resuscitation is a clinical judgment based on the victim's submersion duration, response to resuscitation, duration of the resuscitation, and whether the submersion waters were icy or nonicy. After 25 minutes of resuscitation, survival is very unlikely in the victim submerged in nonicy (≥5°C) waters. No predictors exist for the submersion victim in icy (≤5°C) waters. Chapter 11 includes a further discussion of the management of the hypothermic patient.

ADDITIONAL READING

Rowin ME, Christensen D, Allen EM. Pediatric drowning and near-drowning. In: Rogers MC, Nichols DG, eds. *Textbook of Pediatric Intensive Care,* 3rd ed. Baltimore, Md: Williams & Wilkins; 1996:875-892.

Gillen JP, Vogel MF, Holterman RK, et al. Ventricular fibrillation during orotracheal intubation of hypothermic dogs. *Ann Emerg Med.* 1986;15:412-416.

Graf WD, Cummings P, Quan L, et al. Predicting outcome in pediatric submersion victims. *Ann Emerg Med.* 1995;26:312-319.

Modell JH. *The Pathophysiology and Treatment of Drowning and Near-Drowning.* Springfield, Ill: Charles C Thomas; 1971.

Pearn J, Nixon J, Wilkey I. Freshwater drowning and near-drowning accidents involving children: a five-year total population study. *Med J Aust.* 1976;2:942-946.

Pearn JH, Wong RY, Brown J, et al. Drowning and near-drowning involving children: a five-year total population study from the City and County of Honolulu. *Am J Public Health.* 1979;69:450-454.

Quan L, Gore EJ, Wentz KR, et al. Ten-year study of pediatric drownings and near-drownings in King County, Washington: lessons in injury prevention. *Pediatrics.* 1989;83:1035-1040.

Quan L, Kinder D. Pediatric submersions: prehospital predictors of outcome. *Pediatrics.* 1992;90:909-913.

Wintemute GJ. Childhood drowning and near-drowning in the United States. *Am J Dis Child.* 1990;144:663-669.

Chapter 11

Body Temperature Disturbances

OBJECTIVES

1. Describe basic physiology of temperature regulation.

2. Identify three types of minor heat illness, and describe their management.

3. Differentiate between heat exhaustion and heat stroke, and discuss their management.

4. Discuss the management of mild, moderate, and severe hypothermia.

Body temperature usually is maintained between 36°C and 37.5°C by a balance of heat-generating and heat-dissipating processes. The thermostat regulating temperature is lodged within the preoptic nucleus of the anterior hypothalamus; that center senses the temperature of the perfusing blood and emits nerve signals that ultimately result in heat production or loss. As a consequence, body temperature normally is modulated within a very narrow range. Emergency department equipment should include devices for recording extremes of body temperature.

THERMOREGULATION

Heat is generated in many ways:

- As a byproduct of **basal metabolism**: Approximately 960 calories of heat per square meter of surface area are produced in this manner each day.

- As a consequence of the actions of **catecholamines** and **thyroxine** on cellular processes: For example, some of the additional heat produced during exercise is due to the excess catecholamines that are released.

- As a result of **muscular activity**: Shivering, in particular, generates heat.

- As a byproduct of an **increase in temperature** itself: By accelerating chemical reactions, increases in temperature result in additional heat production.

In contrast, heat is lost from the body surface via:

- **Radiation**: Transfer to the environment in the form of infrared heat waves. This type of heat loss is dependent on the difference of temperature between the environment and the body surface. For example, when one person stands very close to another but does not touch, one can feel the heat from the other body. This thin rim of heat surrounding bodies is the heat lost by radiation. Approximately 55% of heat loss occurs via radiation.

- **Conduction:** Transfer by direct contact with another surface.
  When a person places a hand on a cold surface, the hand begins to get cold because of heat loss through conduction. This accounts for only 2% to 3% of heat loss. This can increase 5 times with wet clothing and 25 times with submersion in cold water.
- **Convection:** Conduction to air, which then is carried away by wind currents. Heat also is lost when the air heated by close proximity to the body is removed through air movement. Normally, this accounts for 12% of heat loss.
- **Evaporation:** Heat is lost through conversion of a liquid (sweat or moisture from the lungs) to a gas. Insensible losses account for 30% of heat loss. Greater losses occur in cool, dry environments. Each day, 360 calories of heat per square meter of surface area are lost via evaporation of water from skin surface and lungs. It is important to note that radiation, conduction, and convection prove ineffective when the ambient temperature exceeds 37°C. Only evaporation allows heat wastage in such extreme conditions. Even evaporation failes to dissipate heat effectively when the humidity exceeds 90% to 95%.

When the preoptic nucleus senses a drop in blood temperature, nerve signals are emitted that result in peripheral vasoconstriction and shivering. Because less blood reaches the periphery, more heat is conserved, and shivering produces an additional heat load. Conversely, when the hypothalamus detects a rise in blood temperature, cutaneous vasodilation and sweating ensue, blood flow to the surface increases, and more heat is lost. Sweating dissipates heat through evaporation.

HYPERTHERMIA

Heat-related syndromes are more common in the hot, humid months. They are implicated in >1700 deaths in the United States annually. Heat illness is a spectrum of disease that can range from minor self-limiting syndromes of heat edema and prickly heat to the potentially fatal heat stroke. It is imperative to recognize serious heat illness syndromes and treat them promptly to prevent death or serious morbidity.

Factors that predispose a patient to heat illness are age (infants and the elderly), obesity,

dehydration, abnormalities of the skin, drugs, lack of acclimatization, fatigue, excessive or restrictive clothing, fever and infection, and a previous episode of heat stroke. Some medications are associated with rare syndromes that result in hyperthermia. Malignant hyperthermia is characterized by severe hyperthermia, muscle rigidity, and autonomic dysfunction after exposure to certain anesthetics. A similar syndrome can occur after exposure to neuroleptic medications, such as butyrophenones and phenothiazines.

Infants and small children are at increased risk of serious heat illness because of poorly developed thermoregulatory mechanism. With an increased interest in outdoor sports and competitive athletics, older children and adolescents are more at risk for thermal illness. Practitioners therefore should have a good understanding of the clinical manifestations and treatment of heat illness, and prevention of thermal injury should be an important focus in caring for an athlete.

PATHOPHYSIOLOGY

The body at rest, with no mechanism for cooling, generates sufficient heat to cause a rise in temperature of 1°C/hr. Exercise or hard work will increase heat production by 12-fold. In addition, the body temperature will rise secondary to external sources, when air temperature exceeds body temperature, or when there is a large radiant heat load (eg, bright sunlight, hot tub, sauna).

When the body is faced with an increase in heat load either from an increase in metabolism (eg. exercise) or from the environment (eg. sauna, direct sunlight), the hypothalamus triggers the heat-losing mechanism, including vasodilatation and sweating through the sympathetic nervous system. Cardiac output increases, as does heart rate, stroke volume, and systemic venous pressure. Large amounts of blood are shunted to the surface to aid in heat dissipation. The individual body's ability to lose heat has a maximum rate. Once this rate is exceeded, the core body temperature will rise.

Young children are less effective than adults in thermoregulation. The temperature at which children begin to sweat is higher than that in adults. They produce more heat for a given exercise than do adults and have a lower rate of sweating. Their body surface area per weight is higher, thereby making them more susceptible to the extremes of the temperature of the environment. Children also have a slower rate of acclimatization. **Acclimatization** is a physiologic adaptive process to hot environments that occurs over time. The time required varies but approximates exercising for 100 min/day for 10 days (14 days in children). Acclimatization is thought to occur via activation of the renin-angiotensin-aldosterone system. Eventually, there will be a small rise in temperature for the same work load and a decrease in cardiac output, cutaneous blood flow, and energy expenditure. There is an increase in extracellular and plasma volumes.

MINOR HEAT ILLNESSES

Heat Edema

Heat edema is a minor heat illness in which the hands and feet become edematous. Heat edema usually occurs within the first days of exposure to a hot environment. The pathophysiology is thought to be secondary to cutaneous vasodilatation and possibly an increase in antidiuretic hormone secretion. Heat edema is self-limited, and treatment consists of moving the patient to a cooler environment.

Heat Cramps

Heat cramps are severe cramps of heavily exercised muscles that occur after exertion. They usually occur in patients who have been sweating in large amounts and taking in hypotonic fluids. It is important not to confuse heat cramps with the muscle rigidity of malignant hyperthermia or neuroleptic malignant syndrome, which can be fatal if unrecognized. The pathophysiology of cramps is uncertain but thought to be due to decreased sodium, secondary to dilution with hypotonic oral solutions. Management consists of removing the patient from the heat stress and providing rest and oral fluids (electrolyte drinks, not salt tablets) or intravenous fluids and salt replacement.

Heat Syncope

Heat syncope is a syncopal episode during heat exposure occurring in unacclimatized people in the early stages of heat exposure. There is a decrease in vasomotor tone, venous pooling, anad hypotension, with mild dehydration. Heat syncope is self-limited, and treatment consists of moving the patient to a cooler environment. The patient should regain consciousness once supine or placed in the Trendelenburg position. Intravenous saline, lactated Ringer's, or oral hydration fluids should be provided.

MAJOR HEAT ILLNESSES

Heat Exhaustion

Heat exhaustion is a precursor to heat stroke and must be differentiated from other illnesses, especially heat stroke. The symptoms of heat exhaustion include a temperature up to 39°C, malaise, headache, nausea, vomiting, irritability, tachycardia, and dehydration. Mental function remains intact. Liver function tests (SGOT, SGPT, LDH) are not significantly elevated.

In heat exhaustion, there is vasodilatation with blood shunted toward the periphery. Sweating increases, thereby increasing water and sodium loss. There is a decrease in central circulating blood volume. A compensatory increase in heart rate and stroke volume occurs, as well as a decrease in renal blood flow. Temperature-regulatory mechanisms remain intact.

Management of heat exhaustion initially consists of moving the patient to a cool environment. Intravenous fluids should be administered to treat dehydration. Initially, 20 mL/kg normal saline or lactated Ringer's should be infused, and then projected losses should be replaced. Laboratory studies should include a complete blood count, electrolytes, blood urea nitrogen, creatinine, and urinalysis. Vital signs should be followed closely. The patient should be observed in the emergency department until normal or hospitalized for observation. If at any time there is doubt, the patient should be treated for heat stroke. Long-term sequelae usually do not occur.

Heat Stroke

Heat stroke is a life-threatening emergency in which normal thermoregulatory mechanisms are no longer functioning. Patients with exposure to heat stress usually present with rectal temperatures of >41°C and altered mental status that can range from bizarre behavior to seizures and coma.

There are two types of heat stroke: exertional and nonexertional (classic). **Exertional** heat stroke can be found in the unacclimatized athlete. There usually is a rapid onset of severe prostration with headache, ataxia, syncope, seizures, and coma. Tachycardia, tachypnea, and hypotension are present. The sweating mechanism usually is intact. **Nonexertional** or **classic** heat stroke is of slower onset and more common in infants and the elderly. Marked dehydration usually is present. Symptoms include anorexia, nausea, vomiting, malaise, dizziness, confusion, seizures, coma, tachycardia, tachypnea, and hypotension. Sweating may be absent.

In heat stroke, all temperature regulation is lost, and there is a precipitous rise in core body temperature. The pathology that ensues involves every organ. The damage to the organ is dependent on the body temperature, exposure time, work load, tissue perfusion, and individual resistance. Patients may exhibit myocardial damage with an elevation of creatine phosphokinase-MB, cerebral edema, intravascular coagulation and thrombocytopenia, hepatocellular degeneration, cholestasis, acute tubular necrosis, interstitial nephritis, or myoglobinuria.

Initial management of the patient with heat stroke begins like the management of all other types of patients: airway, breathing, and circulation. Cooling should be initiated promptly because it is the cornerstone of therapy. Optimum cooling should be ≥0.1°C/min. Stop cooling at 39°C. Remove the patient's clothing and move to an air-conditioned room if possible. The rectal temperature should be monitored continuously.

Methods of cooling vary in their effectiveness and practicality. One of the most effective and practical ways of cooling a patient is to continuously spray water over the body surface and, with fans, create air movement. Ice packs can be applied to the groin and axilla. The use of peritoneal lavage, ice enemas, and ice gastric lavage has not been well studied in humans. Cold intravenous solutions add little to the cooling process and can cause arrhythmias. Cold inhaled oxygen has been studied in the animal model and found to be ineffective. Submersion in cold water has been used by the military with excellent success but may be impractical in an unstable patient. Antipyretics are ineffective in the patient with heat stroke.

The laboratory evaluation includes a complete blood count, urinalysis, electrolytes, blood urea nitrogen, creatinine, glucose, calcium, liver function tests, coagulation studies, creatine phosphokinase, arterial blood gas, and a blood culture (if sepsis is suspected).

Simultaneous with cooling, intravenous lines should be placed. Fluid replacement should begin with a bolus of 20 mL/kg of normal saline or lactated Ringer's and repeated as needed to maintain perfusion and urine output. A central venous line and Foley catheter should be placed for fluid monitoring. Hypoglycemia should be treated with 250 to 500 mg/kg glucose.

Once initial treatment of the patient has been initiated, differential diagnosis can be considered. Head trauma, cerebrovascular accident, thyroid storm, malignant hyperthermia, neuroleptic malignant syndrome, drug ingestion, or heat exhaustion with syncope must be considered.

The complications from heat stroke are numerous. If **seizures** occur, they should be treated with benzodiazepines and then phenobarbital. **Hypotension** that is unresponsive to fluids and cooling should be treated with inotropes such as dopamine or dobutamine. **Incipient renal failure** can be treated with furosemide and mannitol. **Dysrhythmias** are seen in those with heat stroke and can include a variety of abnormalities; cooling usually treats the abnormality. Unfortunately, there is no treatment for the central nervous system and thermoregulatory control abnormalities that occur.

Prognosis of the patient with heat stroke is dependent on the duration of coma, severity of coagulopathy, severity of liver function abnormalities, duration of high temperature, and presence of a preexisting illness.

Heat stroke can be prevented by educating parents and coaches. It is recommended that exertion be avoided during sunlight in hot weather, especially when the temperature is >80°F and humidity approaches 70%. Light clothing should be worn, and adequate intake of an electrolyte solution should be consumed before exercise. Athletes should take frequent water breaks during exercise and not wait until they are thirsty. Salt supplements in the form of salt pills should not be used. Athletes and those working outdoors should permit a period of acclimatization before heavy work or exercise. Symptoms of heat illness should be recognized early, and the athlete or worker should be moved to a cool environment. Athletes and those working outdoors should permit a period of acclimatization before heavy work or exercise.

HYPOTHERMIA

Hypothermia is defined as a core temperature of ≤35°C (95°F). Neonates are predisposed to the development of hypothermia because of their underdeveloped thermoregulatory system, relatively large body surface-to-body mass ratio, and decreased subcutaneous fat. The neonate is most prone to hypothermia just after delivery due to conductive heat losses from being covered with amniotic fluid. Thus, it is important to dry and cover the neonate to prevent heat loss. Infants and young children may develop hypothermia from a simple exposure to cold with inadequate clothing for the environmental conditions. Hypothermia can occur in all seasons of the year. Most cases of accidental hypothermia in children are associated with near-drowning accidents in cold or icy water environments.

Factors that have been found to predispose individuals to the development of hypothermia include the following:

- Endocrine or metabolic derangements (hypoglycemia)
- Infection (meningitis, sepsis)
- Intoxication (alcohol, opiates)
- Intracranial pathology (traumatic, congenital, other)
- Submersion injury
- Environmental exposure
- Dermatologic (burns)
- Iatrogenic (cold intravenous fluids, exposure during treatment)

The mortality from hypothermia is related directly to the associated underlying disorder and is highest for submersion injury.

Pathophysiology

When the core body temperature begins to drop, the preoptic anterior hypothalamus senses blood cooling and immediately initiates sympathetic neurogenic signals that cause an increase in muscle tone and metabolic rate. This is most evident in the **shivering reflex**, which is an attempt by the body to increase heat production through involuntary muscle contraction. Heat production can be increased to approximately four times the normal rate by these mechanisms. Neonates, however, lack the ability to shiver. The sympathetic nervous system also causes cutaneous vasoconstriction, thereby shunting blood toward the vital organs and defending against further heat loss. As the body cools, metabolic rate is reduced, which is reflected by a decrease in CO_2 production and slowing of the heart rate. Situations that create heat loss through convection and conduction, such as high winds or wet clothes, greatly accelerate the development of hypothermia. The most profound effects occur during submersion in cold water, and in this environment, rapid heat loss is intensified by movement. Apnea and asystole can occur very quickly.

Clinical Presentations

The clinical findings of progressive hypothermia in children and adolescents depend on the degree of hypothermia, which can be categorized as mild, moderate, or severe.

Mild Hypothermia (32° to 35°C) (89.6° to 95°F)

Slowing of mental status, which produces slurred speech and mild incoordination, and inappropriate judgment or behavior may be the only manifestations of mild hypothermia. The shivering reflex is preserved in this temperature range.

Moderate Hypothermia (28° to 32°C) (82.4° to 89.6°F)

There is a progressive decrease in the level of consciousness in this temperature range. Coma is likely at temperatures of <30°C. The victim appears cyanotic and will develop tissue edema. Shivering is replaced by muscle rigidity. Respiratory activity may be difficult to detect, and pulses frequently are difficult to palpate. The classic ECG change of a J wave may be apparent (Figure 11-1).

Severe Hypothermia (<28°C) (<82.4°F)

The victim is comatose with dilated and unresponsive pupils. It may be impossible to detect any vital signs, and the distinction between death and profound hypothermia may be difficult to make. Respiratory arrest and ventricular fibrillation occur in older patients at temperatures of <28°C.

Management

As with all severely ill or injured patients, the hypothermic patient must be assessed from head to toe, with particular attention paid to assessment of vital functions, followed immediately by resuscitation as indicated. No prospective controlled studies comparing the various rewarming modalities have been done in human beings. The following recommendations are therefore based on clinical experience.

Methods of Rewarming

There are two types of rewarming: passive and active. **Passive rewarming** involves the use of warm blankets, heat lamps, and heated humidified oxygen.

Active rewarming involves the use of a number of invasive techniques:

- Intravenous fluids are heated to 40° to 42°C and delivered through a fluid warmer. It is a good idea to keep intravenous fluid bags in a blanket warmer at all times. If heated fluid is not available immediately, fluid can be heated rapidly in a microwave oven. The bag should be shaken to distribute warmth evenly.
- Acceptable techniques include gastric lavage with a nasogastric tube or rectal lavage with an enema tube using warmed electrolyte solutions heated to 40° to 42°C.
- Peritoneal lavage with warmed electrolyte solutions heated to 40° to 42°C also is effective. Lavage is carried out with a standard peritoneal lavage kit.

- When the patient has been intubated and is being ventilated, increasing the humidifier temperature on the ventilator to 44°C is a very effective way of core rewarming.
- Extracorporeal blood rewarming with a modified form of cardiopulmonary bypass is the fastest method of restoring body temperature and cardiac output, but this technique often is not readily available.

Treatment of Mild Hypothermia

Mild hypothermia often can be treated with passive rewarming, provided the patient is stable and there is no underlying pathology causing the hypothermia. Patients with core temperatures of >32°C usually are conscious with spontaneous cardiac activity, unless the hypothermia is associated with other significant illness or traumatic injury such as submersion. Mildly hypothermic patients who respond well to rewarming may not warrant laboratory assessment.

Treatment of Moderate to Severe Hypothermia

As with all ill or injured patients, the hypothermic patient must be assessed from head to toe with particular attention to the ABCs. Securing the airway and ensuring that ventilation is adequate is the first concern. This should be followed by an assessment of heart rate and blood pressure. At

FIGURE 11-1.
Example of a J wave in a hypothermic patient.

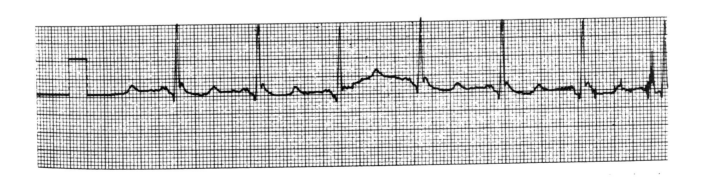

From Cooper MA, Danzl DF. Hypothermia. In: Hamilton GC, Sanders AB, Strange GR, et al, eds. *Emergency Medicine: An Approach to Clinical Problem-Solving*. Philadelphia, Pa: WB Saunders; 1991:411. Reprinted with permission.

temperatures of <30°C, the myocardium is resistant to defibrillation and pharmacologic agents. If the patient has a nonperfusing rhythm, along with monitor evidence of ventricular fibrillation or ventricular tachycardia, then defibrillation should be attempted only once. If unsuccessful, CPR should be continued until the patient's temperature is >30°C, when repeat defibrillation should be performed.

All moderately or severely hypothermic patients should have continuous temperature monitoring with either a rectal or an esophageal probe. If a rectal probe is used, be sure any cold feces is removed before probe placement. These patients must be treated aggressively with active and passive rewarming. This usually involves warm blankets or a heat lamp, warm humidified oxygen, warmed intravenous fluids, and various lavage techniques. Patients with moderate to severe hypothermia may have large amounts of fluid sequestration. Rewarming the victim must be accompanied by fluid resuscitation to prevent cardiovascular collapse. An initial fluid bolus of 20 mL/kg in the form of either crystalloid or colloid solution is indicated. Insert an indwelling catheter to monitor urinary output. Unless needed, defer insertion of a central venous pressure line until a core temperature of 30°C is obtained to prevent precipitation of ventricular fibrillation. The goal should be to raise the temperature by 1° to 2°C/hr.

With rewarming, peripheral vasodilation occurs, and the cold extremities are perfused. This causes the circulating blood to become colder as it passes through the cold extremity and then returns to the central organs, leading to a phenomenon known as **core temperature afterdrop**. Core temperature afterdrop can cause additional problems with mental status, breathing and particularly, cardiac dysrhythmias. These effects usually are transient; nevertheless, rewarming of cold extremities with hot packs should be avoided.

The cold myocardium is resistant to defibrillation and drugs. If initial treatment fails to establish a rhythm, CPR must continue until a core temperature of ≥30° C is reached. At this point, if a perfusing cardiac rhythm has not been established, follow standard life support drug protocols in an attempt to restore a viable cardiac rhythm.

In moderate to severe hypothermia, laboratory studies should include serum electrolytes, blood gases and pH, hemoglobin, white blood cell count, and tests for renal and hepatic function. In profoundly hypothermic patients, thought must be given to the presence of an underlying disease process that predisposes to the development of hypothermia, such as endocrine disturbances, drug and alcohol intoxication, and trauma. It is important to exclude hypoglycemia by measuring the blood glucose, and a blood and urine sample also should be taken for toxicology screening. The presence of any underlying head or spinal cord injury should be excluded, and the possibility of sepsis as a cause of the hypothermia must be addressed in younger children. Resuscitation efforts should continue until the body temperature is >35°C (>95°F) or greater. Children have a remarkable ability to withstand hypothermia, particularly submersion, through induction of the diving reflex, which results in shunting of blood to the brain and heart and is thought to contribute to intact survival after submersion in very cold water.

DISPOSITION

Admit all patients with core hypothermia for observation. Children who present with core temperatures of <32°C, altered mental status, or multisystem failure should be admitted to the intensive care unit for continuous cardiac monitoring until rewarming is accomplished. Underlying problems frequently will be discovered during the observation period. Children with core temperatures as low as 14°C have survived with full neurologic recovery.

ADDITIONAL READING

Hyperthermia

Bracker MD. Environmental and thermal injury. *Clin Sports Med.* 1992;11:419-436.
Costrini A. Emergency treatment of exertional heatstroke and comparison of whole body cooling techniques. *Med Sci Sports Exerc.* 1990;22:15-18.
Heat-related illness and deaths–United States, 1994-1995. *MMWR Morb Mortal Wkly Rep.* 1995;44:465-468.
Squire DL. Heat illness. Fluid and electrolyte issues for pediatric and adolescent athletes. *Pediatr Clin North Am.* 1990;37:1085-1109.
Sterba JA. Thermal problems: prevention and treatment. In: Bennett PB, Elliott DH, eds. *The Physiology and Medicine of Diving,* 4th ed. London: WB Saunders; 1993.
Strange GR. Heat illness. In: Strange GR, Ahrens WR, Lelyveld S, et al. *Pediatric Emergency Medicine: A Comprehensive Study Guide.* New York, NY: McGraw-Hill; 1996:613-615.

Tek D, Olshaker JS. Heat illness. *Emerg Med Clin North Am.* 1992;10:299-310.

Thompson AE. Environmental emergencies. In: Fleisher GR, Ludwig S, eds. *Textbook of Pediatric Emergency Medicine*, 3rd ed. Baltimore, Md: Williams & Wilkins; 1993:802-823.

Hypothermia

Jolly BT, Ghezzi KT. Accidental hypothermia. *Emerg Med Clin North Am.* 1992;10:311-327.

Shields CP, Sixmith DM. Treatment of moderate-to-severe hypothermia in an urban setting. *Ann Emerg Med.* 1990;19:1093-1097.

Sterba JA. Thermal problems: prevention and treatment. In: Bennett PB, Elliott DH, eds. *The Physiology and Medicine of Diving*, 4th ed. London: WB Saunders; 1993.

Steele MT, Nelson MJ, Sessler DI, et al. Forced air speeds rewarming in accidental hypothermia. *Ann Emerg Med.* 1996;27:479-484.

Strange GR, Cooper MA. Cold illness. In: Strange GR, Ahrens WR, Lelyveld S, et al, eds. *Pediatric Emergency Medicine: A Comprehensive Study Guide*. New York, NY: McGraw-Hill; 1996:616-622.

Thompson AE. Environmental emergencies. In: Fleisher GR, Ludwig S, eds. *Textbook of Pediatric Emergency Medicine*, 3rd ed. Baltimore, Md: Williams & Wilkins; 1993:802-823.

Chapter 12

Child Abuse

OBJECTIVES

1. Recognize common presentations of physical abuse, sexual abuse, and neglect.

2. Describe laboratory evidence that should be collected in child abuse cases.

3. Explain the practitioner's responsibility in notifying authorities of suspected abuse.

More than 2.9 million cases of child maltreatment were reported in 1994. More than 1 million cases were confirmed, and more than 1100 deaths from child abuse were substantiated. These data indicate an increase over the 1990 US Department of Health and Human Services statistics. For each case of child maltreatment reported, it is projected that there probably are one or two cases that go unrecognized. According to the American Humane Society, maltreatment of children is defined as harm resulting from inappropriate or abnormal child-rearing practices. It includes physical abuse, sexual abuse, emotional abuse, and neglect. Child abuse is a symptom of family dysfunction.

Because the emergency department is the point of entry for many children into the health care system and because some children with minor abuse subsequently may be severely injured or killed, the practitioner working in this area must have a high level of suspicion for signs and symptoms associated with inflicted trauma. *The possibility of abuse should be considered with every traumatic injury treated.* The practitioner should be alert to the possibility of maltreatment by any unexplained or poorly explained injury, evidence of neglect, delay in seeking appropriate medical care, or contradictory histories.

A multidisciplinary approach in which the practitioner works in cooperation with hospital-based nurses and social workers and with community-based child protective service workers, police, and personnel from other agencies benefits the abused child. In a cooperative multidisciplinary milieu, the child benefits most by having the knowledge of a broad range of experts, by avoiding duplication, and by avoiding many issues that result from the work of agencies in isolation. The essential value judgments and decisions are more easily made by multidisciplinary teams.

This section reviews in detail three of the four major categories of abuse: physical abuse, sexual abuse, and neglect. In the emergency department, it is difficult to diagnose the fourth major category of abuse —psychological/emotional abuse. However, psychological abuse occurs frequently by itself, and it is bound to every intentional physical injury and act of sexual abuse. It is the psychological injury that is responsible for the most serious long-term morbidity and the cyclic intergenerational pattern of abuse.

PHYSICAL ABUSE

Assessment

Recognition of physical abuse is important for two reasons: to accurately diagnose and manage the inflicted trauma and to prevent further injuries or death.

Abuse occurs in all segments of the population and is suggested by the following:

- Unusual aspects of the medical history: Encourage the toddler or older child to describe in his or her own terms what happened. If the history from the child or parent is inconsistent with the physical examination or there is a discrepancy between stories, consider abuse. If the history just does not make sense, consider abuse.
- History describing a minor mishap that is inconsistent with a major injury
- History inconsistent with the developmental capability of the child: Infants younger than 6 months rarely injure themselves. Even minor bruising in an infant is a red flag. Common sense and a basic knowledge of motor milestones for infants and children will help in determining the likelihood that the injury occurred in the stated manner.
- Delay in obtaining medical care, or the use of only sporadic routine health care.

To adequately evaluate abuse, the physician should follow the guidelines of listen, look, explain, evaluate, record, and report.

Listen

In addition to the historical factors highlighted above, there are other cues that the child may have been abused. Obtain a careful history, including the small details of how the injury occurred from both the caretaker and the child. Conflicting, vague, or evasive answers and changing histories suggest abuse. Does the child accuse the caretaker, or does the caretaker inappropriately blame the child, a sibling, or a third party for causing the injury? This should raise suspicion of abuse. Is the child unusually fearful or withdrawn, or overly friendly or trusting? Such patterns of behavior often suggest abuse. Does the child engage in pseudomature or seductive behavior, or does he or she voice age-inappropriate sexual verbalizations? This should raise suspicion of sexual abuse. Most importantly, is the history consistent with the injuries?

Look

Perform a thorough external physical examination looking for fresh and old bruises, lacerations, fractures, burns, sores, and scars. Evaluate the abdomen for tenderness and the urine for blood. Examine the rectum and genitalia for lacerations, bruises, warts, sores, bleeding, and discharge. Rectal and/or vaginal examination to search for poor sphincter tone and/or internal lacerations also is necessary if there is any possibility of sexual abuse.

Explain

What are the circumstances surrounding the injury? When did the injury occur? And when did the caretaker seek medical help? Who brought the child to the hospital? Failure of the caretaker to accompany the child to the hospital, especially if the caretaker cannot be located, should raise suspicion of abuse. Has the child been examined by his or her regular physician? Often, the abused child has been seen by many different physicians to avoid raising suspicion. Has the child had previous injuries or ingestions? Multiple prior injuries or a history of being "accident prone" should raise suspicion of child abuse.

Evaluate

What is the behavior of the caretaker? Does this person seem high, intoxicated, or bizarre in affect? This should raise suspicion of abuse. Does this person show appropriate concern for the condition of the child? Both lack of concern and excessive concern for minor injury should raise suspicion of child abuse. Does this person seem overly aggressive, unusually hostile, or excessively critical or demanding of the child or the practitioner? Such patterns of behavior often suggest abuse. Does this person admit to being abused as a child? A statement by the caretaker that he or she was abused as a child should be interpreted as a plea for help and may be a confession.

Record

Carefully describe the appearance and location of all bruises, bites, lacerations, punctures, burns, sores, signs of choking (eg, strangulation marks), or restraint (eg, rope burns). Use legible handwriting, and make appropriate diagrams as necessary. Suspicious skin lesions should be photographed using good color-balanced photographic technique. Also record the verbatim statement of the child and parents. Exact record-keeping will become very important if the case comes under scrutiny of the legal system.

Report

Reporting of the case to the appropriate child welfare authorities should be done immediately on the basis of suspicion. Determining whether abuse actually has occurred is not the responsibility of the physician but rather of child welfare workers, who are specially trained for this task. Filing a written report of suspected child abuse is required by law. If there is suspicion of child abuse, the child may need to be admitted to the hospital for protection, and a complete evaluation for fractures (ie, skeletal survey) and internal injuries must be performed.

Injuries Related to Abuse

Bruises and Bites

The physically abused child may have injuries of the skin, soft tissue, bones, central nervous system, or internal organs. Ninety percent of such children have only superficial injuries such as bruises, bites, lacerations, puncture marks, burns, or signs of strangulation. Common locations for bruises caused by abuse include the buttocks and lower back (from punishment such as paddling), genitalia and inner thighs (from punishment for masturbation or toilet training accidents), cheeks (from slapping), upper lip and frenulum of the tongue (from forced feeding or bottle jamming), neck (from strangulation), and ear lobes and pinnae (from boxing, pinching, and slapping). Human hand and fingertip marks may appear as oval bruises, linear marks from the fingers, or actual outlines of handprints.

Human bites or teeth marks have a characteristic oval appearance; it can be determined whether the perpetrator was a child or an adult by measuring both the width of the dental mark and the width of the individual teeth. It also is possible to distinguish human from animal bite marks. Scars, marks, and bruises with specific shapes may have been inflicted by recognizable objects such as belts, belt buckles, or doubled-over cords. Circumferential rope marks on the ankles or wrists and gag marks about the mouth are seen in children who have been tied in an effort to restrain them.

It is important to distinguish birthmarks, accidental injuries, and bruises caused by coagulopathies from inflicted trauma. Accidental bruises usually occur over bony prominences, especially the knees, shins, and foreheads of toddlers. Mongolian spots occur on the buttocks, back, and upper arms in many infants, particularly African Americans, Asians, Native Americans, and Hispanics. They are normal birthmarks and not bruises. In addition, people of certain cultures, such as southeast Asians, may have folk remedies that may produce lesions that appear abusive (resembling ecchymoses or hematomas and referred to as *Cai gao*) but are well intentioned and are not fundamentally harmful. Occasionally, excessive bruising may be due to bleeding dyscrasias such as idiopathic thrombocytopenia or von Willebrand's disease. Coagulation studies must be obtained on all children with extensive bruises.

Bruises in various stages of resolution can be expected over bony prominences, but if bruises are located in other areas, such as cheeks and fleshy parts of the arms, buttocks, and abdominal wall, suspect abuse. Observance and documentation of the color and appearance of a bruise will assist in matching it with the history. Although the appearance of a bruise cannot be used to accurately date the age of the injury, a rough estimate of time of injury can be made. In general, bruises 1 to 5 days old are reddish-blue, whereas those 5 to 7 days old usually have turned green. Bruises that are 7 to 10 days old appear yellow, and by 10 to 14 days after the injury, the area begins to appear brown.

Burns

Approximately 10% of physical abuse cases involve burns, most commonly from hot objects (eg, hot plates, radiators, and heating grates) and hot water. Other burn injuries are caused by matches and cigarettes. Inflicted scald injuries from forced hot water immersion commonly occur on the buttocks or perineum, especially in children who have had toilet training accidents. Inflicted extremity burns conform to a symmetric glove-and-stocking distribution. Accidental hot water burns usually are asymmetric and have associated splash lesions.

Head Injuries

Inflicted head injuries are the most serious form of physical abuse and often may be life threatening. Subdural hematomas are associated with a significant mortality. Initially, the affected infant may be irritable and vomiting; later, there may be respiratory depression, seizures, or coma. Suspect subdural hematomas in any child with overt cranial injuries, bulging fontanel, scalp swelling and bruises, retinal hemorrhages, or skull fracture.

Violent shaking also can produce subdural hematomas. Grip marks and retinal hemorrhages in an irritable or comatose infant suggest subdural hematomas secondary to shaking. Subdural hematomas are never spontaneous and are indicative of abuse until proved otherwise. Other head injuries that may suggest abuse include subarachnoid hemorrhages, subgaleal hematomas, traumatic alopecia, and periorbital ecchymoses.

Abdominal Injuries

Abdominal injuries are the second most common cause of death in battered children and result from blunt trauma such as kicks and punches. There may be no bruising of the overlying skin. Massive blood loss with shock and death can occur with splenic, hepatic, renal, or major blood vessel injury. Hematuria may be associated with renal trauma. Acute peritonitis can result from intestinal perforation. Intramural hematomas of the duodenum or proximal jejunum may lead to acute intestinal obstruction. Trauma is the leading cause of pancreatitis in children; suspect abuse if there is no history of an accident. Obtain liver enzymes and amylase levels and abdominal imaging studies for suspected injuries.

Bone Injuries

More than 20% of abused children have radiologic evidence of bone trauma. Such trauma includes long-bone fractures, chip and bucket-handle fractures of the metaphyses, subperiosteal bleeding and calcification, multiple fractures at different stages of healing, repeated

fractures at the same site, and fractures of the ribs, scapulae, or sternum (Table 12-1).

Laboratory Assessment

A complete blood cell count, including a smear and differential count, as well as coagulation studies (bleeding time, partial thromboplastin time, and prothrombin time) may be needed in patients with multiple bruises to rule out a coagulopathy. These studies may be a critical factor in a later trial. Cultures of the bases of burns are important because bullous impetigo can resemble scald lesions.

Obtain skeletal radiologic surveys in all young children in whom abuse is suspected to determine whether there are occult skeletal injuries. Obtain computed tomography scans in any infant with retinal hemorrhages or cranial injuries or if there is suspicion of subdural hematoma (Table 12-2).

Management

Manage acute problems such as head, abdominal, and skeletal injuries in an expeditious manner, paying careful attention to the ABCs of initial assessment and resuscitation. Many infants with such injuries require hospitalization in an intensive care unit. Seek appropriate medical and surgical consultation. Notify children's protective services. Law enforcement agencies may also be notified in appropriate cases.

SEXUAL ABUSE

Sexual abuse is defined as the involvement of children or adolescents in sexual activities that are inappropriate for their age, developmental level, or role in the family by an older, more mature person. Children may agree to the activity because of threats, force, or the use of bribes. Sexual abuse accounted for 30% of reported cases of abuse in 1994 compared with ≈13% in 1980. It is estimated that 25% of females and 10% of males were sexually

TABLE 12-1.
Dating of bone injuries.

Age of Injury	Radiographic Bone Appearance
0-2 days	Fracture, soft tissue swelling
0-5 days	Visible fragments
10-14 days	Callus, periosteal new bone
8 weeks	Dense callus after fracture

TABLE 12-2.
Laboratory aids for diagnosing abuse.

Findings	Differential Diagnosis	Test
Bruising	Trauma	History, physical examination, social evaluation
	Hemophilia	PT, PTT, platelet count, bleeding time
	von Willebrand's	Bleeding time
	Anaphylactoid purpura	Rule out sepsis, platelet count
	Purpura fulminans	Rule out sepsis, platelet count
Dehydration/failure to thrive	Organic	History, physical examination, BUN, creatinine, urine SG
	Nonorganic	
	Mixed type	
Abdominal injury	Trauma	History, physical examination, social evaluation
	Tumor	Urinalysis, liver enzymes
	Infection	Amylase, abdominal ultrasound, cultures
Fractures	Trauma	History, physical examination, social evaluation
	Osteogenesis imperfecta	Radiography/blue sclerae, wormian bones
	Rickets	Nutrition history, radiography
	Birth trauma	Birth history
	Hypophosphatasia	Alkaline phosphatase
	Leukemia	CBC, bone marrow
	Neuroblastoma	VMA, CT scan
	Status post osteomyelitis or septic arthritis	History, CBC, sedimentation rate
	Neurogenic sensory deficit	Physical examination
Metaphyseal or epiphyseal lesions	Trauma	History, physical examination, social evaluation
	Scurvy	Radiography, nutrition history
	Rickets	Nutrition history, radiography
	Menke's syndrome	Deceased Cu, ceruloplasmin
	Syphilis	Serology
	Little league elbow	History
	Birth trauma	History
Subperiosteal ossification	Trauma	History, physical examination, social evaluation
	Osteogenic malignancy	Radiography, biopsy
	Syphilis	Serology
	Infantile cortical hyperostosis	No metaphyseal irregularity, response to aspirin
	Osteoid osteoma	Radiography
	Scurvy	Nutrition history, radiography
CNS injury	Trauma	History, physical examination, social evaluation, CT scan
	Aneurysm	CT scan
	Tumor	MRI

abused before reaching adulthood.

Victims who are to be evaluated fall into one of two categories: acute molestation or chronic molestation. Rape is a legal term meaning unlawful forced sexual contact, with penetration to any degree by the male genitalia into or on the female genitalia. The sexual assault victim seen shortly after the incident may have signs of physical injury associated with the use of force. The perpetrator may be a stranger, but more often he or she is well known to the family. Most often, children are the victims of chronic molestation and are usually seen months or years after the onset of the abuse. The average duration of the abuse in chronic cases before disclosure is 3.5 years. The perpetrator often is a close family member or a person well known to the child.

There has been a growing trend to separate cases in the emergency department based on the time of the last contact. If the child has had contact with a perpetrator within 72 hours, then the examination should be performed in the emergency department. If the contact is more distant than 72 hours, many practitioners will calm the "social emergency" of the disclosure while deferring the physical examination and complete assessment until the child can be seen at a recognized child abuse evaluation center.

Assessment

The **medical history** should include the specific details of the molestation episodes: who did what, and when and where it was done. Those details more often are elicited after an acute molestation. In chronic molestation, the victim frequently will be reluctant to disclose the details and may even deny that anything happened. There are many reasons for such reluctance. Victims of sexual abuse may have been threatened with harm if they reveal anything about the molestation, may have been told they will not be believed, or may have received gifts or rewards for having participated.

Obtain a history of medical and behavioral disturbances related to the chronic abuse, including urinary tract symptoms such as dysuria, recurrent infections, and enuresis; vaginal bleeding or discharge; stooling problems such as constipation, hematochezia, encopresis, fissures, hemorrhoids, and use of suppositories or enemas; sleep disturbances such as nightmares or night terrors;

refusal to attend school or clinginess; poor school performance; anorexia or bulimia; suicidal behavior; promiscuity; sexual acting out; and excessive masturbation. Question adolescents about their age at menarche, their menstrual history, the type of sanitary protection they use, consensual sexual activity, and contraceptive measures. Obtain information regarding previous surgical procedures, particularly any instrumentation of the genitourinary or rectal areas.

Physical Condition. Record the stage of development of secondary sexual characteristics in all children. Perform a general physical examination with special attention to the genital findings. Those findings may differ in acute and chronic molestation. In both instances, note abnormalities in the genital and anal areas.

Acute Injury. In general, there is no need to perform an internal pelvic examination on any prepubescent girl unless there is concern about penetrating vaginal or rectal injuries. If there is vaginal bleeding and no external source can be identified, then the child must be referred to a gynecologist or pediatric surgeon for an examination while under anesthesia. Careful external inspection often reveals any acute injury or the chronic abnormal findings described below. There may be extragenital bruises and injuries, especially in cases of acute molestation. These may involve grip marks on the forearms where the child was held or lacerations on the inner lip if the child was struck on the face in an effort to quiet her or him. Look for bruising around the genital or anal area. There may be abrasions, lacerations, edema, and petechiae. The vagina and rectum may be in spasm after acute trauma. In ≥50% of cases, there may be no physical signs after acute anal penetration.

Chronic physical findings in a child who is a victim of chronic molestation also may be absent or subtle. Changes in the genital or anal area will depend on the activity engaged in by the child or perpetrator. Exposure, fondling, and oral-genital contact may produce no changes. Chronic/recurrent penile or digital penetration usually will disrupt the hymen. There often are healed tears (transections) that appear as irregularities or scars in the hymen. The hymen itself will lose its thin, fine appearance and will appear thickened. The edge of the hymen will be rounded, and there may be rounded hymenal remnants that resemble the hymenal tags seen in the neonatal period. Bands of scar tissue (synechiae) may form between the hymen and perihymenal tissue. Note the coloring of the genital tissues; new blood vessels (neovascularization) form in areas of previous trauma. A gaping introitus that allows easy visualization of the vaginal rugae also may be apparent and may be a sign of chronic penetration. Some investigators have estimated that the average normal transhymenal diameter is 4 mm, but there is great variation depending on the age, relaxation state, and method of measurement.

Chronic anal penetration leads to scarring and observable changes in the anal area in 50% of victims. The skin in the perianal area may be thickened, hyperpigmented, and lichenified from chronic frictional irritation. The adiposity in the perianal area may be lost, leading to a funneled appearance. Fissures may be noted with ongoing abuse. Such fissures may have a characteristic wedge-shaped appearance, being external to the external sphincter and wider distally than proximally. As fissures heal, they may form scars or tags of hypertrophied tissue. The appearance of the rugae in the perianal area changes; they become fewer in number, thickened, and more prominent, extending a greater distance from the anus. The anal tone changes with chronic anal penetration. Observe relaxation and gaping of the external sphincter with separation of the buttocks. In addition, the anal wink, a normal protective reflex, may be lost or diminished.

Colposcopy is a useful adjunct to the evaluation of a child for chronic sexual abuse. The instrument allows for 5X to 20X magnification of the area being examined and may reveal evidence of scars or abnormalities in the vascular pattern that are not visible to the naked eye.

Carefully record normal as well as abnormal findings. Diagrams and photographs are helpful in documenting the findings.

Laboratory Assessment

The laboratory assessment is especially important in cases of acute molestation; collect specimens that will serve as evidence. Details for the proper collection of specimens are usually included in **sexual assault kits** that often are kept in emergency departments or supplied by the police who accompany a sexual assault victim to the hospital.

In general, collect any loose pubic hairs and samples of the victim's pubic and scalp hair. A medicine dropper or nonbacteriostatic saline-moistened (not dry) cotton-tipped applicator may be used for specimen collection. Obtain specimens of semen if present; place on a glass slide and air-dry for acid phosphatase determination. Place permanent smears in PAP fixative. Semen will fluoresce under Wood's light, as will urine until it dries. When semen is detected on a nongenital body area, remove dried semen samples with cotton swabs using lactated Ringer's solution. Perform a pregnancy test on any sexual abuse victim who is at risk.

Obtain specimens to detect **sexually transmitted diseases** from the throat (gonorrhea), rectum (gonorrhea), and vagina or urethra (gonorrhea and *Chlamydia*) in victims of acute or chronic molestation when signs and symptoms suggest the need. Obtain a serologic test for syphilis. In addition, test any patient with a vaginal discharge for *Gardnerella vaginalis* and *Trichomonas vaginalis* (Table 12-3). With proper consent, try to establish

TABLE 12-3.
Evidence of child sexual abuse.

Child's history in detail

History of observers

Documentation of general physical examination
Note signs of force (eg, bruises)
Documentation of genital injury
Colposcopy
Documentation of sexual contact
Presence of sperm or semen (on patient's clothing or linens)
Sexually transmitted disease
Pregnancy
Foreign material
Documentation of penetration
Sperm: motile/nonmotile
Seminal fluid
    Genetic marker (blood group antigens)
    Acid phosphatase
P30 glycoprotein
Blood
Hair analysis
DNA matching

From DeJong AR, Finkel MA. Sexual abuse of children. *Curr Probl Pediatr.*1990;20:489-567. Adapted with permission.

the HIV status of both the patient and perpetrator.

For some children, there will be tremendous fear generated by the examination and the obtaining of laboratory specimens. It is very important that the examiner not produce more fear in the child. Try to gain the child's cooperation by having the child be aware of what is happening and about to happen. The child often can be instructed to obtain her or his own cultures under direct supervision. If the child is uncooperative or out of control, suspend the evaluation.

Avoid the Second Sexual Assault. It is always better to suspend the evaluation and try again the next day, perhaps in a more quiet setting under more calm circumstances. If the child is bleeding from the site of injury, then the child will have to be examined while under anesthesia. On completion of the evaluation, summarize the findings. Table 12-4 presents a scheme for summarizing the information and setting a course of action.

Management

Both prepubertal and postpubertal victims of molestation may have sexually transmitted diseases and need appropriate diagnostic evaluations and therapy, unless the patient or family objects. The possibility of pregnancy should be discussed, and treatment with Ovral ("morning-after pill") should be offered to patients at risk. The dose is 2 tablets stat and 2 in 12 hours. An antiemetic before use is recommended.

Reassure victims of molestation, both chronic and acute, that they are all right and that their bodies have not been damaged in any way.

Referral to counseling agencies is recommended for all victims of both acute and chronic sexual misuse. Notify law enforcement and children's services of the physical findings of sexual abuse.

The practitioner is obligated by law to report all cases of suspected child abuse. Although the specifics of reporting differ from state to state, in general, practitioners must make a report by

TABLE 12-4.
Overall assessment of the likelihood of sexual abuse.

Class 1: No evidence of abuse
Normal examination, no history, no behavioral changes, no witnessed abuse
Nonspecific findings with another known etiology, and no history or behavioral changes
Child considered at risk for sexual abuse, but gives no history and has nonspecific behavior changes

Class 2: Possible abuse
Class 1, 2, or 3 findings in combination with significant behavioral changes, especially sexualized behaviors, but child unable to give history of abuse examination
Child has made a statement, but not detailed or consistent
Class 3 findings with no disclosure of abuse

Class 3: Probable abuse
Child gives a clear, consistent, detailed description of molestation, with or without other findings present
Class 4 findings in a child, with or without a history of abuse, in the absence of any convincing history of accidental penetrating injury
Culture-proven infection with *Chlamydia trachomatis* (child older than 2 years) in a prepubertal child. Also culture-proven herpes type 2 infection in a child or documented *Trichomonas* infection.

Class 4: Definite evidence of abuse or sexual contact
Finding of sperm or seminal fluid in or on a child's body
Witnessed episode of sexual molestation. This also applies to cases in which pornographic photographs or videotapes are acquired as evidence.
Nonaccidental, blunt penetrating injury to the vaginal or anal orifice
Positive, confirmed cultures for *Neisseria gonorrhoeae* in a prepubertal child or serologic confirmation of acquired syphilis

From *Adolesc Pediatr Gynecol* 1992;5:73-75. Reprinted with permission of Springer-Verlag, New York.

telephone immediately to law enforcement and children's services. Follow this oral report with a timely written report, preferably immediately but always within 3 days.

Confronting a family about child abuse may be difficult. It is important to keep in mind the important role of the reporting practitioner as an advocate for the child who is being evaluated. In addition, the abusive parent often is seeking help for himself or herself when bringing in the injured child. The practitioner thus may be able to help not only the child but also the troubled parent.

Consultation with other professionals (eg, social workers or psychologists) may be helpful in completing the evaluation and disposition planning.

NEGLECT

The most common form of child abuse is neglect, yet it is the least often reported. Neglect of children is insidious. It has many profoundly negative consequences and often goes unreported for months or years because of the lack of either positive physical findings or a specific crisis point. The forms of neglect seen most often in the emergency department are abandonment, medical neglect, and nonorganic failure to thrive (FTT).

Abandonment

Abandonment refers to the parent or parents leaving a child without proper care or supervision in a situation in which harm may come to the child. There are no specific lengths of times or conditions dictated by society; thus, there must be value judgments made by the health care team in deciding when to initiate a report. Children who are abandoned must be thoroughly examined, assessed for signs of neglect, such as starvation and dehydration, and reported to child welfare authorities. If there are no provisions for community-based emergency foster care, the child should be admitted to the hospital for protective care.

Medical Neglect

Medical neglect is a term indicating that despite appropriate instructions from a health care provider, a parent refuses to provide or obtain health services for a child. Because of the parental neglect, the child sustains injury, develops an illness, or has worsening of a condition. A common

form of medical neglect is substantial delay in obtaining or deliberate ignoring of the need for appropriate immunizations for a child. Cases of medical neglect are very difficult to document. When encountered, filing a report of the incident with a child welfare (protection) agency is required.

Failure to Thrive

FTT is a disorder characterized by impairment of physical, emotional, and intellectual growth that occurs because of disturbances in the manner in which an infant or child is nourished and nurtured. The hallmark of the disorder is impairment of growth, with height or weight below the fifth percentile or normal height with low weight. Because many chronic medical disorders lead to impairment of physical growth, differentiate the child whose growth is related to environmental factors from the child with a medical problem.

Patients with FTT often present to the emergency department with complaints unrelated to the growth retardation. They also may be victims of physical or sexual abuse. They frequently have intercurrent illnesses related to malnutrition, particularly gastroenteritis. An astute practitioner will appreciate that a child is malnourished or too small for his or her chronologic age. In all cases, refer to the growth chart.

The physical examination of infants may reveal findings of malnutrition, such as diminished subcutaneous tissue, thin extremities, and prominent ribs. A child's head may appear disproportionately large because weight and length are more greatly affected than head circumference. The examination may also reveal signs of dehydration. Infants with nonorganic FTT exhibit distinct behavioral characteristics. They often have a watchful, wary, wide-eyed gaze and avoid eye contact. They are hypertonic and dislike close interpersonal interactions, pulling away from the examiner. Observe mother-infant interactions to determine whether these are disturbed. Little vocalization occurs between such a mother and a nonthriving infant. Vocalization that does occur may be negative. A mother frequently may hold an infant at arm's length or leave the child unattended in an infant seat, on the floor, or on the examining table.

For infants and children suspected of having FTT, admit to the hospital or arrange appropriate management and investigative procedures in an outpatient setting. That will allow sufficient time to perform an appropriate assessment. From 90% to 95% of infants and children with nonorganic FTT gain weight as expected after intervention. Some children with nonorganic FTT also may be reportable under state child abuse reporting laws.

SUMMARY

The problems of child abuse and neglect are complex multifactorial issues of individual behavior, family function, and societal stresses. The physician cannot be expected to treat child abuse the way an infectious illness might be managed; the management of abuse more closely resembles the treatment of a chronic disease, one that often requires many different "therapists" from different professional backgrounds and varied hospital-based and community agencies. However, no therapy can begin without recognition and reporting of the problem. In these tasks, the emergency department practitioner is unique and bears a heavy responsibility for being alert and sensitive and for having the courage to speak up on behalf of the child. Failure to do so unwittingly condones the abuse and positions the child for further injury both physically and psychologically. The overriding principle to remember is that suspicion equals reporting and reporting equals help.

ADDITIONAL READING

Ablin D, Greenspan A, Reinhart M, et al. Differentiation of child abuse from osteogenesis imperfecta. *AJR Am J Roentgenol.* 1990;154:1035-1046.

American Academy of Pediatrics, Section on Radiology. Diagnostic imaging of child abuse. *Pediatrics.* 1991;87:262-264.

American Academy of Pediatrics. *Focus on Child Abuse. Resources for Prevention, Recognition and Treatment CD-ROM.* Elk Grove Village, Ill: American Academy of Pediatrics; 1996.

American Academy of Pediatrics, Committee on Child Abuse and Neglect. Guidelines for the evaluation of sexual abuse of children. *Pediatrics.* 1991;87:254-260.

Bays J, Chadwick D. Medical diagnosis of the sexually abused child. *Child Abuse Negl.* 1993;17:91-110.

Child homicide–United States. *MMWR Morb Mortal Wkly Rep.* 1982;31:292-294.

Coant PN, Kornberg AE, Brody AS, et al. Markers for occult liver injury in cases of physical abuse in children. *Pediatrics.* 1992;89:274-278.

Council on Scientific Affairs, American Medical Association. Adolescents as victims of family violence. *JAMA.* 1993;270:1850-1856.

De Jong AR, Finkel MA. Sexual abuse of children. *Curr Probl Pediatr.* 1990;20:489-567.

De Jong AR, Rose M. Frequency and significance of physical evidence in legally proven cases of child sexual abuse. *Pediatrics.*1989;84:1022-1026.

Duhaime AC, Alario AJ, Lewander WJ, et al. Head injury in very young children: mechanisms, injury types, and ophthalmologic findings in 100 hospitalized patients younger than 2 years of age. *Pediatrics.* 1992;90:179-185.

Gordon S, Jaudes PK. Sexual abuse evaluations in the emergency department: is the history reliable? *Child Abuse Negl.* 1996;20: 315-322.

Gutman LT, Herman-Giddens ME, McKinney RE. Pediatric acquired immunodeficiency syndrome: barriers to recognizing the role of child sexual abuse. *Am J Dis Child.*1993;147:775-780.

Kempe CH, Silverman FN, Steele BF, et al. The battered-child syndrome. *JAMA.* 1962;181:17-24.

Kleinman PK. *Diagnostic Imaging of Child Abuse.* Baltimore, Md: Williams & Wilkins; 1987.

Kleinman PK, Marks SC, Blackbourne B. The metaphyseal lesion in abused infants: a radiologic-histopathologic study. *AJR Am J Roentgenol.* 1986;146:895-905.

Ludwig S, Kornberg AE, eds. *Child Abuse: A Medical Reference.* New York, NY: Churchill Livingstone; 1992.

Schwartz AJ, Ricci LR. How accurately can bruises be aged in abused children? Literature review and synthesis. *Pediatrics.* 1996;97:254-257.

Wissow LS. Child abuse and neglect. *N Engl J Med.* 1995;332:1425-1431.

Emergencies with Altered Level of Consciousness

Chapter 13

Altered Level of Consciousness

OBJECTIVES

1. Describe the possible etiologies of altered level of consciousness in children.

2. Outline the appropriate sequence of diagnostic and therapeutic interventions for children presenting with altered level of consciousness.

3. Describe the initial evaluation and management of patients with specific presumptive diagnoses

The child presenting with altered mental status is one of the most difficult diagnostic and management problems. The gravity of the situation, need to move quickly to avoid irreversible damage, and rather wide array of the possible diagnoses call for a calm, orderly approach to the problem at hand. The initial management includes immediate attention to the ABCs to sustain life and prevent loss of brain function.

PATHOPHYSIOLOGY

Altered level of consciousness (ALC) refers to any deviation from a child's normal age-appropriate responsiveness to environmental stimuli. There is a spectrum of alterations of mental status, ranging from disorders in perception (eg, confusion or delirium) to states of decreased awareness (eg, lethargy, obtundation, and, ultimately, coma).

Coma generally is indicative of either diffuse or bilateral impairment of cerebral functions, failure of brainstem-activating mechanisms, or both. This can be caused by supratentorial lesions affecting deep diencephalic structures, subtentorial lesions affecting the brainstem, or metabolic disorders diffusely affecting neuronal function. Unilateral hemispheric lesions generally do not cause stupor or coma unless they secondarily affect other areas, particularly the diencephalon.

Both traumatic and nontraumatic causes of coma can lead to cerebral edema and resultant herniation of cerebral structures through the foramen magnum (see Chapter 6). Two major patterns of supratentorial herniation occur: **rostrocaudal (central) herniation**, characterized by an orderly progression of brainstem dysfunction, and **uncal herniation**, often heralded by a unilaterally fixed dilated pupil caused by compression of the oculomotor nerve by the medial portion of the temporal lobe (uncus). If left untreated, supratentorial herniation generally follows a rostrocaudal progression with increasing brainstem dysfunction. This progression is not seen so clearly in lesions primarily affecting the brainstem, in which prompt loss of consciousness usually is the rule. Rough guidelines for differentiating classes of coma are presented in Table 13-1.

ETIOLOGY

The etiologic possibilities are diverse. The mnemonic **TIPS from the VOWELS** has been a useful method for organizing the diagnostic possibilities.

   T — Trauma, which is a major cause of ALC and the leading cause of death in the first four decades of life. Head injuries leading to hypoxia, and blood loss leading to shock have significant effects on the level of consciousness.

   I — Insulin/hypoglycemia. Although known diabetics obviously are at risk for unintentional insulin overdoes, occasionally toddlers ingest another family member's oral hyoglycemic agent or inject their insulin.

Ketotic hypoglycemia, probably the most common cause of hypoglycemia in childhood, comprises a number of disease processes. Extensive diagnostic testing may be required to establish a specific diagnosis. Specimens should be drawn and frozen for potential later use in determining levels of cortisol, insulin, growth hormone, and medium-chain aldol dehydrogenase. Children with this problem are often young (18 months to 5 years) and often have histories of low birth weight. Attacks are episodic, most apt to occur in the morning and after prolonged fasting, and frequently are associated with ketonuria. Hypoglycemic episodes, resulting from an inappropriate response to a prolonged fasting state, respond promptly to the administration of glucose.

   I — Intussusception, caused by the prolapse of a portion of small intestine into an adjacent loop, not uncommonly presents with mental status changes before the development of abdominal findings. In the child younger than 3 years with unexplained lethargy or loss of consciousness, this diagnosis should be entertained, with careful and repeated examination of the abdomen and testing of the stool for blood.

   I — Inborn errors of metabolism. These are important disorders to keep in mind, particularly when the onset of symptoms occurs within the first few months of life. Presenting signs include vomiting and seizures. Presentation often is triggered by an otherwise innocuous viral illness. The two major groups of inborn errors of metabolism that produce ALC are associated with hyperammonemia or metabolic acidosis. Tests conducted in the emergency department should include serum ammonia and arterial blood gases. Specimens for lactate, pyruvate, and organic acids can be drawn, but only serum lactate is available stat in most centers. Specimens for serum lactate must be drawn carefully from a free-flowing venous source (without tourniquet), an arterial stick, or an indwelling catheter. Establishment that a metabolic acidosis with a normal lactate level is present should lead to strong consideration of an inborn error of metabolism.

   P — Psychogenic. Although factitious ALC is rare in young children, it is a cause worth considering in older children and adolescents. Careful neurologic examination often will reveal abnormalities inconsistent with an organic etiology.

TABLE 13-1.
Differentiating characteristics of structural and metabolic coma.

Supratentorial Lesions	Infratentorial Lesions	Toxic, Metabolic, or Infectious Processes
Initial signs focal	Brainstem abnormalities often are initial signs	Confusion/stupor often precedes motor signs
Rostrocaudal progression seen	Sudden onset of coma	Symmetric examination
Asymmetric examination often	Cranial nerve abnormalities often seen; respiratory pattern often altered	Pupillary reactions preserved; respiratory rate often altered

S — Seizures. Postictal states are common causes of ALC, and an actively seizing infant may appear to be in coma until close observation reveals continued subtle seizure activity.

S — Stroke, shock, and other cardiovascular causes. Poor brain perfusion due to hypovolemia may lead to altered sensorium in the presence of an otherwise normal central nervous system. Cardiovascular abnormalities, such as arteriovenous malformations, present only rarely in childhood, resulting in focal neurologic deficits or ALC.

S — Shunt. Patients with ventriculoatrial or ventriculoperitoneal shunts may present with ALC when the shunt is blocked or infected. Rapid evaluation of the shunt is necessary.

A — Alcohol, which is more commonly encountered in adolescents than in younger pediatric patients; however, it is not an infrequent cause of accidental ingestion in the young child. Young children may exhibit ALC at serum levels of <100 mg/dL and also may be obtunded from concurrent hypoglycemia.

A — Abuse. Child abuse must be considered in any child presenting in coma, particularly when the history and physical examination findings are not congruent. The practitioner must look for subtle physical signs of trauma, including bruising, cranial tenderness or swelling, and retinal hemorrhages. The shaken baby syndrome can result in ALC not associated with external signs of physical abuse.

E — Electrolytes. Any condition causing abnormal fluid losses can cause ALC due to abnormalities in electrolytes such as Na^+, K^+, Ca^{2+}, and Mg^{2+}. This also can be the result of disorders such as adrenal insufficiency and the syndrome of inappropriate antidiuretic hormone. General inspection should include a search for ambiguous genitalia or hyperpigmented scrotum, as evidence of congenital adrenal hyperplasia.

E — Encephalopathy. Reye's syndrome, although decreasing in incidence, is a consideration in any child presenting with a history of pernicious vomiting leading to altered mental status, particularly when there is a history of an antecedent varicella or a flu-like illness. A history of salicylate use should be sought.

Like other hepatic encephalopathies, Reye's syndrome usually is associated with an elevated serum ammonia level. Other causes of hepatic encephalopathy include valproate toxicity, late-phase acetaminophen toxicity, acute viral hepatitis, and partial urea cycle defect.

Lead encephalopathy, although unusual, continues to be a concern in the pediatric age group, particularly in children living in older buildings in which leaded paint may still be present. Children can have rapid increases in blood lead levels through ingestion of loose paint chips or mouthing of items contaminated with lead paint, dust, and soil. An antecedent history of fatigue, vomiting, or abdominal pain in a child living in an older dwelling should alert the practitioner to the possibility of this diagnosis. Screening tests include blood lead, free erythrocyte protoporphyrin, and complete blood cell count. Occasionally, radiopaque lead chips will be found on abdominal radiographs. Treatment involves chelation therapy.

I — Infection. Meningitis and encephalitis are more common in the pediatric patient than in adults. Infections outside the central nervous system, particularly sepsis, also can cause ALC if associated with cerebral hypoperfusion.

O — Overdose/ingestion. Ingestion always is a strong consideration in the young child with an unexplained alteration in consciousness. A complete history of medications in the household should be obtained early in the evaluation of these patients.

U — Uremia, which usually is slow in onset. Hemolytic uremic syndrome is a multisystem disorder characterized by a prodromal phase of gastroenteritis or upper respiratory infection followed by acute onset and rapid progression of renal failure, microangiopathic hemolytic anemia, and thrombocytopenia. Other causes of chronic renal impairment in childhood also may lead to markedly elevated blood urea nitrogen levels and uremic encephalopathy.

EVALUATION

Immediate Considerations

The initial approach to the child in coma is to ensure that the brain is receiving adequate oxygen, glucose, and blood flow to maintain viability. The practitioner must assess vital signs and simultaneously address and support the status of the airway, breathing, and circulation. A bedside assessment of blood glucose is obtained.

An abbreviated, targeted history often is indicated at this point. The practitioner should determine whether the child has had any chronic or recent illness, antecedent fever, pernicious vomiting, or trauma.

An assessment of the rapidity of onset of the change often is helpful. A history of all medications in the household should be obtained. Naloxone (0.1 mg/kg IV) is given for suspected narcotic intoxication in children <5 years of age; the dose for children >5 years of age is 2 mg IV.

Secondary Considerations

The level of consciousness can be assessed and quantified with use of the Glasgow Coma Scale (see Chapter 6). In addition, four pathophysiologic variables help determine the nature of the lesion affecting the brain, functional level of involvement, and rate and extent of progression of the disease process; these functions include the pattern of respiration, size and reactivity of the pupils, spontaneous and induced eye movements, and motor responses.

Respiratory Pattern

Control of ventilation is governed by centers located in the lower pons and medulla and modulated by cortical centers located mainly in the forebrain. Respiratory abnormalities signify either metabolic derangement or neurologic insult. Several characteristic patterns exist (and are presented in order of rostrocaudal involvement). **Postventilation apnea** generally is characterized by brief periods of apnea lasting 10 to 30 seconds, followed by voluntary deep breathing. It usually is representative of forebrain involvement. **Cheyne-Stokes respirations** constitute a pattern of breathing in which phases of hyperpnea regularly alternate with apnea. The depth of breathing waxes in a smooth crescendo and then, once a peak is reached, wanes in an equally smooth decrescendo. Cheyne-Stokes respirations usually imply dysfunction of structures deep within both cerebral hemispheres or in the diencephalon. This pattern of ventilation commonly occurs in metabolic encephalopathy.

Central neurogenic hyperventilation is manifested by sustained regular and rapid respirations despite normal PaO_2 and low $PaCO_2$. This is both a rare and serious finding and points to midbrain dysfunction. **Apneustic breathing** is characterized by brief inspiratory pauses lasting 2 to 3 seconds, often alternating with end-expiratory pauses. Clinically, this pattern is characteristic of pontine infarction but occasionally can be seen in anoxic encephalopathy or severe meningitis.

Eye Findings

The eye examination tells much about both the level of the lesion and the prognosis of the patient. Specific eye findings to evaluate include pupillary size and responsiveness, spontaneous and induced eye movements, and results of funduscopic examination.

Pupillary Signs. The pupillary reactions — **constriction** and **dilatation** — are controlled by the sympathetic and parasympathetic nervous system. Because brainstem areas controlling consciousness are adjacent to those controlling the pupils, pupillary changes often are informative. In addition, because pupillary pathways are relatively resistant to metabolic insult, the presence or absence of a reaction to light is the most important physical finding distinguishing structural from metabolic disease. Most metabolic conditions affecting the central nervous system lead to pupils that are constricted but remain reactive to light. At times, the pupils are so small they appear to be light-fixed, but reactivity is readily apparent when a bright light is used and the pupils are visualized with a magnifying glass. Pupillary findings are invalid if atropine has been administered.

Pupillary responses to structural lesions depend on the site of the primary disturbance and on secondary effects of increased intracranial pressure.

Selected pupillary abnormalities are presented in Figure 13-1.

Induced Eye Movements. Two specific eye maneuvers are helpful in evaluating the comatose child. The **oculocephalic**, or **doll's eye, reflex** is performed by holding the eyelids open and briskly rotating the head from side to side. This test is contraindicated in any child in whom cervical spine injury is a possibility. The normal, or positive, doll's eye response is conjugate deviation of the eyes contrary to the direction in which the head is turned. The stimulus for this reflex involves the vestibular system, proprioceptive afferents in the neck, or both.

The **oculovestibular reflex,** better known as **caloric testing,** is performed by elevating the patient's head to 30 degrees and slowly injecting 50 mL of cool water through a catheter placed in the external auditory canal. This technique causes vestibular stimulation. In the normal awake patient, with brainstem intact, the response to ice water testing is nystagmus, with the slow component toward the irrigated ear and the fast nystagmus away from the irrigated ear. In the unconscious patient whose brainstem is intact, the fast nystagmus is abolished, and the eyes move toward

the stimulus and remain tonically deviated for ≥1 minute, before slowly returning to the midline. This test is contraindicated if tympanic membranes are not intact or there is suspicion of basilar skull fracture.

Deviation of the eyes at rest also is of great diagnostic significance. With cerebral lesions, conjugate deviation is noted toward the side of the lesion, whereas with brainstem lesions, conjugate deviation is away from the lesion. The "setting sun" sign, characterized by downward deviation of the eyes, is associated with upper midbrain lesions. Third nerve paralysis generally causes the eye to point downward and outward.

Ophthalmoscopic Examination. A brief ophthalmoscopic examination should be performed to assess the presence or absence of papilledema or retinal hemorrhages. Although not usually an early finding, papilledema is suggestive of increased intracranial pressure and merits efforts aimed at its control. Retinal hemorrhages, thought to be highly

FIGURE 13-1.
Pupillary abnormalities in the patient with coma.

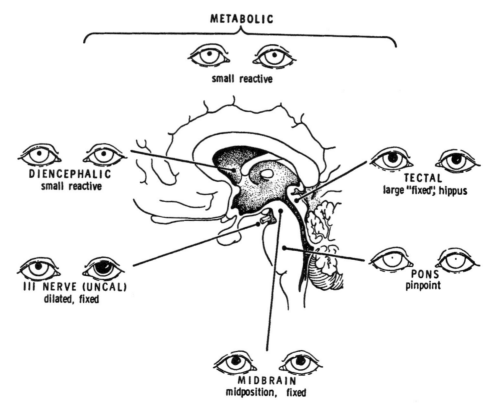

From Plum F, Posner JB. *The Diagnosis of Stupor and Coma.* Philadelphia, Pa: FA Davis; 1982:46. Reprinted with permission.

suggestive of abuse, have also been postulated to result from aggressive resuscitative efforts.

Motor Examination

The motor examination of the comatose patient consists of eliciting various responses to stimuli, either auditory or physical. Muscle strength, tone, and deep tendon reflexes should be assessed for normality and symmetry. The ability of the patient to localize, as well as the presence or absence of abnormal posturing (Figure 13-2), also helps assess the severity of involvement. **Decorticate posturing** (flexion of the upper extremities with extension of the lower extremities) suggests involvement of the cerebral cortex and subcortical white matter with preservation of brainstem function. **Decerebrate posturing** (rigid extension of the arms and legs) generally represents added brainstem involvement, usually at the level of the pons.

The flaccid patient with no response to painful stimuli has the most grave prognosis and generally has sustained injury deep into the brainstem.

FIGURE 13-2.
Motor responses in the unconscious patient.

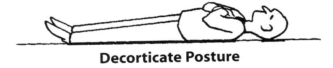

Decorticate Posture

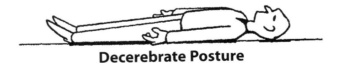

Decerebrate Posture

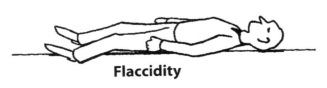

Flaccidity

From Pellock JM, Myer EC, eds. *Neurologic Emergencies in Infancy and Childhood,* 2nd ed. Stoneham, Mass: Butterworth-Heinemann; 1993:183. Reprinted with permission.

DIAGNOSTIC AIDS

Laboratory evaluation of the patient with altered mental status can be divided into the routine and the specific. Suggested laboratory tests for the patient with altered mental status of undetermined etiology include complete blood cell count, electrolytes, blood urea nitrogen, creatinine, and immediate bedside and serum glucose levels. When a metabolic cause for coma is suspected, liver function testing, serum ammonia, measured and calculated serum osmolality, and toxicology screens should be considered. Arterial blood gases are useful in monitoring the adequacy of ventilation and oxygenation and in assessing acid-base status. Metabolic acidosis without elevated lactate level suggests an organic acidemia (inborn error) or ingestion. Focal abnormalities or signs of increased intracranial pressure (ICP) usually mandate a computed tomography scan once the patient is stabilized. In the patient who remains an enigma, a stat EEG should be considered because nonmotor status epilepticus at times is not clinically obvious. Performance of a lumbar puncture evaluates clinical suspicion of meningitis and can be done if no signs of increased ICP are present. Additional laboratory tests to consider, when clinically indicated, include blood alcohol level, thyroid function tests, blood lead level, blood culture, skeletal survey, and barium or air enema.

MANAGEMENT

Primary Survey

The initial task is to assess the adequacy of the patient's airway, degree of ventilation, and circulatory status.

Airway and Breathing

Ensure the patency of the airway while protecting the cervical spine if there is a possibility of cervical spine trauma. Open the airway using the chin lift or jaw thrust maneuver. Avoid extension of the neck because it can occlude the airway in an infant. Insert a nasal airway as needed; oral airways are best avoided in the lightly comatose patient because of the risk of inducing vomiting and aspiration. Provide supplemental oxygen. If the child is apneic or has markedly impaired respirations, assist ventilatory efforts with bag-valve-mask ventilation or intubation. If the patient has an inadequate gag reflex, intubation will be necessary. If respirations are present but noisy, suction and inspect for foreign material. Controlled ventilation to a $PaCO_2$ of 30 to 35 mm Hg is indicated if there are signs of increased ICP. Hyperventilation to $PaCO_2$ levels of <30 mm Hg should be limited to use in patients with clear evidence of transtentorial herniation, primarily unilateral pupillary dilatation.

Cardiovascular Status

The patient's skin perfusion and capillary refill best estimate circulatory status. Measure the pulse and blood pressure, and place the child on a monitor. Achieve venous or intraosseous access, draw diagnostic blood specimens, and perform a rapid estimate of blood sugar. The state of hydration as indicated by physical examination should dictate the fluid selection and rate. Shock should be treated as described in Chapter 3. Check oxygen saturation with pulse oximetry. Only after the ABCs are addressed can attention be directed to the neurologic and general examination.

Disability (Neurologic Status)

Perform an objective evaluation of the child's level of consciousness using either the AVPU system or the Glasgow Coma Scale (see Chapter 6). Note pupillary size and reactivity. Look for evolving signs of increased ICP, such as alterations in vital signs (including Cushing's triad of bradycardia, hypertension, and irregular respirations), pupillary responses, respiratory pattern, or ophthalmoscopic examination. Treat patients with clinical evidence of increased ICP as detailed in Chapter 6. Save a tube of blood for later laboratory study. Infuse glucose (250 to 500 mg/kg IV) for documented hypoglycemia. Use 2.5 to 5 mL/kg $D_{10}W$ for neonates, 1 to 2 mL/kg $D_{25}W$ for infants up to age 2, and 0.5 to 1 mL/kg $D_{50}W$ for older children. If the child improves, a continuous infusion of 10% dextrose in balanced saline solution should be initiated at the child's maintenance rate. If intravenous access cannot be obtained, administer glucagon intramuscularly (0.025 mg/kg up to 1 mg). Infuse naloxone (0.1 mg/kg IV) up to a maximum dose of 4 mg to reverse a potential narcotic-induced alteration in mental status.

Exposure

Remove the patient's clothing, splints, and other items that hinder full evaluation and replace them as needed after an adequate examination.

Secondary Survey

Once the immediate life-threatening concerns have been addressed, an abbreviated targeted history should be obtained. The practitioner should determine whether the child has had any chronic or recent illness, antecedent fever, rash, pernicious vomiting, or trauma. Explore any recent exposure to infection, medications, or intoxicants. Immunization history, past medical history, and family history should be obtained when time permits. Be alert for any inappropriate responses and delays in seeking care that may arouse the suspicion of child abuse.

The observations in the secondary survey should attempt to uncover signs of occult infection, trauma, or toxic or metabolic derangements. Important areas to evaluate include the fundi, extraocular movements, oculocephalic or oculovestibular responses, anterior fontanel, and neck for stiffness. Many afebrile toddlers with altered mental status may have an unknown ingestion. Signs suggestive of a specific toxidrome should be sought.

DISPOSITION

The above approach may delineate a specific cause of ALC. When a presumptive diagnosis is confirmed, carry out specific management. Definitive therapy can be initiated in the emergency department. Admit or transfer to a pediatric intensive care unit any patient not responding to therapeutic intervention who will require ongoing monitoring or intensive therapy or in whom the diagnosis is still in question after the initial management.

PROGNOSIS

In general, the prognosis of the pediatric patient in a coma is much better than that of his or her adult counterpart. Particularly in relation to traumatic etiologies, age appears to be a major independent factor affecting both mortality and morbidity. Be cautiously optimistic about the potential for recovery in most children presenting with significant altered mental status.

ADDITIONAL READING

Barkin RM, Rosen P. Coma. In: Barkin RM, Rosen P, eds. *Emergency Pediatrics: A Guide to Ambulatory Care.* St Louis, Mo: Mosby; 1990:101-107.

Fuchs S. Altered mental status and coma. In: Strange GR, Ahrens WR, Lelyveld S, et al, eds. *Pediatric Emergency Medicine: A Comprehensive Study Guide.* New York, NY: McGraw-Hill; 1996:220-224.

Gauthier M, Guay J, Lacroix J, et al. Reye's syndrome. A reappraisal of diagnosis in 49 presumptive cases. *Am J Dis Child.* 1989;143:1181-1185.

Isaacman DJ. Coma and altered mental status. In: Barkin RM, ed. *Pediatric Emergency Medicine: Concepts and Clinical Practice.* St Louis, Mo: Mosby–Year Book; 1992:893-899.

Packer RJ, Berman PH. Coma. In: Fleisher GR, Ludwig S, eds. *Textbook of Pediatric Emergency Medicine,* 3rd ed. Baltimore, Md: Williams & Wilkins; 1993:122-134.

Plum F, Posner JB. *The Diagnosis of Stupor and Coma.* Philadelphia, Pa: FA Davis; 1982.

Vannucci RC, Wasiewski WW. Diagnosis and management of coma in children. In: Pellock JM, Myer EC, eds. *Neurologic Emergencies in Infancy and Childhood,* 2nd ed. Boston, Mass: Butterworth-Heinemann; 1993:103-122.

Yager JY, Johnston B, Seshia SS. Coma scales in pediatric practice. *Am J Dis Child.* 1990;144:1088-1091.

Chapter 14

The Septic-Appearing Infant

OBJECTIVES

1. Describe conditions that can simulate sepsis in an infant.

2. Select appropriate diagnostic procedures for use in the evaluation of septic-appearing infants.

3. Outline a management approach for the infant who is presumed to be septic.

For the purpose of the current discussion, a septic-appearing infant is an infant younger than 1 year who looks ill and has ashen color, pallor, or cyanosis. The baby may be irritable or lethargic and normothermic, febrile, or hypothermic. Most septic-appearing infants have tachycardia and tachypnea and may be poorly perfused or hypotensive. Parents of such infants usually report the baby has been fussy, anorectic, and perhaps sleeping more than usual.

When confronted with an ill-appearing infant, the physician always should consider sepsis as the etiology. Although it is correct to begin immediate management for sepsis, life-threatening conditions other than sepsis can produce a similar appearance in a young infant and also should be considered. A detailed history, careful physical examination, and appropriate laboratory tests will help establish the definitive diagnosis.

PATHOPHYSIOLOGY

Septic infants will have poor perfusion due to the effect of **toxins** on the vascular system. However, infants also may be poorly perfused due to **hypovolemia** or **cardiac failure** as well. **Respiratory failure** and **increased intracranial pressure** also can be responsible for a toxic appearance. (In other chapters, the pathophysiology of many of these conditions is discussed in greater detail.)

DIFFERENTIAL DIAGNOSIS

There are numerous disorders that cause an infant to appear quite ill (Table 14-1). This chapter focuses on infants in the first 2 or 3 months of life who appear to be "septic."

Infection

Sepsis should always be considered as the diagnosis when an infant appears toxic. In some infants, the history may reveal sudden onset of illness, whereas others may have been ill for days before presentation. Symptoms may include lethargy, irritability, diarrhea, vomiting, fever, or poor feeding. Physical examination may reveal pallor, cyanosis, or ashen appearance. The baby may be febrile or hypothermic (common in septic infants in the first few months of life). There usually is extreme tachycardia and tachypnea. Hypotension may be noted. The baby may be irritable or lethargic. The skin may be cool and mottled and have petechiae or purpura if disseminated intravascular coagulopathy has developed. If the infection has seeded specific sites, other findings may be present, such as otitis media or joint swelling or tenderness in an extremity. (The most common bacterial causes of sepsis are listed in

TABLE 14-1.
Differential diagnosis of the septic-appearing infant.

Cardiac Disease
Congestive heart failure
Ductal-dependent lesions
Left heart obstruction
Pericarditis/myocarditis
Supraventricular tachycardia
Child Abuse
Shaken baby syndrome
Endocrine Disorders
Congenital adrenal hyperplasia
Gastrointestinal Disorders
Appendicitis
Gastroenteritis
Hirschsprung's enterocolitis
Incarcerated inguinal hernia
Intussusception
Pyloric stenosis
Necrotizing enterocolitis
Volvulus
Hematologic Disorders
Anemia
Methemoglobinemia
Infectious Diseases
Bacterial sepsis/meningitis
Congenital syphilis
Viral infections (enterovirus, RSV, herpes simplex)
Metabolic Disorders
Cystic fibrosis
Dehydration (hyponatremic, hypernatremic, and isotonic)
Hypoglycemia
Toxins (alcohol, aspirin)
Urea cycle defects
Neurologic Disease
Infant botulism
Genitourinary Disorders
Posterior urethral valves, other obstructive uropathies
Pyelonephritis

Table 3-3).

Overwhelming **viral infections** also may result in sepsis in young infants. Enteroviral infections in the neonate frequently cause respiratory distress and bleeding of the gastrointestinal tract. Abdominal distention, splenomegaly, and/or icterus may be found. Myocarditis and encephalitis with resultant seizures are more serious complications that contribute to the high mortality for enteroviral infections in the neonate. These infections often cannot be distinguished clinically from bacterial sepsis except that bacterial cultures eventually prove to be negative and the offending organism may be found in viral isolates from stool, nasopharynx, or cerebrospinal fluid.

Another viral infection to consider is **respiratory syncytial virus (RSV)**. This is a common infection in winter, and young infants with this infection may present with apnea, cyanosis, and respiratory distress. Wheezing may not appear until later in the course. Those born prematurely or those with underlying pulmonary or cardiac diseases are especially susceptible to respiratory failure, apnea, and death from this infection.

Herpes simplex virus can cause encephalitis, leading to high morbidity and mortality. Infants can present with fever, septic shock, apnea, coma, fulminant hepatitis, pneumonitis, disseminated intravascular coagulation, and seizures that are difficult to control. Ocular findings, such as conjunctivitis and keratitis, may occur. Neurologic findings may be focal. Signs and symptoms usually are noted at 7 to 21 days of life. Typical vesicular skin lesions are helpful diagnostically but present in only one third to one half of patients. A history of maternal genital herpes should make the physician highly suspicious, but in the majority of cases, the mother is completely asymptomatic.

Pneumocystis carinii **pneumonia** is an opportunistic infection that has become more common in pediatric patients due to therapeutic advances in the management of immunologic and neoplastic diseases. *P. carinii* pneumonitis generally presents with a relatively sudden onset of respiratory distress, hypoxia, fever, and a diffuse interstitial pattern on chest radiograph, although it can be insidious and cause wheezing, mild cough, and dyspnea that slowly worsens. The chest radiograph may show hyperinflation or may be normal. Typically, the alveolar-arterial gradient is

>30 mm Hg, and the serum lactate dehydrogenase level tends to be markedly elevated. For the ill-appearing child with respiratory symptoms, with or without a positive chest radiograph, trimethoprim-sulfamethoxazole for *P. carinii* pneumonia should be started. Treatment for suspected *P. carinii* pneumonia should not be delayed because of the fear of interfering with the diagnostic work-up.

Congenital syphilis is another infection that can mimic sepsis. Neonates may present with extreme irritability, jaundice, pallor, hepatosplenomegaly, or edema. The irritability often is due to painful limbs. The infants also may have pneumonia, aseptic meningitis, rash, and snuffles. Although infants with syphilis appear quite ill, the history typically reveals that they have had chronic symptoms, unlike the septic infant. Certainly, if the mother has a history of infection during pregnancy, this diagnosis should be considered.

Cardiac Diseases

Congenital heart disease (CHD) can produce congestive heart failure and clinical findings similar to those of sepsis. Patients with lesions such as valvular insufficiency, coarctation of the aorta, ventricular septal defect, or hypoplastic left heart syndrome may develop tachycardia, tachypnea, pallor, cyanosis, or mottled skin, especially when complicated by simple upper respiratory infection. Hypotension and weak pulses also may be present. A complete history and physical examination may distinguish shock due to most types of CHD from sepsis, but the signs and symptoms of left heart obstructive lesions may be very similar to those of sepsis. A history of poor weight gain and laborious, prolonged feeding suggests heart disease. The presence of a cardiac murmur suggests a structural lesion. A gallop rhythm and hepatomegaly also point to cardiac disease rather than sepsis. Rales, rhonchi, wheezing, and intercostal retractions may be present with both sepsis (due to pneumonia) and heart failure, so such findings may not be diagnostic. Likewise, an infant with anomalous coronary arteries can develop myocardial infarction. These infants may have dyspnea, sweating, cyanosis, vomiting, pallor, and other signs of heart failure. The rather sudden onset of symptoms can easily be confused with sepsis.

Certain dysrhythmias, such as **supraventricular tachycardia (SVT),** may cause an infant to look septic. This dysrhythmia is idiopathic in half the cases but may be associated with CHD. It also may be related to fever or infection, so it can easily be confused with sepsis. Often, young infants with SVT have been fussy and feeding poorly, with slightly rapid breathing, for a few days before presentation. Eventually, if untreated, they develop congestive heart failure, with signs of shock. A careful physical examination reveals extreme tachycardia (250 to 300 beats/min), perhaps with hepatomegaly, making the diagnosis of SVT more likely than sepsis.

Cardiac infections also should be considered. Suppurative pericarditis is a very rare infection, often caused by *Haemophilus influenzae* and *Staphylococcus aureus.* Although infants with this infection appear critically ill with fever, tachypnea, and tachycardia, they differ from septic infants in that they may have hepatomegaly, neck vein distention, and friction rub. A friction rub is not heard when the condition is severe. Heart sounds may seem distant if a pericardial effusion is present. Similarly, those with myocarditis due to *Mycoplasma, Neisseria meningitidis,* or Coxsackie B viral infection may look septic yet have a gallop rhythm or tachycardia out of proportion to the degree of fever present. They, too, may have other signs of heart failure.

Kawasaki disease with coronary artery aneurysms may be seen in older infants and children. For the diagnostic criteria, see Table 4-6.

Endocrine Disorders

Infants with **congenital adrenal hyperplasia (CAH)** may present in the first few weeks of life with vomiting, lethargy, or irritability. Examination will show signs of marked dehydration with tachycardia and hypothermia. More careful history may distinguish this condition from sepsis, because these infants have chronic feeding problems and progressive symptoms over a few days. Physical examination may reveal ambiguous genitalia or hyperpigmentation of the areola and scrotum. Laboratory evaluation may reveal hyponatremia, hyperkalemia, and hypoglycemia.

In the acute situation, the child should be hemodynamically stabilized and started on steroids, followed by referral to a pediatric endocrinologist or other physician experienced in the management of this disease.

Genitourinary Disorders

Urinary tract infection is a common cause of sepsis in infants and may be the only clinical finding in the septic neonate. Renal failure in the young infant also can mimic sepsis. This could be due to **posterior urethral valves** causing bladder outlet obstruction. This condition is more common in males, and approximately one third of cases are diagnosed in the first week of life. However, approximately half the cases go undetected for the first few months of life. Parents usually report that the baby has been vomiting or anorectic, but there often are more chronic symptoms such as poor growth or abdominal swelling. Physical examination may reveal findings unusual for sepsis such as hypertension or abdominal mass due to hydronephrosis or urinary ascites.

Metabolic Disorders

Hypoglycemia is common, and it can be catastrophic if not detected and treated promptly. A bedside screening test for blood glucose should be obtained on all severely ill infants and followed with a serum glucose measurement.

Dehydration with or without electrolyte disturbances and acid-base abnormalities can cause an infant to appear quite ill. The degree of dehydration is assessed through evaluation of mental status, urine output, skin character, and vital signs. Young infants who have diarrhea or vomiting can develop marked **hyponatremia** from water intoxication. They will be extremely lethargic, with slow respirations, hypothermia, and possibly seizures. Likewise, dehydrated infants with **hypernatremia** may be irritable or lethargic with muscle weakness, seizures, or coma. In addition, some infants with persistent vomiting have cardiac dysfunction or weakness due to hypokalemia and hypochloremic alkalosis. In addition to gastroenteritis, a cause of hyponatremic dehydration to consider is **cystic fibrosis**. In these cases, the history may be unhelpful initially, except that the infant may reportedly get very ill in hot weather. Such babies may also have poor growth, recent poor intake, or lethargy. There may be a history of cough, tachypnea, or previous pneumonia. More specific questioning may reveal that the baby's skin "tastes salty" or that the baby

had delayed stool production or prolonged jaundice as a newborn. Physical examination shows dehydration, which may be difficult to distinguish from sepsis without laboratory tests.

Rare inborn errors of metabolism, such as inherited urea cycle defects, may cause vomiting, lethargy, seizures, and coma. A common time for these problems to present is when the infant starts to sleep through the night.

Certain **toxins** such as alcohol and salicylates can cause similar problems. Because physical examination will not distinguish poisoned infants from those with sepsis, history of exposure to medications is crucial. Toxic ingestions are discussed in detail in Chapter 9.

Hematologic Disorders

An infant with severe **anemia** caused by blood loss, congenital blood dyscrasia, aplastic disease, or hemolysis will look quite ill. Also, disorders of hemoglobin, including **methemoglobinemia**, can cause an infant to appear toxic. This may result from an inherited disorder or environmental toxicity from oxidizing agents, such as nitrites found in some specimens of well water. Methemoglobinemia also has been described in young infants with severe gastroenteritis and metabolic acidosis. It is thought that the infectious agent that caused the diarrhea or the secondary metabolic acidosis produces the oxidant stress that leads to methemoglobin formation. These infants present with cyanosis, poor feeding, failure to thrive, vomiting, diarrhea, and lethargy. On examination, they appear toxic with hypothermia, hypotension, tachypnea, and tachycardia. The cyanosis is not affected by oxygen administration. Methemoglobinemia is confirmed through specific measurement of methemoglobin in the serum.

Gastrointestinal Disorders

Salmonella or *Shigella* **gastroenteritis** can produce shock in a young infant due to dehydration or sepsis. A history of mucoid or bloody diarrhea may suggest this diagnosis. Fluid resuscitation may improve the infant's appearance and make dehydration the most likely cause for the moribund appearance, but sepsis often must be ruled out through appropriate laboratory studies. The picture may be complicated in *Shigella* infections because secretion of toxin can produce central nervous symptoms.

Pyloric stenosis also can cause severe vomiting, usually in a male infant 4 to 6 weeks old. An infant with pyloric stenosis may present with lethargy and dehydration but usually without fever. A thorough history shows that vomiting, often projectile, is the predominant feature of the illness. There may be a positive family history for pyloric stenosis. Physical examination may reveal an abdominal mass (olive) in 25% to 50% of cases. Ultrasonography or upper gastrointestinal series will further strengthen the diagnosis of pyloric stenosis.

Intussusception also can cause vomiting, irritability, fever, and signs of abdominal pain such as withdrawal of the legs into a flexed position at the hips. Intussusception rarely occurs in infants younger than 5 months old, but it has been reported in some infants aged 2 or 3 months. Infants with this disorder may have spasms of pain followed by periods of lethargy, apathy, and listlessness. Diarrhea without blood may be seen, but blood-streaked or red "currant jelly" stool may point to intussusception rather than sepsis. Physical examination may show an abdominal mass, and bloody stool may be detected on digital examination of the rectum.

Midgut volvulus with or without strangulation may present with emesis, which is usually bilious; abdominal distention; and peritoneal findings. Presentation most commonly occurs in the first week of life. Symptoms and findings may be intermittent. With ischemia, heme-positive or frankly bloody stools will develop. Diagnosis is made on the basis of upper gastrointestinal series. Emergency pediatric surgery consultation and early surgery are required to prevent bowel infarction.

Incarcerated hernias are a leading cause of obstruction in the first 6 months after delivery and may cause an infant to appear septic. A thorough abdominal and groin examination is indicated to prevent this serious problem from being missed.

Hirschsprung's enterocolitis and necrotizing enterocolitis are other gastrointestinal disorders that will cause an infant to appear very ill. **Necrotizing enterocolitis**, which is more common in preterm infants, can occur in the first 10 days after delivery in full-term babies who have had anoxic episodes at birth or other neonatal stresses. These infants present with lethargy, anorexia, irritability, distended abdomen, and, often, bloody stools.

Radiographs that show free air, air in the bowel wall, or air in biliary tree will help make the diagnosis. **Appendicitis** is quite rare but must be considered in the septic-appearing infant with a distended abdomen.

Neurologic Disease

Infant botulism often causes an infant to appear very ill, but they usually maintain normal perfusion and are not tachypneic. This illness is produced by neurotoxins from *Clostridium botulinum*. The history helps distinguish this from sepsis in that infants have a gradual progression of symptoms that include weakness, especially a weak cry; lethargy; and constipation. The disease often is associated with the ingestion of honey or living in a rural environment. On physical examination, the infants usually are afebrile, quite hypotonic, and hyporeflexic. They have a weak cry and may be dehydrated. They may have increased secretions and drooling due to bulbar muscle weakness. Moreover, they may have facial droop, ophthalmoplegia, and diminished gag reflex, which helps distinguish them from infants with sepsis. Apnea also may occur.

Child Abuse

Intracranial hemorrhage resulting from child abuse may occur as part of the **shaken baby syndrome**. Hemorrhage occurs when a young infant is shaken vigorously or thrown against a surface. There may be a history of vigorous shaking of the infant, but more likely there is no admitted violence; instead, the caretaker may report respiratory distress of sudden onset. On examination, the infant may appear gravely ill with apnea, seizures, bradycardia, hypothermia, and poor respiratory effort but may not have obvious physical findings. Although respiratory distress is present, there usually is no stridor, rales, or wheezing. The absence of these findings should lead one to consider a central nervous system etiology.

The anterior fontanel may be full or bulging. There may be other neurologic findings that simulate meningitis, such as nuchal rigidity, irritability, coma, opisthotonic posturing, or seizures. However, retinal hemorrhages, found in ≈85% to 90% of cases, strongly suggest trauma instead of meningitis. Bruises elsewhere on the body are seen only infrequently. Further studies help confirm the diagnosis of shaken baby syndrome, which has a high incidence of morbidity and mortality.

DIAGNOSTIC AIDS

Any ill-appearing young infant should have **laboratory evaluation**, which includes complete blood cell count, urinalysis, electrolytes, blood urea nitrogen, creatinine, rapid glucose evaluation and serum glucose, serum calcium, and bicarbonate level. Cultures of blood, urine, and, usually, cerebrospinal fluid (CSF) also should be obtained. Lumbar puncture may be omitted if another diagnosis is obvious or delayed if the infant appears too ill to tolerate the procedure. CSF that shows pleocytosis with both lymphocytes and red blood cells, with elevated protein, may imply Herpes simplex infection. An arterial blood gas also is indicated. A chest radiograph should be taken. Additional laboratory tests should be guided by results of these studies, as well as by the history and physical examination.

In bacterial sepsis, the complete blood cell count classically shows a leukocytosis with a left shift, but neutropenia also is a frequent finding. However, such findings are not specific and also may be seen with overwhelming viral infections, shaken baby syndrome, cardiac infections such as myocarditis or pericarditis, and gastrointestinal disorders such as neonatal appendicitis and intussusception. Anemia may suggest hemolysis, blood loss, or inhibition of red blood cell production. If the complete blood cell count shows a normal or low total white count but many bands, *Shigella* should be considered. Thrombocytopenia suggests disseminated intravascular coagulopathy or viral sepsis with bone marrow suppression.

The measurement of **electrolytes** is helpful in many cases. Although no specific abnormalities are expected with sepsis, the associated dehydration may produce mild hypernatremia or hyponatremia. Hyponatremia also should cause the practitioner to consider gastroenteritis, water intoxication, syndrome of inappropriate secretion of antidiuretic hormone, cystic fibrosis, and salicylate toxicity. If such hyponatremia is associated with marked hyperkalemia, congenital adrenal hyperplasia (CAH) should be considered. CAH is confirmed by serum analysis for 17-hydroxy progesterone, renin, aldosterone, and cortisol levels. Also, low serum electrolyte levels in a dehydrated baby, especially without gastrointestinal losses, make cystic fibrosis or meningitis a likely diagnosis. A lumbar puncture or sweat test could confirm these diagnoses. Hypochloremia, hypokalemia, and metabolic alkalosis associated with significant vomiting suggest pyloric stenosis and should lead to confirmation of the diagnosis with an ultrasound or upper gastrointestinal series.

Measurement of **blood glucose** is crucial in a young infant who appears ill. Hypoglycemia can result from overwhelming sepsis or viremia, as glycogen stores are rapidly depleted in the ill infant. However, profound hypoglycemia also may be found with CAH and salicylism, or it can be a marker for metabolic diseases such as inborn errors of metabolism.

Evaluation of **serum bicarbonate** often is helpful. Acidosis or alkalosis can be verified with an arterial blood gas. Acidosis can be expected with sepsis or other conditions that lead to poor perfusion, such as left heart obstruction, dehydration, or CAH with shock. It also may be found with renal failure, inborn errors of metabolism, or salicylism. A severe metabolic acidosis is noted with methemoglobinemia (pH 6.9 to 7.2); in fact, this may precipitate the methemoglobin formation. Although acidosis is a somewhat nonspecific indicator of poor perfusion, alkalosis is less common in ill infants. The finding of alkalosis, especially in the presence of vomiting, hypochloremia, and hypokalemia, should suggest pyloric stenosis. Alkalosis also is found in some metabolic disorders, such as urea cycle defects. Aspirin poisoning can cause alkalosis, so measurement of a salicylate level should be considered.

A **chest radiograph** is necessary in the evaluation of a very ill young infant. It may show pneumonia, which suggests bacterial disease and sepsis. It is not always easy to distinguish an infiltrate from atelectasis, which can be seen with RSV infections or infant botulism. Diffuse patchy infiltrates and atelectasis may point to a viral illness, such as RSV, rather than bacterial pneumonia. Certainly, the chest radiograph is a useful tool for evaluation of possible cardiac disease. The presence of pulmonary edema or cardiomegaly should lead to consideration of problems other than sepsis.

Other diagnostic studies should be obtained if there are specific findings on history or physical examination or the initial tests are abnormal. If a septic-appearing infant has petechiae or purpura, a coagulation profile is indicated to look for disseminated intravascular coagulopathy. If there is localized infection (eg, septic arthritis), fluid should be aspirated for culture and Gram stain.

For patients with vesicular skin lesions, a Tzanck smear or direct fluorescent antibody staining of vesicle scraping may offer a rapid diagnosis of herpes simplex virus. If this condition is suspected, culture skin vesicles, mouth or nasopharynx, eyes, urine, blood, CSF, stool or rectum. A computed tomography scan may be helpful. Antiviral therapy should not be delayed while awaiting results of diagnostic tests.

If wheezing is noted, a rapid slide test and culture for RSV is important. Also, if syphilis is suspected because of the clinical presentation described above, radiographic studies can be obtained to look for characteristic diffuse periostitis of several bones. A serologic test for syphilis is needed to confirm the diagnosis.

When **cardiac disease** is suspected, an ECG or echocardiogram will be helpful in making the diagnosis of congenital heart disease. The ECG often will show right or left ventricular hypertrophy and an abnormal axis. If pericarditis or myocarditis is suspected on the basis of physical examination or the appearance of a large heart on chest radiograph, an ECG may show generalized T-wave inversion and low-voltage QRS complexes, especially when pericardial fluid is present. ST-T wave abnormalities may also be seen. An echocardiogram is essential to confirm the presence or absence of pericardial effusion and evaluate cardiac anatomy and myocardial function. It also is essential in confirming the diagnosis of left heart obstruction. The suspicion of SVT may be confirmed with a rhythm strip showing regular atrial and ventricular beats with 1:1 conduction at a rate usually >220 beats/min. P waves may be retrograde and difficult to see because they often are buried in the T waves.

Cyanosis in the ill infant usually is related to respiratory disease, cardiac shunting, or low cardiac output. As noted above, however, cyanosis with severe diarrhea and metabolic acidosis that does not improve with supplemental oxygen makes methemoglobinemia likely. The PaO_2 will be normal, but the SaO_2 will be low. The blood gas specimen also should be measured for the methemoglobin level, which may be elevated up to 65% (normal 0% to 2%). The blood may appear chocolate brown when exposed to air or placed on filter paper and waved in the air.

In young infants with an **abdominal mass** associated with hypertension and vomiting, posterior urethral valves might be suspected. Serum creatinine and blood urea nitrogen usually are elevated markedly. A suprapubic ultrasound will demonstrate a dilated posterior urethra and bladder, strongly suggesting posterior urethral valves.

Abdominal mass, distention, or tenderness associated with vomiting or bloody stool might lead the physician to obtain an **abdominal radiograph**. This may show evidence of small bowel obstruction in the case of intussusception or volvulus. It may show pneumatosis cystoides intestinalis caused by gas in the intestinal wall with necrotizing enterocolitis, or it may show a paucity of gas in the right lower quadrant, evidence of free peritoneal fluid, or a right abdominal wall thickened by edema with appendicitis. In some cases, **abdominal ultrasound** will add information (ie, assist in the diagnosis of pyloric stenosis). If intussusception is suspected, an air or a barium enema may be diagnostic by showing a filling defect near the ileocecal valve. If bloody diarrhea is found without other significant abdominal pathology, a stool culture and stool smear for leukocytes may be helpful in evaluation of bacterial etiology.

If infant botulism is considered, a stool specimen to identify toxins of *C. botulinum* can be ordered, as can electromyography, which shows decreased muscle action potential with the "staircase" phenomenon in this disease.

If intracranial hemorrhage is suspected, computed tomography scan or magnetic resonance imaging is indicated. If child abuse is suspected, obtain radiographs of the skull, chest, and long bones to look for occult fractures.

MANAGEMENT

Any young infant who is critically ill initially should be presumed to have sepsis. Figure 14-1 summarizes the approach to the septic-appearing infant. Because sepsis is a life-threatening illness that may respond to early treatment, it is imperative to stabilize the child rapidly. While airway, breathing, and circulation are being assessed and managed appropriately, vascular access should be obtained. Unless an alternative diagnosis, as discussed above, is immediately obvious, it is best to draw a blood culture and administer intravenous antibiotics while pursuing alternative diagnoses. A common empiric regimen is ampicillin and gentamicin for infants younger than 4 weeks. Cefotaxime should be substituted for gentamicin in infants 4 weeks to 3 months of age and is used by some in those children younger than 4 weeks

(Table 3-3). Cefotaxime or ceftriaxone is recommended for infants 3 to 24 months of age. Consider the addition of intravenous acyclovir (500 mg/m2 q8h) if herpes simplex infection is suspected. Fluids are administered as outlined in Chapter 3.

A complete history should be obtained by other personnel while the infant is being stabilized. A careful physical examination should be performed once immediate management issues are attended to. Laboratory studies should be ordered, guided by information obtained from the history and physical

FIGURE 14-1.
Initial approach to the septic-appearing child.

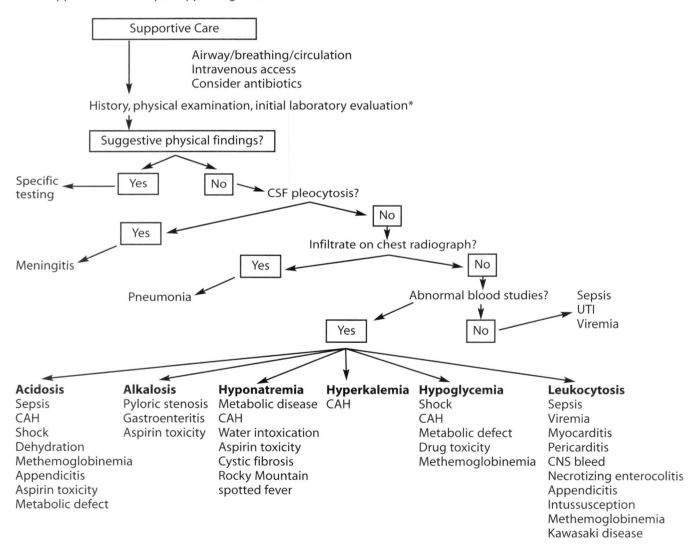

*Initial laboratory evaluation includes culture of blood, urine, usually cerebrospinal fluid, chest radiograph, CBC, urinalysis, electrolytes, rapid and serum glucose, bicarbonate, and possibly arterial blood gases.

examination. A lumbar puncture is performed when the infant is stabilized, but performance of lumbar puncture should not be allowed to delay the administration of antibiotics in the unstable child. When a diagnosis other than sepsis is confirmed, management protocols can be altered and referral to appropriate subspecialists considered.

ADDITIONAL READING

American Academy of Pediatrics. *1997 Red Book: Report of the Committee on Infectious Diseases*, 24th ed. Elk Grove Village, Ill: American Academy of Pediatrics; 1997.

American Academy of Pedatrics, Provisional Committe on Quality Improvement, Subcommittee on Febrile Seizures. Practice parameter: the neurodiagnostic evaluation of the child with a first simple febrile seizure. *Pediatrics.* 1996;97:769-772.

Arvin AM, Prober CG. Herpes simplex virus infections: the genital tract and the newborn. *Pediatr Rev.* 1992;13:107-112.

Avner JR, Henretig FM, McAneney CM. Acquired methemoglobinemia. The relationship of cause to course of illness. Am J Dis Child. 1990;144:1229-1230.Belfer RA. The emergency department evaluation of the febrile infant and child with HIV infection. *AIDS Reader* 1994;Jan-Feb:8-12.

Baraff LJ, Bass JW, Fleisher GR, et al. Practice guideline for the management of infants and children 0 to 36 months of age with fever without source. Agency for Health Care Policy and Research. *Ann Emerg Med* 1992;22:1198-1210.

Byard RW, Edmonds JF, Silverman E, et al. Respiratory distress and fever in a 2-month old infant. *J Pediatr.* 1991;118:306-313.

Crain EF, Gershel JC. Urinary tract infections in febrile infants younger than 8 weeks of age. *Pediatrics.* 1990;86:363-367.

Hall CB. Respiratory syncytial virus: what we know now. *Contemp Pediatr.* 1993;Nov:92-110.

Hampers L, Tunnessen WW. A neonate in extremis. *Contemp Pediatr.* 1995;Jul:91-93.

Hurst DL, Marsh WW. Early severe infantile botulism. *J Pediatr.* 1993;122:909-911.

Press S, Lipkind RS. Acute myocarditis in infants. Initial presentation. *Clin Pediatr.* 1990;29:73-76.

Saez-Llorens X, McCracken GH. Sepsis syndrome and septic shock in pediatrics: current concepts of terminology, pathophysiology, and management. *J Pediatr.* 1993;123:497-508.

Selbst SM. The septic-appearing infant. In: Fleisher GR, Ludwig S, eds. *Synopsis of Pediatric Emergency Medicine.* Baltimore, Md: Williams & Wilkins; 1996; 233-238.

Ward JC. Inborn errors of metabolism of acute onset in infancy. *Pediatr Rev.* 1990;11:205-216.

Chapter 15

Meningitis

OBJECTIVES

1. Describe the clinical signs of life-threatening central nervous system infection.

2. Explain the appropriate sequence and timing of therapeutic intervention.

Practitioners who see children frequently must diagnose and treat pediatric infectious diseases. They must decide which children have relatively benign illnesses and which have septicemia or meningitis. The presentations of serious infections may not be obvious. Practitioners must be able to rapidly recognize and manage meningitis. This diagnosis should be entertained in any child with thermal instability or central nervous system (CNS) dysfunction. Like the surgeon who must perform some negative laparotomies to avoid missing cases of appendicitis, the practitioner managing febrile infants must perform a certain percentage of negative lumbar punctures to avoid missing cases of meningitis.

To help the practitioner make the correct diagnosis, this chapter primarily is concerned with the assessment and emergency interventions appropriate for children with suspected bacterial meningitis. There also is a discussion of lumbar puncture technique with a brief review of interpretation of the results.

PATHOPHYSIOLOGY

Meningitis results from the hematogenous spread of bacteria from distant areas of infection or colonization, most commonly colonization of the nasopharynx. Much less commonly, meningitis occurs secondary to direct extension from a local infection such as sinusitis or orbital cellulitis. Infants and young children particularly are vulnerable because of immature immune responses and lack of previous exposure to the organisms commonly causing meningitis. The **inflammatory response** to both the initial bacterial invasion and the cytokine inflammatory mediators released in response to **antibiotic therapy** results in CNS damage. The goals of meningitis therapy are to control the infection and control the secondary effects of the infection (eg, inflammation, seizures, increased intracranial pressure).

INITIAL ASSESSMENT

The first step in providing appropriate therapy is to recognize signs and symptoms that suggest a high probability of meningitis. The practitioner must pay careful attention to all aspects of clinical assessment because the signs and symptoms can be very subtle. As is true with many other pediatric illnesses, the younger the child, the more nonspecific are the signs and symptoms.

The Neonate

Neonates with meningitis lack specific manifestations; diagnosing these patients can be a formidable problem. Parents may state that the infant feeds poorly or has a fever, but even these signs may be absent. *Fever, restlessness, irritability that is inconsolable, or a listless response to social contact may be the only clues.* Use of subtle observational cues can aid greatly in the detection of sick children, especially infants. Social contact or "playfulness" is a major indicator of health. Appropriate contact with both the examiner and the surrounding environment may be the best predictor of general well-being.

Listless infants may become more lethargic and unresponsive as meningitis progresses. Seizure activity also may be seen. Alterations in respiratory patterns or cardiovascular status are nonspecific and are late manifestations of intracranial infection. Late signs include **Cheyne-Stokes respirations** and **Cushing's reflex**, consisting of progressive systemic hypertension with a widened pulse pressure, bradycardia, and a decreased respiratory rate. Nuchal rigidity, a more specific sign of meningeal irritation, occurs in fewer than a fourth of infants with meningitis. Similarly, a bulging fontanel, diastasis of the sutures, or opisthotonos may be seen infrequently late in the course of meningitis.

A lumbar puncture must be an early consideration. However, inability to obtain an adequate lumbar puncture sample must not delay the prompt administration of intravenous antibiotics. Waiting until late signs present may subject the infant to harm and death.

Infants and Children

In older infants and children, meningitis may be more easily diagnosed on the basis of presenting signs and symptoms. Fever, irritability, disturbances of sensorium, generalized seizure activity, focal neurologic signs, photophobia, anorexia, and vomiting frequently are seen in children with meningitis. Verbal children typically complain of a severe headache. *Children with meningeal irritation often prefer not to be carried or walk but instead remain recumbent, sometimes assuming the fetal position.* After the first year of life, nuchal rigidity is seen reliably in the acute phase of meningitis. It is not seen immediately after seizure activity when both the Kernig and Brudzinski signs also are blunted. The absence of nuchal rigidity at any age, however, does not rule out intracranial infection.

INDICATIONS FOR LUMBAR PUNCTURE

When the subtle manifestations of meningitis in children are recognized, lumbar puncture should be performed. The threshold of clinical suspicion that leads to lumbar puncture should be lower for the following groups of patients: neonates, immunocompromised children, children in close contact with someone who has meningitis, and children with documented bacteremia. *Remember, infants in the first month of life do not manifest the expected clinical signs and symptoms of meningitis.* Extreme lethargy or uncompromising irritability may be the only clinical manifestations in the young febrile infant.

Similarly, the immunocompromised child with neutrophil dysfunction, hyposplenism, or defective cellular or humoral immunity may not exhibit the typical clinical manifestations of serious infection. Focal or disseminated infection in those patients may be characterized by fever, a gradual onset of prodromal symptoms, and an apparent state of well-being that may proceed rapidly to circulatory collapse and death. Children closely exposed to others with meningococcal disease or invasive *Haemophilus influenzae* type b (Hib) disease who have not received adequate Hib vaccination are at risk for intracranial infection. Likewise, children with unexplained fever and a recent diagnosis of bacteremia are at risk for persistent bacteremia and intracranial infection. In other high-risk patients, such as febrile children with skull fracture and leakage of cerebrospinal fluid (CSF) or children with petechial rashes in association with febrile illness, a lumbar puncture should be seriously considered. The old axiom still holds true: *If one seriously considers the diagnosis of meningitis or the need to do a lumbar puncture, then a lumbar puncture should be done.*

Rapid intervention with a lumbar puncture in a

child who has increased intracranial pressure may lead, on rare occasion, to the potentially fatal complication of herniation, as evidenced by sudden changes in vital signs, sudden dilation and nonreactivity of a pupil, or a sixth cranial nerve palsy. In selected cases, a computed tomography (CT) scan may be warranted before lumbar puncture. For example, a child with focal neurologic findings, findings suggestive of increased intracranial pressure, or a ventriculoperitoneal shunt should have a CT scan before lumbar puncture. A lumbar puncture need not be done on every child with a febrile seizure, as long as the source of the fever can be readily identified and the seizure is not prolonged or focal. If the child with an apparent febrile seizure is not typical, ie, exhibits petechiae, nuchal rigidity, focal neurologic signs, inconsolable irritability, or a prolonged postictal state, CSF examination is warranted. In the seriously ill, toxic child in whom bacterial meningitis is suspected, lumbar puncture can be withheld until after stabilization and initiation of appropriate antibiotics.

DIFFERENTIAL DIAGNOSIS

Most patients beyond the neonatal period with bacterial meningitis appear acutely ill. Other etiologies of the child's toxic presentation also must be considered, including septicemia without coexistent meningitis. Septicemia must be ruled out because of its high potential for morbidity and mortality and because of the possibility of coexisting meningitis. Toxic infants with major infections in other areas, such as the lungs and urinary tract, may present with a broad range of nonspecific findings.

Nuchal rigidity always should provoke strong consideration of meningitis. However, in many other conditions patients may present with an apparent "stiff neck," including very serious (eg, pneumonia, peritonsillar abscess, brain tumor) and less serious (eg, cervical adenitis, rotatory torticollis, shigellosis) conditions.

Trauma may complicate the differential diagnosis. Although in most instances the practitioner will know by the history whether the child had a traumatic insult, in the case of child abuse, that clue often will be lacking. Children with head trauma and intracranial hemorrhage, especially those with the shaken baby syndrome,

often present as if they had afebrile meningitis. Retinal bleeding on ophthalmoscopy and bloody CSF on lumbar puncture suggest trauma. If abuse is suspected, a CT scan should be obtained before lumbar puncture.

EVALUATION AND MANAGEMENT

Critical and Unstable Patient

The top priority in management must be stabilization of the patient's vital signs and preservation of cardiopulmonary and cerebral function. These aspects are discussed first.

The unstable patient with meningitis may have respiratory or circulatory failure, increased intracranial pressure, seizure activity, or hypoglycemia. As with all patients requiring emergency care, regardless of the age, first stabilize the patient by following the ABCs. Ensure adequate airway and ventilation. Even if spontaneous and adequate respirations are present, administer supplemental oxygen to all critical, unstable children. If the child's ventilations are shallow or breathing is irregular after simple airway-opening maneuvers have been attempted, initially assist ventilation with the bag-valve-mask. Then perform endotracheal intubation as indicated by clinical assessment or interpretation of arterial blood gases.

Patients who present with altered sensorium may be in shock. Obtain intravenous access to allow rapid infusion of 20 mL/kg volume-expanding fluid such as normal saline or lactated Ringer's. Care should be taken, however to not fluid overload the patient who has meningitis. If blood pressure is normal or high after the initial fluid bolus, further fluid administration should be limited to two thirds of the usual maintenance rate. Insert a urinary catheter to monitor output. Dextrose should be administered if hypoglycemia is demonstrated. Vasopressors may be required, but withhold them at least until adequate ventilations are provided and a trial of volume expansion has been done. Remember, if the patient is febrile, the fluid requirement is increased.

Initiate anticonvulsant therapy if the child is actively seizing, starting with a dose of an intravenous benzodiazepine, which may be repeated if needed, and followed later by intravenous phenytoin (see Chapter 17).

In a patient with meningitis, the presence of

papilledema or other signs of increased intracranial pressure requires immediate therapy. An infant with open sutures may have a full fontanel but does not require therapy unless there are other signs of intracranial pressure. Elevate the patient's head 20 degrees and place it in a midline position. Initiate controlled ventilation so that the $PaCO_2$ is brought down to 30 to 35 mm Hg. Serial arterial blood gas determinations are necessary to confirm adequate therapy.

A glucose oxidase reagent tape should be used to rapidly estimate the child's **blood glucose**. Meningitis often is complicated by metabolic derangements, poor oral intake, and vomiting, all of which can lead to hypoglycemia. If the patient's blood glucose is <40 mg/dL, administer an infusion of glucose at a dose of 250 to 500 mg/kg intravenously (as 10% dextrose for neonates and 25% dextrose for infants younger than 2 years). The glucose content in the intravenous fluids may need to be increased. Watch for glycosuria and osmotic diuresis.

After those supportive measures have been accomplished, other diagnostic tests are ordered, including complete blood cell count, blood cultures, electrolytes, blood urea nitrogen, creatinine, serum glucose, and a portable chest radiograph.

In these severely ill children, it is imperative to start specific intravenous antimicrobial therapy at the earliest opportunity, preferably without waiting for results of laboratory tests or performance of the lumbar puncture. (Further discussion of corticosteroid and intravenous antimicrobial therapy follows.)

Critical but Stable Patient

Many pediatric patients with suspected meningitis have adequate oxygenation and ventilation, normal blood pressure, hemodynamics, and intracranial pressure. In such instances, a time-efficient and orderly diagnostic protocol can be carried out. This diagnostic protocol involves phlebotomy before lumbar puncture (Table 15-1).

Alterations in the total white blood cell count, differential, and red blood cell morphology, although nonspecific, may lend support to the diagnosis of meningitis. Normal parameters, however, do not lower the potential for diagnosis of meningitis in the appropriate clinical setting.

It is important to replenish body fluids in a dehydrated child by supplying sequential 10 to 20 mL/kg boluses of normal saline over 20-minute periods until hypovolemia is corrected. Next, maintain intravenous fluid therapy while waiting for results of the CSF analysis. If the child has a glucose oxidase or serum glucose level of <40 mg/dL, use an electrolyte solution containing 10% glucose. If the child has a normal blood glucose level, then use either normal saline solution (if patient is in shock) or D5 0.5 NS. Keep in mind that overzealous use of intravenous fluids can contribute to the development of cerebral edema. Both cerebral edema from overhydration and the inadequate hydration of a febrile child with meningitis worsen the prognosis.

Urine output is a gauge for adequate fluid therapy with an objective of 0.5 to 1.0 mL/kg per hour. A specimen of urine should be cultured; use the remainder for urinalysis, specific gravity, and

---

TABLE 15-1.
Diagnostic protocol for patients suspected of having meningitis.

Phlebotomy
   Glucose oxidase strip
   Serum glucose level
   Electrolytes, blood urea nitrogen
   Complete blood cell count
   Blood culture
Lumbar Puncture
   Manometrics
   Culture
   Protein, glucose levels
   Cell count and differential
   Gram stain
   Latex agglutination if there has been prior treatment
Intravenous Fluids
   Bolus 10-20 mL/kg normal saline and repeat until perfusion is normalized.
   Push 0.25-0.5 g/kg glucose if serum glucose is <40 mg/dL.
   Maintenance:
      Run 10% dextrose in one-half normal saline if glucose oxidase strip is <40 mg/dL (at three fourths of maintenance rate) or run 5% dextrose in one-half normal saline if glucose oxidase strip is >40 mg/dL (at three fourths maintenance rate).
Miscellaneous
   Urinalysis
   Urine culture
   Blood gas determination
   Chest radiograph

bacterial antigen determinations, such as the latex agglutination test or countercurrent immunoelectrophoresis.

Lumbar Puncture

The procedure for lumbar puncture is described in Appendix 15-1.

When pleocytosis exceeds 500 cells/mL, CSF glucose is <50% of the simultaneously obtained blood glucose level, or the Gram stain shows microorganisms, the diagnosis usually is bacterial meningitis (Table 15-2).

The provisional diagnosis should be bacterial meningitis in any child with a compatible clinical syndrome regardless of the CSF findings. The common CSF findings with viral and bacterial meningitis are listed (Table 15-2). CSF that later grows bacterial pathogens, however, occasionally may have a normal cell count and chemistries, especially in immunocompromised children. Conversely, CSF cellular response and chemistry with viral meningitis may resemble that classically seen with bacterial meningitis. The organisms most commonly responsible for bacterial meningitis are listed in Table 15-3.

Other Tests

The practitioner may want to use other tests to help delineate the specific organism causing the infection. Performance of a Gram stain on the buffy coat of the blood or on a scraping of any petechial lesions may give such information. Patients who have been pretreated with antibiotics may have sterile cultures. Countercurrent immunoelectrophoresis or latex agglutination can be performed on urine, serum, and CSF to detect bacterial capsular antigens such as Hib, *Streptococcus pneumoniae*, and *Neisseria meningitidis*. These tests are expensive, however, and often not helpful in the acute situation.

ANTIBIOTIC AND CORTICOSTEROID TREATMENT

Definitive management of the patient with presumed bacterial meningitis is administration of intravenous antibiotics. If the child has had inadequate vaccination against Hib, corticosteroids are indicated before the first dose of antibiotics. The corticosteroids are believed to blunt the inflammatory response to bacterial cell death after the administration of antibiotics in patients with Hib meningitis. In this fashion, the incidence of hearing loss and other complications of meningitis is diminished. However, only 86 cases of invasive Hib disease in children younger than 5 years were reported in the United States in 1995. Because of the Hib vaccine has virtually eliminated this disease in children, a careful immunization history is mandatory. With other bacterial pathogens, the use of corticosteroids has not been well studied. When

TABLE 15-2.
Common cerebrospinal fluid findings.

	Normal*	Bacterial	Viral
Appearance	Clear	Clear to cloudy	Clear
Cell count (WBCs/mm³)	<10	>100-20,000	>10-500
Differential (% PMNs)	0	>90	0-30†
Glucose (mg/dL)	50-90	<40	50-90
Protein (mg/dL)	15-45	100-500	50-100
Gram stain (bacterial)	Negative	Positive	Negative

*In the neonatal period, these normal values may vary as follows: cell count, <22 WBCs/mm³ with <60% PMNs; glucose, 34-119 mg/dL; and protein, 20-170 mg/dL.
†May be predominantly polymorphonuclear neutrophil leukocytes (PMNs) early in the course of the illness.

TABLE 15-3.
Common bacterial organisms.

The most common bacterial organisms causing meningitis vary with age.

Age	Organism
1st month	Group B *Streptococcus* *Escherichia coli* *N. meningitidis* *Listeria*
2nd month	Group B *Streptococcus* *N. meningitidis* *H. influenzae* type b
3rd month and older	*S. pneumoniae* *N. meningitidis* *H. influenzae* type b

indicated, give dexamethasone in a dose of 0.15 mg/kg IV.

The choice of antibiotic therapy varies with age and possibly with the availability of a laboratory to monitor serum levels of some of the potential antibiotics (Table 15-4). In the first month of life, **ampicillin plus an aminoglycoside** (gentamicin, tobramycin, or amikacin) are the usual drugs of choice, although **ampicillin plus cefotaxime** may be equally effective. For the young infant, in the absence of evidence that suggests the presence of unusual organisms, conventional therapy is **ampicillin and a third-generation cephalosporin.** Beyond the third month of life, **a third-generation cephalosporin alone** will provide adequate antibacterial coverage. The rates of clinical response, eradication of organisms, and most meningitis sequelae are approximately equivalent with single-drug therapy as with multidrug regimens in children.

Therapy should be modified when Gram's stain of the CSF demonstrates a presumptive pathogen (Table 15-5). Resistance of invasive strains of *S. pneumoniae* to penicillin and cephalosporins has increased over the past few years. Because **vancomycin** is the only antibiotic to which all strains of *S. pneumoniae* are susceptible, vancomycin in combination with a **broad-spectrum cephalosporin** is recommended when Gram-positive cocci are identified on Gram's stain of the CSF.

Care after hospital admission should ensure that the pediatric patient receives continuous monitoring of level of consciousness and cardiopulmonary status. Vital signs can change rapidly; some children require care in an intensive care setting to provide monitoring and maintain the crucial intravenous lines. Immediate intervention for life-threatening events must be available at all times.

TABLE 15-4.
Initial dose for empiric antibiotic therapy for meningitis.

Category	Antibiotic	Initial Dose
Neonatal (0-28 days)	Ampicillin **and**	100 mg/kg
	gentamicin	2.5 mg/kg
Infant (29-90 days)	Ampicillin **and**	100 mg/kg
	cefotaxime	50 mg/kg
	OR	
	ampicillin **and**	100 mg/kg
	ceftriaxone	100 mg/kg
	OR	
	ampicillin **and**	100 mg/kg
	chloramphenicol*	25 mg/kg
Child	Cefotaxime **OR**	50 mg/kg
	ceftriaxone **OR**	100 mg/kg
	ampicillin **and**	100 mg/kg
	chloramphenicol*	25 mg/kg

* This choice has been supplanted by the other agents listed but is included as an option for use in locations in which cephalosporins may not be available.

TABLE 15-5.
Recommendations for antibiotic therapy based on Gram's stain of cerebrospinal fluid.

Type of Bacteria on Gram's Stain	Choice of Antibiotic	Recommended Initial Dose
Cocci		
Gram-positive	Vancomycin **and**	15 mg/kg
	cefotaxime	50 mg/kg
Gram-negative	Penicillin G	300,000 units/kg per day
Bacilli		
Gram-positive	Ampicillin **and**	100 mg/kg
	gentamicin	2.5 mg/kg loading dose
Gram-negative	Cefotaxime **and**	50 mg/kg
	gentamicin	2.5 mg/kg loading dose

From Quagliarello VJ, Scheld VM. Drug therapy: treatment of bacterial meningitis. *N Engl J Med.* 1997;336:712. Copyright 1997, Massachusetts Medical Society. All rights reserved.

ADDITIONAL READING

American Academy of Pediatrics, Committee on Infectious Diseases. Therapy for children with invasive pneumococcal infections. *Pediatrics.* 1997;99:289-299.

Progress toward elimination of *Haemophilus influenzae* type b disease among infants and children—United States, 1987-1995. *MMWR Morb Mortal Wkly Rep.* 1996;45:901-906.

Givner LB, Woods CR, Abramson JS. The practice of pediatrics in the era of vaccines effective against *Haemophilus influenzae* type b. *Pediatrics.* 1994;93:680-681. Editorial.

Lelyveld S. Meningitis: In: Strange GR, Ahrens WR, Lelyveld S, et al, eds. *Pediatric Emergency Medicine: A Comprehensive Study Guide.* New York, NY: McGraw-Hill; 1996:263-266.

Nozicka CA. Pediatric meningitis: clinical guidelines, issues and update. *Pediatr Emerg Med Rep.* 1997;2:47-56.

Odio CM, Faingezicht I, Paris M, et al. The beneficial effects of early dexamethasone administration in infants and children with bacterial meningitis. *N Engl J Med.* 1991;324:1525-1531.

Quagliarello VJ, Scheld WM. Bacterial meningitis: pathogenesis, pathophysiology, and progress. *N Engl J Med.*1992;327:864-872.

Quagliarello VJ, Scheld WM. Treatment of bacterial meningitis. *N Engl J Med.* 1997;336:708-716.

Schoendorf KC, Adams WG, Kiely JL, et al. National trends in *Haemophilus influenzae* meningitis mortality and hospitalization among children, 1980 through 1991. *Pediatrics.* 1994;93:663-668.

Wald ER, Kaplan SL, Mason EO, et al. Dexamethasone therapy for children with bacterial meningitis. *Pediatrics.* 1995;95:21-28

Appendix 15-1. Lumbar Puncture Procedure.

Proper performance of the lumbar puncture is necessary to ensure procurement of adequate specimens and minimize the risk of obtaining a "bloody tap." A lumbar puncture may be contraindicated in children who have clotting disorders or evidence of elevated intracranial pressure thought to be due to mass lesion. An effort should be made to visualize the optic discs before the procedure.

Appropriate positioning of the child is vital. Although the lateral recumbent position (**fetal position**) generally is preferred, in neonates, it may be better to have the infant in a sitting position. An assistant who restrains the child must pay close attention to the child's vital signs because airway compromise may be an inadvertent byproduct of positioning. The child also may spontaneously deteriorate during the procedure. The oxygen saturation should be monitored with pulse oximetry during the procedure. All children will benefit from injected or topical local anesthesia.

The best level of the spine for local anesthesia and subsequent puncture is the L4-5 interspace in neonates or the L3-4 interspace in older patients. The L3-4 interspace can be located by drawing an imaginary line transversely between the two posterior iliac crests. (If a difficult or bloody tap is encountered, use the next higher interspace.) Prepare and drape the area; carry out the entire procedure under strict aseptic conditions. The stylet of the needle must be in place whenever advancing the needle to prevent introduction of a fragment of soft tissue into the subarachnoid space. Anesthetize the skin and deep structures in the midline just above the spinous process at the chosen level. Then slowly advance the spinal needle perpendicular to the axis of the spine or slightly cephalad with angulation toward the umbilicus. Stop frequently and remove the stylet to check for the appearance of CSF through the needle lumen as evidence of entry into the subarachnoid space. (The infant's dura mater may not allow the practitioner to feel a "give" as is common with adults.) It may take several seconds for the CSF to migrate down the needle. The entire process must not be rushed. Advancement of the needle too far often is signaled by the appearance of blood in the needle lumen due to penetration of the anterior spinal venous plexus (**a bloody tap**).

Once CSF is obtained, a manometer may be attached if measurement of the opening pressure is desired. Next, allow 0.5 to 1.0 mL of fluid to drip slowly into each of three sterile tubes. Then slowly withdraw the needle with the stylet in place. Be sure to remove all excessive iodine-containing skin preparations because they may cause skin irritation. An adhesive bandage should be placed to protect the puncture site on the skin. Send the tubes of fluid to the laboratory for the tests shown in Table 15-6.

TABLE 15-6.
Recommended order for tubes for cerebrospinal fluid.

Tube 1	Gram's stain, bacterial culture, and sensitivity
Tube 2	Protein and glucose levels
Tube 3 (or clearest tube)	Cell count and differential

A fourth tube may be collected for any of the following: a repeat cell count and differential, especially if the count on tube 1 suggests a bloody tap; countercurrent immunoelectrophoresis; latex agglutination tests; or fungal and viral cultures. Alternatively, this tube can be frozen for later use.

Chapter 16

Diabetic Ketoacidosis

OBJECTIVES

1. Explain the disordered metabolic processes that lead to the ketoacidotic state in a diabetic and the mechanism of reversal of those processes in the acute setting.

2. Outline an appropriate sequence of therapeutic interventions for use during the first hour of management of a child with diabetic ketoacidosis.

3. Identify the common pitfalls encountered in management of diabetic ketoacidosis.

Diabetes mellitus is the most common life-threatening pediatric endocrine disorder. Prevalence of the disease increases to 1 in 60 by age 15. Most children with diabetes have insulin-dependent diabetes, an autoimmune disease that destroys pancreatic β cells and leads to complete dependence on administered insulin. This form of diabetes has also been called **type I**, or **juvenile**, diabetes. Non–insulin-dependent diabetes is synonymous with **type II**, or **maturity-onset**, diabetes.

Children with diabetes often present in **ketoacidosis**. Diabetic ketoacidosis (DKA) is a true medical emergency with an overall mortality rate of 2% to 10%. A substantial percentage of these deaths are preventable if metabolic derangements and complications are recognized and appropriate treatment is administered in a timely manner.

In previously diagnosed patients, DKA may occur as a result of inadequate knowledge of the disease on the part of the patient and family. Psychological and socioeconomic factors may cause poor compliance, resulting in failure on the part of the patient to administer insulin for secondary gain or as a suicidal gesture or resulting in lack of necessary supplies because of the patient's financial difficulties. Acute illness, especially those associated with vomiting, also can alter glucose levels in a previously well-controlled diabetic patient and lead to DKA.

PATHOPHYSIOLOGY

In DKA, lack of insulin prevents glucose from entering the cells, so the cell is unable to meet its metabolic requirements. In response to this, there is a release of counterregulatory hormones (CRHs), epinephrine, glucagon, cortisol, and growth hormone. CRHs cause hepatic glucose production and glycogen breakdown (gluconeogenesis), as well as increased lipolysis within adipose tissue.

The abnormalities in glucose metabolism result in progressive hyperglycemia, but decreased glucose utilization by peripheral tissues persists because of insulin deficiency. Lipolysis releases long-chain fatty acids that are oxidized by the liver, producing ketoacids, primarily β-hydroxybutyrate and acetoacetate. Hydrogen ions released from these acids produce a metabolic acidosis, which causes a shift of potassium to the extracellular fluid, where it is excreted in the urine, leading to total body potassium depletion.

Hyperglycemia leads to osmotic diuresis and fluid loss. **Ketonemia** can cause nausea, vomiting, and abdominal pain, thereby interfering with fluid intake and worsening dehydration.

Elevated catecholamines cause diaphoresis and tachycardia. Metabolic acidosis evokes tachypnea and compensatory respiratory alkalosis. Insensible fluid loss is increased. All of those factors can result in profound dehydration and, ultimately, shock. When this occurs, lactic acidosis produced by anaerobic metabolism will compound the preexisting ketoacidosis.

ASSESSMENT

Signs and Symptoms

The classic presentation of DKA includes weight loss, polyuria, polydipsia, polyphagia, weakness, vomiting, and abdominal pain with the characteristic "fruity" acetone breath and the deep, regular sighing breathing pattern known as **Kussmaul respirations**. Alteration in level of consciousness varies.

Mild forms of DKA can present with symptoms that are vague and difficult to diagnose. Symptoms of vomiting, malaise, anorexia, low-grade fever, or abdominal pain can occur alone or in combination. The patient can present with tachycardia, tachypnea, fever, dehydration, or mental status changes. Ketoacidosis should be considered in any diabetic patient presenting with any of the above symptoms.

Dehydration

The child in severe DKA always is dehydrated. The exact amount of the dehydration can be difficult to determine because most children will compensate well with tachycardia and peripheral vasoconstriction. When compensatory mechanisms are exhausted, vascular collapse may occur quite suddenly. Hyperosmolarity causes fluid to be drawn from the cells into the intravascular space, thereby preserving the intravascular volume in the face of severe total body fluid deficit. The dehydrated child generally will have dry oral mucous membranes and sunken eyes and may complain of thirst. If a

TABLE 16-1.
Diagnostic tests for assessment of diabetic ketoacidosis.

Question Asked	Immediate Diagnostic Tests: Permit Initiation of Therapy	Delayed-Result Diagnostic Tests: Refine Therapy
Hyperglycemia?	Blood and urine glucose oxidase reagent strips	Blood glucose
Metabolic acidosis?	Arterial, venous, or capillary blood gas for pH determination	Electrolytes (bicarbonate, anion gap)
Ketosis?	Urine dipstick, acetest	Serum ketones or serum β-hydroxybutyrate
Dehydration?	Urine specific gravity, hemoglobin from blood gas	Electrolytes, blood urea nitrogen, complete blood cell count
Potassium level?	ECG	Serum potassium
Infection?		Chest radiograph, blood culture and sensitivity, urinalysis, culture and sensitivity
Other?		Serum magnesium, phosphorus, osmolality

previous weight is available, weight loss may be used to quantify the percent dehydration. Although the initial deficits in severe DKA vary from patient to patient, some useful estimates are 100 mL/kg water, 9 mEq/kg sodium, and 6 mEq/kg potassium.

LABORATORY EVALUATION

Laboratory evaluation of the patient with suspected DKA is best thought of in two phases: immediate and delayed (Table 16-1).

The immediate phase of laboratory evaluation includes determinations that will guide immediate therapy. A rapid bedside determination of blood glucose, urine glucose, and urine ketones should be performed. Arterial blood gas determinations will rapidly confirm and quantify the acidosis, and the T wave on the 12-lead ECG is evaluated to detect evidence of hyperkalemia that would preclude the replacement of potassium before the availability of the serum potassium value.

Blood for delayed-result studies is drawn simultaneously with immediate studies, but results typically will not be available for 30 to 60 minutes. Other laboratory and radiologic studies, such as blood cultures and chest radiographs, are ordered as clinically indicated.

There are several pitfalls in the interpretation of laboratory results in the patient with DKA. Hyperglycemia falsely lowers the serum sodium determination. To compensate, add 1.6 to the serum sodium value for every 100 mg/dL blood glucose over 100 mg/dL. For example, if the blood glucose is 400 mg/dL and the serum sodium is 140 mEq/L, the corrected serum sodium concentration will actually be 144.8. A high serum lipid level also will contribute to lower serum electrolyte concentrations. Laboratories usually report serum that is grossly lipemic, suggesting the need to reinterpret electrolyte values.

Total body potassium and magnesium stores always are depleted in the patient with DKA.

However, initial determinations may not reflect this. Acidosis causes extracellular shifts of both potassium and magnesium, and dehydration produces hemoconcentration. Treatment with fluids, insulin, and bicarbonate dramatically lowers serum levels of both potassium and magnesium to potentially symptomatic levels. If the initial serum potassium and magnesium levels are noted to be above normal, delay replacement of these cations but perform repeat determinations immediately after therapy is initiated.

Ketone determinations are difficult to interpret and not essential. Usually, the ratio of β-hydroxybutyrate to acetoacetate is 3:1; however, the ratio may be as high as 30:1 in a severely acidotic patient. Because both the dipstick and laboratory determinations measure only acetoacetate, they may profoundly underestimate the serum (and urine) ketone concentrations.

MANAGEMENT

Fluid Replacement

Volume restoration is the first priority. Even if no other therapy is pursued, volume replacement will lower the blood glucose by as much as 15% to 20% and improve pH. If the child is in shock, 20 mL/kg normal saline is given by intravenous push as rapidly as possible. Repeat this fluid challenge until the child shows signs of resolution of shock. If the patient is not in shock, administer 10 to 20 mL/kg normal saline over the first hour. Then administer one-half normal saline. If corrected serum sodium is dropping, continue the patient on normal saline until stable. Volume restoration must be adequate, but the risk for development of cerebral edema must be kept in mind; therefore, conservative fluid replacement is recommended. The degree of dehydration is estimated and the volume deficit calculated. Deficits are corrected over a period of 48 hours (Tables 16-2 and 16-3). Ongoing fluid and electrolyte losses secondary to glycosuria should be

TABLE 16-2.
Example of fluid and electrolyte calculations in diabetic ketoacidosis based on a 25-kg (1-m²) patient.

	Deficit	Maintenance (24 hr)
Water	25 kg X 10% = 2.5 kg (2500 mL)	1600 mL
Sodium	9 mEq/kg = 225 mEq	3 mEq/100 mL H$_2$O = 48 mEq
Potassium	6 mEq/kg = 150 mEq	2 mEq/100 mL H$_2$O = 32 mEq

factored into the replacement calculation.

Potassium

If potassium values can be obtained from the laboratory within 30 to 60 minutes, adding this cation in the intravenous fluids can be delayed until laboratory results are available. If the results are not available in a timely manner, it is prudent to initiate replacement after assurance that T waves on the ECG show no evidence of hyperkalemia and that the child has urinated. A common approach is to add 40 mEq of potassium to the second liter of IV fluids. When laboratory determinations are available, continue to add 40 mEq ofpotassium to each liter of normal saline as long as the level is at or below the normal range. If the levels are elevated, monitor the potassium hourly to determine the proper time for supplementation. Potassium replacement may take the form of potassium chloride alone or half may be given as potassium chloride and half as potassium phosphate. The latter approach reduces the possibility of over-replacement of chloride, leading to a hyperchloremic acidosis, and addresses the theoretical problems associated with inadequate supplies of phosphate, although the clinical significance of hypophosphatemia in the setting of DKA has not been demonstrated.

Continued Reassessment

A flow sheet is essential in following a patient with DKA and should be initiated in the emergency department. Unless the patient can be moved to an inpatient unit within 1 hour of initiation of treatment, repeat sampling and laboratory determinations will be needed to properly monitor the response to therapy. A heparin lock is useful for facilitating frequent blood sampling. In addition to monitoring laboratory data, closely follow the patient's vital signs, input, output, and mental status.

Insulin and Glucose

Numerous treatment protocols have been described, including subcutaneous, intramuscular, and either intermittent or low-dose continuous intravenous infusion. Subcutaneous insulin therapy requires high doses, and absorption from the subcutaneous space may be affected by peripheral tissue perfusion and therefore may vary in the early resuscitation phase of DKA. This route generally is not used except in the mildest cases. Intramuscular injections are useful in most children, but there may be delayed absorption in the face of vascular collapse. Low-dose continuous intravenous infusion delivered with a constant infusion pump provides a more controlled method of treating DKA. It provides a more predictable and regular (linear) decline in blood glucose level that helps prevent hypoglycemia and hypokalemia from occurring during treatment. If the blood glucose level drops rapidly, the infusion can be discontinued without

TABLE 16-3.
Example of replacement procedure in diabetic ketoacidosis based on a 25-kg (1-m^2) patient.

	Volume	Solution
Stat if in shock*	20 mL/kg and repeat PRN	Normal saline
First 30-60 min	20 mL/kg = 500 mL	Normal saline
Next 8 hr	One-half deficit = 1250 mL 8-hr maintenance = 530 mL Run at 225 mL/hr Total = 1780 mL	0.5 normal saline + 40 mEq/L potassium (chloride or half chloride and half PO$_4$ Add 5% dextrose when blood sugar ≤250-300 mg/dL

*Rapid restoration of volume is indicated for hypovolemic shock, followed by replacement of calculated deficit and provision of maintenance fluids. Serial assessments are indicated to evaluate patient response and prevent volume overload.

continued decline in blood glucose because the half-life of intravenous regular insulin is only 6 to 8 minutes. The goal of treatment is to decrease the blood glucose level by 75 to 100 mg/dL per hour and to avoid dropping the level below 180 mg/dL.

Historically, a loading or priming dose of 0.1 U/kg has been given, followed by a continuous infusion of 0.1 U/kg per hour (Table 16-4). However, the loading dose is not necessary, and treatment can be initiated with the infusion. Fifty units of regular insulin may be mixed in 500 mL of normal saline to provide a solution that delivers 0.1 U/mL. Thus, infusion of this solution at a rate of 1 mL/kg per hour will provide 0.1 U/kg per hour insulin. It is important to use a pump to regulate the rate. It is safer to give the insulin through a separate line so the rate of insulin infusion can be regulated without affecting the rate of fluid and electrolyte replacement.

If the blood glucose level is >1000 mg/dL, some investigators suggest that the infusion rate be lowered to 0.05 U/kg per hour because a slower decline in blood glucose level may be desirable in hyperosmolar states. The corrected serum sodium should be followed closely to prevent rapid shifts.

When the blood glucose level reaches ≈250 to 300 mg/dL, the infusion rate can be decreased to 0.05 U/kg and the fluid changed to a solution containing 5% dextrose. Alternatively, the rate of insulin infusion can be maintained and the glucose supplemented by the use of a 10% infusion.

TABLE 16-4.
Insulin use in diabetic ketoacidosis based on a 25-kg (1-m^2) patient.

Priming Dose
 0.1 U/kg = 2.5 U intravenous push, if desired

Continuous Infusion
 0.1 U/kg per hour
 Mix 50 U regular insulin in 500 mL normal saline solution

 Rate: 25 mL/hr (2.5 U/hr)

Insulin infusion is replaced by subcutaneous injections when the glucose is < 200 mg/dL, pH has normalized, and ketones have cleared.

Bicarbonate

The use of bicarbonate in the therapy of DKA generally is not recommended. Fluid therapy alone has been demonstrated to raise pH effectively. Increased circulating volume decreases the production of lactic acid and promotes the generation of bicarbonate in the distal renal tubules. Insulin therapy decreases the amount of ketoacids. There is evidence to suggest that type I diabetics treated with insulin and fluids alone do as well and have fewer complications than those who receive bicarbonate. It is clear that patients receiving bicarbonate are at an increased risk of hypokalemia, hypomagnesemia, and excessive alkalinization. Rapid alkalinization has been associated with paradoxical cerebrospinal fluid acidosis and cerebral edema in children.

Some practitioners still believe that bicarbonate is beneficial in certain situations. It is recognized that at pH ≤7, myocardial contractility decreases, respirations are depressed, and hypotension may result. Although rarely indicated, sodium bicarbonate may be administered when the pH is below this level. When used, sodium bicarbonate (1 to 2 mEq/kg) is administered over ≥2 hours, along with the other resuscitation fluids. *Never "push" the bicarbonate, and do not administer bicarbonate to correct a pH >7.1.*

COMPLICATIONS

Hypoglycemia is a common complication of therapy and tends to occur after several hours of treatment. It is less likely to occur with low-dose continuous insulin infusion. Hourly laboratory monitoring of the initial response to therapy and the use of a flow sheet will reduce the likelihood of development of hypoglycemia. When the serum glucose levels have fallen to 250 to 300 mg/dL, glucose must be added to the infusion, if necessary, and the rate of insulin infusion decreased to avoid hypoglycemia.

Hypokalemia is very likely to occur unless early potassium replacement is initiated. Total body potassium levels essentially are always depleted, and there is a shift of potassium into the extracellular space as a result of the acidosis. As this is corrected, the potassium will move back into the intracellular space, and serum levels will plummet. Replacement should be started as early as possible.

Cerebral edema is a rare but deadly complication. It usually occurs as the patient's metabolic parameters are improving and is heralded by the onset of headache, dizziness, and somnolence. Although the exact mechanism of development is unclear, it probably is related to rapid shifts in osmolarity. Preventive measures include gradual reduction in the serum glucose level, maintenance of corrected serum sodium level, cautious replacement of fluid over 48 hours, and avoidance of the use of sodium bicarbonate. It has been recommended that fluid replacement not exceed 4 L/m^2 per 24 hours. Treatment consists of fluid restriction, controlled hyperventilation, and mannitol, usually associated with intracranial pressure monitoring.

DISPOSITION

Patients with DKA as the initial presentation of diabetes should be considered for admission. However, established patients with very early ketoacidosis do not always require hospital admission. They may present with nausea, malaise, and ketones in the urine but only mild acidosis and dehydration. These patients may be treated with intravenous fluids, and after establishment of the level of hyperglycemia, regular insulin can be administered subcutaneously in an amount equal to 10% to 20% of the usual daily dose. This amount may be repeated in 4 hours. If there is a good response to this therapeutic trial and adequate support systems at home, the child can be followed closely on an outpatient basis. Children who have persistent vomiting or fail to respond are admitted.

All children with moderate to severe DKA require admission to the hospital. Those with shock, severe acidosis, or persistently altered sensorium will benefit from observation in a pediatric intensive care unit.

ADDITIONAL READING

Bonadio WA. Pediatric diabetic ketoacidosis: pathophysiology and potential for outpatient management of selected children. *Pediatr Emerg Care.* 1992;8:287-290.

Chase HP, Garg SK, Jelley DH. Diabetic ketoacidosis in children and the role of outpatient management. *Pediatr Rev.* 1990;11:297-304.

Ellis EN. Concepts of fluid therapy in diabetic ketoacidosis and hyperosmolar hyperglycemic nonketotic coma. *Pediatr Clin North Am.* 1990;37:313-321.

Fleckman AM. Diabetic ketoacidosis. *Endocrinol Metab Clin North Am.* 1993;22:181-207.

Linares MY, Schunk JE, Lindsay R. Laboratory presentation of diabetic ketoacidosis and duration of therapy. *Pediatr Emerg Care.* 1996;12:347-351.

Wood EG, Go-Wingkun J, Luisiri A, et al. Symptomatic cerebral swelling complicating diabetic ketoacidosis documented by intraventricular pressure monitoring: survival without neurologic sequela. *Pediatr Emerg Care.* 1990;6:285-288.

Chapter 17

Status Epilepticus

OBJECTIVES

1. Define status epilepticus.

2. Describe the common causes of status epilepticus by age.

3. Discuss the possible central nervous system complications of prolonged status epilepticus.

4. Explain the mechanism of non–central nervous system complications in status epilepticus.

5. Describe the initial stabilization of all children presenting in status epilepticus.

6. Select appropriate anticonvulsant medications and dosages.

7. Identify the therapeutic interventions in a patient with refractory status epilepticus.

A **seizure** is a clinical entity associated with an involuntary alteration of consciousness or motor activity, secondary to the abnormal, rapid electrical discharge of a group of cerebral neurons. Illness, injury, or genetic factors may act separately or together to produce seizures. Repetitive or continuous seizures lasting >30 minutes without recovery of consciousness may be defined as **status epilepticus**. Most seizures in children end spontaneously or can be controlled before meeting the definition of status. Therefore, early recognition, initial stabilization of vital functions, and therapy directed at controlling the seizure and treating the underlying cause can prevent death and neurologic injury.

PATHOPHYSIOLOGY

Generalized **convulsive status epilepticus** (seizures associated with abnormal motor activity and altered mental status) is associated with pathophysiologic changes in two categories: cerebral and systemic.

Cerebral Alterations

Cellular studies of brain tissue demonstrate rapid loss of energy substrates (ATP and phosphocreatine) and progressive lactic acidosis during seizure activity. Because cellular utilization of glucose is rapid and transport of glucose into the brain lags behind the actual requirement, there is a relative cerebral hypoglycemia. A marked decrease in cerebral energy metabolites occurs as the process becomes self-sustaining.

Cerebral alterations in status epilepticus include an increase in blood flow, oxygen and glucose consumption, and carbon dioxide production. During status epilepticus, in which cerebral metabolic requirements exceed the availability of metabolic substrates, neuronal destruction occurs. Cerebral blood flow ceases to be autoregulated and can become pressure dependent. After 30 to 60 minutes of continuous seizure activity, neuronal damage may occur despite the presence of adequate oxygen, glucose, and other metabolic substrates.

Systemic Alterations

Initial systemic physiologic changes result from a massive autonomic sympathetic system discharge; this leads to hypertension, tachycardia, and hyperglycemia. The initial systemic hypertensive response may actually maintain or increase cerebral flow despite the loss of autoregulation.

The prolonged increase in skeletal muscle metabolic activity and decrease in pulmonary ventilation lead to lactic acidosis, hyperkalemia, hypoxia, hypercarbia, elevated temperature, and hypoglycemia. Causes of hypoxia are multifactorial and include increased metabolic demand and inhibition of medullary respiratory centers.

ETIOLOGY AND EARLY ASSESSMENT

The etiology of status epilepticus in children differs with age (Table 17-1). Common toxins and medications that may cause seizures are listed in Table 17-2. Most commonly, children who present with status epilepticus are those with epilepsy whose anticonvulsant levels are not therapeutic. Important immediate concerns, however, are stabilization of the patient regardless of etiology and early antibiotic administration if meningitis is likely.

Obtain a pertinent history, especially regarding prescribed medications and compliance. Perform a directed physical examination, which should include all vital signs (Table 17-3). Laboratory studies should be obtained based on the age of the child and likely etiologies.

Although central nervous system infection, tumor, bleed, or head trauma may cause seizures, these also may be associated with increased intracranial pressure (ICP). Increased ICP with impending cerebral herniation may present as decerebrate posturing with stiffening, opisthotonos, extension, and internal rotation of the extremities. **Posturing** often is mistaken for a seizure and requires immediate management of ICP rather than anticonvulsants. If increased ICP is suspected, direct the initial stabilization toward reduction in ICP (intubate and hyperventilate) to prevent further brain herniation and death, rather than solely toward anticonvulsant therapy.

All children should be stabilized before undergoing a diagnostic lumbar puncture or computed tomography scan of the head.

The child who has a history of recurrent status epilepticus and is poorly controlled on chronic anticonvulsants may not require as many studies at the time of initial stabilization. Because anticonvulsant toxicity also may cause increased seizure activity, blood for drug levels should be drawn before further administration of the same anticonvulsant.

MANAGEMENT

The management of status epilepticus in children begins with ensuring a patent airway, administering 100% oxygen, establishing vascular access, restoring and stabilizing circulation, monitoring the child's cardiorespiratory status, and concurrently assessing for the etiology of seizures. An aggressive, organized approach to generalized convulsive status epilepticus with appropriate stabilization and therapy improves morbidity and mortality (Table 17-4).

TABLE 17-1.
Etiology of status epilepticus by age.

Neonatal (First Month)
Birth injury (anoxia, hemorrhage)
Congenital abnormalities
Inborn errors of metabolism (lipidoses, amino acidurias)
Infection (meningitis)
Metabolic disorders (hypoglycemia, hypocalcemia, hyponatremia)
Early Childhood (≤6 yr)
Birth injury
Cerebral degenerative diseases
Fever
Idiopathic
Infection
Metabolic disorders
Neurocutaneous syndromes
Post-trauma
Toxins
Tumor
Childhood and Adolescence
Birth injury
Cerebral degenerative diseases
Cerebral hemorrhage (arteriovenous malformation)
Epilepsy with inadequate drug levels
Idiopathic
Infection
Toxins
Trauma
Tumor

STABILIZATION

Oxygenation and Ventilation

Provide a patent airway by positioning the child's head and suctioning any secretions. Always administer 100% supplemental oxygen by face mask. A rigid large-bore suction catheter should be available immediately. Oral or nasal airways are useful adjuncts. Force should not be used to open clenched jaws during convulsive status epilepticus or undue trauma may result. Oral or nasogastric decompression of the stomach contents should be performed as early as possible to prevent emesis and secondary aspiration. If the patient has no gag reflex, endotracheal intubation should precede gastric intubation. If there is a possibility of trauma, perform in-line cervical spine immobilization before further interventions (see Chapter 7). If there is no likelihood of trauma, the child may be placed in a left lateral decubitus position to help prevent aspiration of gastric contents.

Monitor for poor oxygenation or hypoventilation by pulse oximeter (O_2 saturation <90%) or by arterial blood gas (PaO_2 <65 mm Hg, $PaCO_2$ >50 mm Hg). Assist ventilation as necessary with bag-valve-mask or endotracheal intubation. Indications for endotracheal intubation include inability to adequately oxygenate and ventilate with use of bag-valve-mask technique, increased ICP that requires treatment with controlled oxygenation and hyperventilation, and refractory status epilepticus that requires general anesthesia. Intubate the child's trachea with the technique of rapid sequence induction (see Chapter 2). If the child is intubated and paralyzed, closely monitor the child's EEG and cardiorespiratory status. Continued electrical seizure activity as documented by EEG monitoring requires additional anticonvulsant intervention.

TABLE 17-2.
Toxins and medications that may cause seizures.

Anticonvulsant overdose
Belladonna alkaloids
Camphor
Carbon monoxide
Cocaine
Cyanide
Cyclic antidepressants
Heavy metals (lead)
Hypoglycemic agents (insulin, ethanol)
Isoniazid
Nicotine
Pesticides (organophosphates)
Phencyclidine (PCP)
Sympathomimetics (amphetamines, phenylpropanolamine)
Theophylline
Topical anesthetics (lidocaine)

TABLE 17-3.
Directed history and physical examination.

History
  Head injury
  Meningitis
  Intoxication or toxic exposure
  Preceding illness
  Prior history of epilepsy
  Anticonvulsant use and compliance
  Ventriculoperitoneal shunt
  Current medications
  Birth history
  Development
  General health
  Other past medical history
Physical Examination
  Vital signs (heart rate, respirations, blood pressure, Cushing's triad)
  Temperature
  Ventilatory status
  Cardiovascular status
  Status of fontanels
  Pupillary size, reactivity, symmetry
  Meningismus
  Posturing
  Evidence of head injury
  Evidence of other trauma
  Toxicologic syndromes
  Evidence of skin lesions
    Petechiae or purpura
    Herpetic vesicles
    Marks of neurocutaneous syndromes

Circulation and Vascular Access

Monitor for clinical signs of poor perfusion, including thready peripheral or central pulses, delayed capillary refill time, and cool extremities. Early administration of isotonic fluids for

---

TABLE 17-4.
Management protocol for status epilepticus.

Stabilization
Provide patent airway; suction airway
Cervical spine immobilization if indicated
Supplemental 100% oxygen by face mask
Oral or nasopharyngeal airway
Establish vascular access (intravenous or intraosseous)
Consider endotracheal intubation
- Protect airway
- Support ventilatory effort
Consider nasogastric tube; left lateral decubitus position

Therapy for all Unresponsive/Unconscious Patients
Glucose 250-500 mg/kg
Naloxone 0.1 mg/kg

Anticonvulsant Therapy
Intravascular access (intravenous or intraosseous) established
- Lorazepam 0.05-0.10 mg/kg q10-15min (maximum, 4 mg/dose)
  or
  Diazepam 0.1-0.3 mg/kg q2min (maximum, 10 mg/dose)
  and followed by
- Phenytoin (or fosphenytoin) 10-20 mg/kg by slow infusion (1 mg/kg per minute; maximum, 50 mg/min) (up to 3 mg/kg per minute for fosphenytoin)
  or
- Phenobarbital 20 mg/kg by slow infusion (1 to 2 mg/kg per minute; maximum, 100 mg/min)
- Repeat lorazepam-or-diazepam or phenobarbital doses if needed
Unable to establish intravascular access
- Intramuscular midazolam 0.20 mg/kg
- Rectal diazepam 0.5 mg/kg (maximum dose, 20 mg)

Therapy for Refractory Status Epilepticus
General anesthesia induced by:
- Barbiturates
- Inhalation anesthetics
Cardiorespiratory support
- Endotracheal intubation
- Muscle relaxants
Continuous monitoring
- Cardiorespiratory monitor
- Pulse oximeter
- Electroencephalogram

---

hypovolemia is crucial.

Establish intravascular access immediately for the administration of fluids and anticonvulsants. Vascular access is of paramount importance because most of the available and effective anticonvulsants are administered only via an intravenous or intraosseous route. Obtaining intravenous access in the infant or young child with active seizure activity often is difficult, and the intraosseous route may be the only obtainable vascular access. This is a satisfactory alternative for anticonvulsant medication administration.

ANTICONVULSANT THERAPY

Status epilepticus generally responds well to an appropriately administered anticonvulsant. The goal of anticonvulsant intervention is to achieve effective therapeutic effect as quickly as possible, ideally within 30 to 60 minutes of presentation. Once an anticonvulsant is administered, the treating physician should allow adequate time (Table 17-5) for the anticonvulsants to reach therapeutic levels in the brain.

The anticonvulsants commonly available for the treatment of status epilepticus fall into three categories: benzodiazepines, phenytoin, and barbiturates (Tables 17-5 and 17-6).

The **benzodiazepines** are highly effective in the treatment of patients with generalized convulsive status epilepticus. Lorazepam, midazolam, and diazepam have rapid onsets of action (within 1 to 5 minutes) and should be titrated for clinical response. **Diazepam** may be administered rectally if intravenous access is not rapidly obtainable. After initial control with diazepam, seizures often recur because of its very short duration of action, and the administration of an additional longer-acting anticonvulsant, such as phenytoin or phenobarbital, is required. **Lorazepam** has anticonvulsant activity that lasts from several to 48 hours and therefore is preferred to diazepam due to its significantly longer duration of action and only slightly less rapid onset of action. Doses of both lorazepam and diazepam may be repeated, if needed, in 10 to 15 minutes.

If the child is not already intubated, cardiorespiratory status must be monitored carefully, and the physician should be prepared to assist ventilation with a bag-valve-mask if necessary.

Although intravenous **midazolam** has no demonstrated advantage over diazepam or lorazepam, it is clearly efficacious as an intramuscular anticonvulsant, when intravenous or intraosseous access is not immediately available. Currently, midazolam is the only anticonvulsant with a rapid onset of action that can be safely administered as either an intravenous or intramuscular injection. A dose of 0.20 mg/kg IM appears to be clinically efficacious in >90% of children in status epilepticus.

Phenytoin is most effective for idiopathic generalized tonic-clonic, focal, posttraumatic, and psychomotor seizures. It is minimally effective for absence seizures or status epilepticus due to alcohol withdrawal and not effective for febrile seizures. Peak activity of phenytoin in the brain occurs in 10 to 30 minutes after infusion.

The proper administration of phenytoin is critical. Infuse phenytoin in saline; it is poorly soluble in water and precipitates in dextrose-containing solutions. Intravenous phenytoin must be infused with the use of constant infusion pump at a rate of <1.0 mg/kg per minute in children and <50 mg/min in adults. The maximum infusion should be 1 g in children and up to 1.5 g in adolescents. **Fosphenytoin** is a new formulation that is metabolized to phenytoin after infusion. It can be infused much faster than phenytoin because injection site complaints are less common and the incidence of cardiac conduction abnormalities and hypotension should be decreased because toxic diluents are not present. The pharmacokinetic profile in pediatric patients is similar to that in adults, but approval for use in children younger than 5 years is pending. Concomitant hemodynamic monitoring during infusion of either phenytoin or fosphenytoin is imperative. Rapid administration may result in hypotension, sinus bradycardia, other cardiac dysrhythmias, and asystole.

In a patient with known epilepsy maintained on phenytoin, a blood level should be determined.

Phenobarbital has a high degree of efficacy against most seizures, especially in the treatment of febrile and neonatal status epilepticus. Peak activity after an intravenous loading dose occurs within 10 to 20 minutes. The rate of administration should not exceed 1 to 2 mg/kg per minute in children and 100 mg/min in adults. The maximum single dose is 1 g. The main disadvantages of phenobarbital are that it significantly depresses mental status and has a somewhat slower onset of action. Phenobarbital can be used safely in patients already maintained on the drug, but a level should be drawn before administration.

TABLE 17-5.
Anticonvulsants in the treatment of status epilepticus.

Class of Drug	Drug	Onset of Action	Duration	Cardiorespiratory Effects*	CNS Effects†	Drug Interactions
Benzodiazepines	Lorazepam	2-3 min	12-48 hr	+	+	+
	Diazepam	1-3 min	5-15 min	+	+	+
	Midazolam	1.5-5 min	1-5 hr	+	+	+
Hydantoins	Phenytoin	10-30 min after infusion	12-24 hr	+	–	–
	Fosphenytoin‡	10-30 min after infusion	12-24 hr	±	–	–
Barbiturates	Phenobarbital	10-20 min	1-3 days	+	+	+

*Cardiorespiratory side effects include hypotension, respiratory depression, bradycardia, cardiac conduction defects, and dysrhythmias.
†CNS side effects include drowsiness, decreased level of consciousness, and lethargy.
‡Approval for use in pediatrics pending.

ALTERNATE ROUTES OF ADMINISTRATION

All anticonvulsants may be administered via the intraosseous route when the child has no intravenous access. The doses are the same as for the intravenous route, although higher doses of phenytoin may be needed to overcome possible marrow retention of the drug.

Intramuscular administration of midazolam (0.2 mg/kg) is preferable to no therapeutic intervention in a patient with no intravenous or intraosseous access. Intramuscular phenobarbital is suboptimal, and intramuscular phenytoin is not recommended because of potential muscle necrosis, as well as variable and unpredictable absorption. Fosphenytoin may, however, be administered intramuscularly.

Rectal administration of diazepam appears to be effective at an initial dose of 0.5 mg/kg (maximum of 20 mg). The parenteral preparation of diazepam is injected into the lower rectum with a 1-mL syringe, feeding tube, or 6-cm catheter advanced 4 to 6 cm. In the prehospital setting, rectal diazepam should be considered for the child in status epilepticus who has no vascular access.

TREATMENT OF SPECIFIC CAUSES OF STATUS EPILEPTICUS

Certain etiologies of status epilepticus produce seizures that are difficult to control without treating the cause; these include intracranial hemorrhage (therapy is evacuation), hypoglycemia, hyponatremia, hypernatremia, hypocalcemia, hypomagnesemia, pyridoxine deficiency (therapy is replacement of pyridoxine at 50 to 100 mg IV), and theophylline, isoniazid, or carbon monoxide intoxications.

Consideration of these entities, when the seizures are not controlled with initial therapy, may help to direct definitive therapy.

TREATMENT OF REFRACTORY STATUS EPILEPTICUS

If the child continues to seize for >60 minutes despite adequate trials of effective doses of the major anticonvulsants (benzodiazepines, phenytoin, or phenobarbital), control of the seizures with

TABLE 17-6.
Intravenous doses of anticonvulsants.

	Dose (IV, IO)	Rate	Maximum Dose	Effective Serum Concentration
Lorazepam	0.05-0.10 mg/kg Repeat q10-15min if needed	<2 mg/min	4 mg/dose	Not applicable
Diazepam	0.1-0.3 mg/kg* Repeat q2min if needed	<2 mg/min	10 mg/dose 40 mg/24 hr	Not applicable
Midazolam	0.05-0.2 mg/kg† Repeat q10-15min	<2 mg/min	5 mg/dose	Not applicable
Phenytoin	10-20 mg/kg	<1 mg/kg per minute	1000 mg <50 mg/min	10-20 µg/mL
Fosphenytoin	10-20 mg PE‡/kg	<3 mg PE‡/kg per minute <150 mg PE‡/min	1000 mg PE‡	10-20 µg/mL
Phenobarbital	20 mg/kg	<100 mg/min <1-2 mg/kg per minute	1000 mg	15-40 µg/mL

*May be administered rectally at dose of 0.5 mg/kg (maximum, 20 mg).
†May be administered intramuscularly at dose of 0.2 mg/kg.
‡PE = phenytoin equivalents.

general anesthesia should follow. Intracerebral hemorrhage, hypoxic injury, meningoencephalitis, hypertensive encephalopathy, or idiopathic causes are more commonly associated with refractory seizures. Children with refractory status require intensive management with general anesthesia induced by inhalation anesthesia or barbiturate coma and hypothermia (30° to 31°C) during induction. Barbiturate coma commonly is induced with pentobarbital (5 to 10 mg/kg loading dose followed by a constant infusion of 0.5 to 3.0 mg/kg per hour) or phenobarbital (5 to 10 mg/kg repeated every 20 minutes). All children requiring general anesthesia should be paralyzed and intubated, have continuous EEG and cardiorespiratory monitoring, and have pharmacologic cardiovascular support as needed. They should be treated in the critical care setting, under the care of a pediatric anesthesiologist and critical care staff who are familiar with the risks and complications of these agents.

FURTHER STUDIES

An emergency computed tomography scan is indicated in any child if there is a suspected head injury or increased ICP by history or on initial physical examination. Intracranial hemorrhage is an uncommon cause of status epilepticus but may cause death if not promptly diagnosed and evacuated.

Lumbar puncture for cerebrospinal fluid analysis and culture is indicated if the child has symptoms of CNS infection and no signs of ICP or intracranial mass lesion and is hemodynamically stable. Obtaining cerebrospinal fluid for analysis or a computed tomography scan of the head should not delay the treatment for suspected CNS infection.

DISPOSITION

Once the child is stabilized and seizure activity is controlled, the cause of the seizure should be investigated. Consultation with the neurologist or neurosurgeon may be helpful. Half of all episodes of status epilepticus in children have no known cause. Half of these "idiopathic" episodes occur in febrile patients between 6 months and 3 years of age. Children who have a persistent altered mental status after control of seizure activity or who present with prolonged status epilepticus should be admitted to the pediatric critical care unit for continued observation, evaluation, and treatment.

ADDITIONAL READING

American Academy of Pediatrics, Committee on Drugs. Drugs for pediatric emergencies. *Pediatrics*. 1998;101:1-11.

Chamberlain JM, Altieri MA, Futterman C, et al. A prospective randomized study comparing intramuscular midazolam with intravenous diazepam for the treatment of seizures in children. *Pediatr Emerg Care*. 1997;13:92-94.

Donovan PJ, Cline D. Phenytoin administration by constant intravenous infusion: selective rates of administration. *Ann Emerg Med*. 1991;20:139-142.

Gross-Tsur V, Shinnar S. Convulsive status epilepticus in children. *Epilepsia*. 1993;34(suppl 1):S12-S20.

Lacroix L, Deal C, Gauthier M, et al. Admissions to a pediatric intensive care unit for status epilepticus: a 10-year experience. *Crit Care Med*. 1994;22:827-832.

Maytal J, Shinnar S, Moshe SL, et al. Low morbidity and mortality of status epilepticus in children. *Pediatrics*. 1989;83:323-331.

Pellock JM. Fosphenytoin use in children. *Neurology*. 1996;46(suppl 1):S14-S16.

Pellock JM. Status epilepticus in children: update and review. *J Child Neurol*. 1994;9(suppl 2):27-35.

Ramsay RE. Treatment of status epilepticus. *Epilepsia*. 1993;34(suppl 1):S71-S81.

Rashkin MC, Youngs C, Penovich P. Pentobarbital treatment of refractory status epilepticus. *Neurology*. 1987;37:500-503.

Rivera R, Segnini M, Baltodano A, et al. Midazolam in the treatment of status epilepticus in children. *Crit Care Med*. 1993;21:991-994.

Tunik MG, Young GM. Status epilepticus in children: the acute management. *Pediatr Clin North Am*. 1992;39:1007-1030.

Walsh-Kelly CM, Berens RJ, Glaeser PW, et al. Intraosseous infusion of phenytoin. *Am J Emerg Med*. 1986;4:523-524.

Wasterlain CG, Fujikawa DG, Penix L, et al. Pathophysiological mechanisms of brain damage from status epilepticus. *Epilepsia*. 1993;34(suppl 1):S37-S53.

Working Group on Status Epilepticus. Treatment of convulsive status epilepticus. Recommendations of the Epilepsy Foundation of America's Working Group on Status Epilepticus. *JAMA*. 1993;270:854-859.

Pediatric Emergency Management Issues

Chapter 18

Pain Management and Sedation in Acute Care

OBJECTIVES

1. Explain the principles of pain conduction.

2. Describe the selection of agents and methods for prevention or relief of localized pain.

3. Discuss the advantages and disadvantages of the various narcotic agents.

4. Discuss the use of non-narcotic sedatives and analgesics.

5. Recognize the need for sedation, principles of monitoring the sedated patient, and criteria for discharge after sedation.

Pain and anxiety are prominent concerns for any child undergoing emergency treatment. Unfortunately, the focus of medical care too often centers entirely on the physiologic components of a child's problem, and the emotional or painful aspects of a child's treatment are ignored. The lack of attention to this aspect of a child's needs is not intentional but stems from a number of misconceptions on the part of health care providers. Difficulty in assessing pain or anxiety in a child, misconceptions concerning children's perception of pain, and a lack of appropriate education of medical professionals all contribute to this problem. There is no evidence that any child, regardless of age or neurologic development, is any less sensitive to painful stimuli than an adult. In addition, children are not more easily addicted to narcotics and, with the exception of the first few months of life, are not more prone to respiratory depression than adults. A child's memories of pain appear to be as vivid as those of any adult, and children deserve the same considerations for pain management as any other patient.

NEUROANATOMY AND NEUROPHYSIOLOGY

Perception of pain is the result of the transmission of painful stimuli from peripheral nerves to the central nervous system. Pain receptors originate as free nerve endings within the dermatones enervated by individual neurons. These pain receptors, also known as **nociceptors**, initiate pain signals from the periphery by converting mechanical, thermal, or chemical stimulation into electrical activity. The cell bodies of these sensory neurons are located within the dorsal horns of the spinal cord, where they synapse with second-order neurons. These nerve fibers then cross to the contralateral side of the spinal cord as they ascend via the spinal thalamic track to the brainstem. From the brainstem, these neurons conduct impulses through to the thalamus and cerebral cortex, where the sensation of pain is perceived.

There are two types of nerve fibers in the periphery that detect stimuli: A-Δ and C fibers. Transmission of impulses along peripheral nerve fibers occurs as a result of sequential depolarization of the axon via the opening and closing of sodium and potassium channels in the cell membrane. The A-Δ fibers are composed of myelinated axons that transmit the sharp localized pain perceived immediately after an injury (first pain). C fibers, in contrast, contain unmyelinated axons and transmit dull or burning sensations (second pain). These fibers conduct much slower than A-Δ fibers and are associated with the throbbing, aching sensation of a painful injury. The neurons for both of these types of pain fibers are located in the dorsal horn area of the gray matter in the posterior aspect of the spinal cord. This area is specifically involved in the integration, modification, and relay of peripheral sensory input to the brain and cerebral cortex. As the spinal cord ascends from the lumbar to the cerebral region, the pain fibers are organized into layers, or **laminae.**

Beginning in the spinal cord and continuing through to the cerebral cortex, painful stimuli are modified by several chemical mediators. The nature of the mediator and its site of action determine whether the effect produced is excitatory, enhances the perception of pain, or is inhibitory, minimizing a painful sensation. The most significant modifiers of pain are the endogenous opioid substances: **endorphins, enkephlins,** and **dynorphins.**

Opioid analgesics, whether **intrinsic,** as the endorphins, or **extrinsic,** as narcotic drugs, produce their effects through binding to specific opioid receptors. Currently, there are six known opioid receptor types recognized in the central nervous system (CNS): $\mu 1$, $\mu 2$, δ, κ, σ, and ε. The physical receptors appear to be composed of combinations of these different receptor types. Stimulation of different receptors produces different effects depending on the composition and location of the receptor within the CNS. For example, μ receptor stimulation in the periaqueductal gray area of the midbrain produces profound analgesia, whereas κ receptor activation produces the same effect in the spinal cord proper. The major actions of δ receptors appear to be respiratory depression, whereas σ receptors tend to initiate dysphoria. The exact mechanism by which these receptors modify pain perception is multifactorial and has not been clearly elucidated. Receptor stimulation does change ion channels in the cell membranes, resulting in hyperpolarization of the membrane and modification of other cell membrane proteins.

Most of the pharmacologic actions of the narcotic analgesics seem to result from stimulation of the μ and κ receptors.

In addition to intrinsic analgesic capabilities, the brain possesses inherent feedback mechanisms to control neuronal stimulation and reentry excitation. Without such an inhibitory system, a seizure would result every time a neuron depolarized. The major neuroinhibitor in the CNS is γ-aminobutyric acid (GABA). This small organic acid binds to a specific GABA receptor, opening a chloride channel in the neuron and hyperpolarizing the cell membrane. The receptor itself is a five-protein complex composed of three different protein subunits. One of these proteins serves as the actual GABA receptor, one binds benzodiazepines, and the third binds barbiturates. This is why the benzodiazepines and barbiturates have such similar actions.

ROUTES OF ADMINISTRATION

The preferred route of administration of any sedative or analgesic depends on the child's age, clinical condition, and nature of the underlying problem. **Oral** agents are most appropriate in relatively healthy children who require minimal sedation for a painful procedure or analgesia for a mildly uncomfortable condition. Some agents may be given transmucosally through the **nasal, oral,** or **rectal mucosa.** Higher serum levels of a medication can be achieved with smaller doses when the transmucosal route is used. Because the drug is absorbed directly into the systemic circulation, it bypasses the initial first-pass metabolism of the liver that occurs with drugs administered through the gastrointestinal tract. However, because mucosal absorption also is dependent on contact time and exposed surface area, this route can be more erratic than oral administration.

Intramuscular administration of medications provides more consistent and higher levels of medications than either the oral or transmucosal route. However, this method of drug administration requires a child to undergo a painful needle puncture to deliver the medication. If the drug being given is a one-time injection, then this may not be a concern; however, if multiple doses of a medication are anticipated, a different route should be ordered.

Intravenous administration is the optimal method of either analgesic or sedative administration in a child who requires repeated drug administrations or titration of the action of a drug. Intravenous medications may be administered directly into the child's bloodstream, producing a rapid onset along with an ability to augment the amount of medication if a desired effect is not achieved with the initial dose. Intravenous access also allows the child to use a patient-controlled analgesia (PCA) apparatus. These devices permit patients to titrate continuously the amount of analgesic they require; lock-out devices within the electronics of the pumps prevent inadvertent overdoses. Any child with an ongoing painful condition who is old enough to understand how to use a PCA device should be presented with this option. Most children older than 9 or 10 years usually can use a PCA device without difficulty. Children who are candidates for PCA devices should have the device instituted as quickly as possible, preferably in the emergency department or post anesthesia recovery area.

MONITORING

Any child receiving analgesics or sedatives to produce an alteration in level of consciousness must undergo some form of cardiovascular or respiratory monitoring. Children receiving simple analgesics that do not produce a significant change in their cognitive abilities do not require continuous monitoring. Children undergoing controlled manipulation of their state of awareness should be monitored with continuous pulse oximetry. Depending on the degree of sedation or analgesia required, continuous cardiac monitoring, noninvasive blood pressure monitoring, or continuous capnometry also may be included. Any child who requires monitoring for a given procedure should have such monitoring continued until he or she returns to the normal state of awareness. Many sedatives and analgesics will produce a loss of normal coordination, and children should be observed until minimal motor functions return. Table 18-1 contains the discharge criteria for a child undergoing iatrogenic modification of level of consciousness.

ASSESSMENT OF PAIN

Children by their very nature make it more difficult to assess painful or anxiety-producing situations. The complexities of childhood behavior often make it almost impossible for the clinician to distinguish a truly terrified child from one attempting to manipulate a situation through a tantrum. The subtleties of assessing childhood discomfort are exaggerated in extremely young or preverbal children.

Assessment Technique by Age Group

Infants and Toddlers

The nonverbal state of most of these children makes it extremely important for the clinician to be cognizant of the potential for pain or anxiety to exist. It certainly is safe to assume that any procedure performed in an adult that requires sedation or analgesia requires the same considerations in children of this age group; this includes lumbar puncture, fracture manipulation, intravenous line placement, and wound and burn care.

Preschool Children

Verbal self-reporting is the best indication of pain in this age group. Children 3 to 7 years of age may be intimidated by the activities of an emergency department or acute care setting and not verbalize their conditions readily. Do not wait for the child to complain spontaneously. Ask specifically, "Do you have pain?" It is also more appropriate to offer analgesics directly to a child this age and not expect the child to request a pain medication. Visual-analog scales help children this age to express discomfort, and their use in pain assessment should be encouraged. Visual-analog scales that have proved to be clinically useful

TABLE 18-1.
Discharge criteria after sedation.

Stable vital signs (pulse, temperature, respirations, blood pressure, pulse oximetry)
Intact protective airway reflexes
Ability to take sips from a cup or to take a bottle
Return to baseline verbal skills*
   — Understands commands
   — Verbalizes at level equal to that before sedation
Return to baseline motor skills*
Has reliable caretaker who has received and understands discharge instructions

*These abilities may need to be modified depending on the child's presenting problem.

include the Ocher scale, poker chip tool, ladder scale, color scale, pediatric pain questionnaire, and behavioral observation scales.

School-Aged Children and Adolescents

Children aged 7 years and older are in the developmental cognitive stage that allows them to begin to understand and report an abstract phenomenon such as pain. Even though these children are more verbal, they also should be questioned specifically about pain and their analgesic needs. Visual-analog scales also should be used in these patients because they are more accurate and allow the treating health care providers to assess more objectively the patient's degree of pain.

PRINCIPLES OF PAIN MANAGEMENT

Pain should be treated aggressively and prevented whenever possible. Even in instances in which it is not practical to eliminate all pain, some pain relief is almost always possible. It also is important to identify and provide increased attention to children who may have difficulty in communicating their pain as a result of cognitive impairment, psychiatric disorders, or difficulties with the native language.

The optimum approach to pain management depends not only on the nature of the patient, but also on the cause of the patient's pain. Pain originating from an extremity or a well-localized peripheral site may be best managed with a regional anesthesia approach that completely eliminates the sensation of pain. Pain originating from a more generalized problem or multiple sites that cannot be

successfully anesthetized is best managed through a centrally acting pharmacologic agent that decreases the child's perception of pain. In addition to pharmacologic interventions, techniques that distract the child or in some way change the perception of pain may be used.

NONPHARMACOLOGIC MODALITIES

Table 18-2 contains a summary of the mechanism of action and level of pain modulation for various nonpharmacologic pain management techniques.

Application of Cold

The application of ice packs to an area of acute inflammation and swelling, such as a fractured extremity, helps reduce painful sensation by reducing inflammation in the area and in some instances directly suppresses neuronal excitability. Caution must be used with this technique because thermal injuries secondary to extended low temperatures can occur.

Vigorous Vibration

With this technique, pain originating from an extremity is masked through vigorous stimulation of the nerve endings in the skin fibers of the area. This technique is used inherently, as exemplified by rubbing the scalp after a head bump. The physiologic basis for the success of this technique is that the spinal cord dorsal roots and the cerebral cortex have a limited ability to sense and distinguish multiple simultaneous stimuli. By aggressively rubbing the skin, a flood of stimuli is presented to the dorsal roots, essentially closing the gates of the large myelinated A fiber neurons. This gate closure effectively prevents these neurons from relaying impulses from the painful stimuli because they are so overwhelmed with sensations coming from the vigorous rubbing. Dentists frequently use a similar technique when performing injections. To mask the pain of the puncture, they grasp the lip and tug quickly on the skin just before an injection. This maneuver prevents the patient from sensing the needle amid the flood of stimuli from the pinched lip.

Transcutaneous Nerve Stimulation

As with vigorous vibration, transcutaneous electrical nerve stimulation can saturate sensory nerve fibers, creating a low-amplitude, high-volume

TABLE 18-2.
Nonpharmacologic pain management.

Technique	Action
Cold application	Decreased inflammatory response
Vigorous vibration and transcutaneous nerve stimulation	Gate closure in dorsal horn neurons through overstimulation of afferent axons
Behavior modification and hypnosis	Cognitive diversion and reinterpretation of pain stimuli

stimulatory wave that overwhelms the sensation of any painful stimuli. This type of therapy seems to be most effective for patients with chronic pain.

Behavior Modification

These approaches also have been used successfully in all age groups. Relaxation techniques, including desensitization through gradual exposure to anxiety-producing stimuli, positive reinforcement, rewards, and guided imagery or fantasy work particularly well. Hypnosis also has been used effectively in children; the effectiveness of this technique seems to be related to the extreme susceptibility of children to suggestion. In patients who are good subjects, hypnosis has been used very effectively to reduce the anxiety of such procedures as lumbar puncture and bone marrow aspirations.

PHARMACOLOGIC MODALITIES

Local Wound and Peripheral Extremity Techniques

Topical Anesthesia

Laceration repairs frequently are a source of anxiety in children of all ages. Frequently, on arrival in the emergency department or other acute care setting, the child is no longer experiencing any pain from a wound but is extremely anxious over its potential repair. Because of the slightly thinner stratum corneum of a child's skin and the improved blood supply, children are excellent candidates for the use of topical anesthetic agents as opposed to infiltrative anesthesia. Many different combinations of **lidocaine**, **epinephrine**, **tetracaine**, **bupivacaine**, and **cocaine** have been used successfully for topical anesthesia of lacerations and wounds in children. All these agents appear to be most effective on the face and scalp, although they also have been used with some success on the extremities. When using these solutions, it is important to allow at least 20 to 30 minutes for the medications to diffuse into the wound and produce anesthesia. Because all these agents contain vasoconstrictors, their use should be avoided in any lacerations that involve end-organ blood supplies, including the tip of the nose, fingers, toes, and penis. Solutions that contain cocaine should not be used around mucosal surfaces in which inadvertent absorption of the

cocaine may occur. Seizures and deaths have been reported secondary to systemic absorption after the inappropriate application of cocaine solutions to mucosal surfaces or extensive abrasions or burns.

Infiltrative Anesthesia

Both **lidocaine** and **bupivacaine** may be used to infiltrate the subcutaneous tissue surrounding a wound to induce anesthesia. Both of these agents produce their effect by blocking sodium channels in the axons of the sensory nerves and inhibiting transmissions of nerve impulses to the central nervous system. Most wounds can be anesthetized adequately with local infiltration with 1% or 2% lidocaine with or without epinephrine. The maximum dose of plain lidocaine is 4.5 mg/kg and, for lidocaine with epinephrine, the maximum dose is 7 mg/kg. Solutions with epinephrine should not be used in regions supplied by end arteries (eg, fingers, toes, lips, nose, ears, genitalia). Lidocaine has a rapid onset of action and duration of 30 to 120 minutes. The onset of action of bupivacaine is intermediate, and the duration of action is 2 to 6 hours.

Multiple techniques have been shown to decrease the pain of local infiltration of these anesthetics. Most prominent among these is the **buffering** of the anesthetic solutions. Adjustment of the pH closer to 7.4 allows more rapid absorption of the anesthetic into the axonal fibers and more rapid blockade of the sodium channels. Lidocaine solutions are buffered by the creation of a 9:1 lidocaine/bicarbonate solution. These solutions can be prepared by removing and replacing 1 mL of lidocaine with 1 mL of 8.4% $NaHCO_3$ (1 mEq/mL) for every 10 mL of a standard lidocaine solution. For a fresh 30-mL bottle of lidocaine, this would require removal of 3 mL of lidocaine and replacement with 3 mL of the standard bicarbonate solution. Alternate therapies that also may decrease the pain of local infiltration include the use of a small-gauge needle (27 to 30 gauge), slow infiltration, maintenance of solution temperature close to body temperature, and subdermal rather than intradermal infiltration.

The properties of lidocaine and bupivacaine are summarized in Table 18-3.

Regional Anesthesia

Selective **blockade of peripheral nerves** may

provide excellent pain relief in a child with an injury to a specific body area. **Digital nerve blocks** are particularly effective in children with crush injuries to the fingers. These blocks are best applied immediately on arrival without waiting for formal registration to be completed. If the digit is anesthetized quickly while the child is still upset over the injury, the child may not even notice the puncture associated with the placement of the block. These children then will calm down rapidly once the finger no longer hurts. Other nerve blocks that are effective include median, ulnar, and radial nerve blocks at the wrist for more extensive anesthesia of the entire hand. Supraorbital, infraorbital, and mental nerve blocks can provide regional anesthesia of the face, whereas tibial, sural, and peroneal nerve blocks at the ankle can anesthetize the plantar surface of the foot. Femoral nerve blocks are extremely effective in children with femur fractures and should be considered in any child presenting with this injury.

Patients with extensive injuries to an isolated upper or lower extremity can be managed through the use of **intravenous regional anesthesia.** Use of this technique should be limited to personnel skilled in its use.

Special Anesthetic Situations

Ophthalmic anesthetics are safe and useful for children with corneal abrasions or ocular foreign bodies. Both **tetracaine** and **proparacaine** produce excellent topical anesthesia for anterior eye injuries. Topical nasal anesthesia may be obtained from a 4% cocaine solution, which provides both local anesthesia and vasoconstriction for nasal mucosa.

Even with good regional or local anesthesia, some children will be too excited to undergo a specific procedure. In these instances, the local anesthesia must be supplemented with some form of sedation to protect the child and allow safe completion of a needed intervention.

Systemic Analgesics

The indications for centrally acting analgesics include patients with undefined pain or pain that cannot be managed easily through the use of peripheral or regional anesthesia.

Narcotic Analgesics

The cornerstone of centrally acting analgesics are the **narcotic analgesics.** This class of drugs produces its effect by mimicking the intrinsic analgesics through binding to CNS opioid receptors. Most narcotics used clinically in medicine produce their effects through actions on both the μ and κ receptors. Narcotic agonists bind and stimulate both sites; narcotic agonists/antagonists stimulate one site and block the other, and narcotic antagonists block both sites. Commonly used opioid agonists or narcotics are summarized in Table 18-4. All of the narcotics may be given orally or parenterally, although for effective pain relief, parenteral titration probably is the optimum means of administration. Fentanyl also may be given transmucosally.

Morphine sulfate is the prototypical high-potency narcotic and the standard by which most other narcotics are measured. It is most effective when administered intravenously, although intramuscular and subcutaneous administrations have been used effectively. The disadvantage of intramuscular or subcutaneous administration is that a child must undergo a painful needle stick to acquire an analgesic for relief of pain. Like other narcotics, morphine can produce dose-dependent respiratory depression. Although generally

TABLE 18-3.
Infiltrative anesthetics.

Drug	Maximum Dose	Onset	Duration
Lidocaine	4.5 mg/kg	2-3 min	1-2 hr
Bupivacaine*	1.5 mg/kg	3-5 min	4-8 hr

Calculation of dosage. A 1% solution of an anesthetic contains 1 g of anesthetic in 100 mL of solution. This translates into 10 mg/mL. A 0.25% solution contains 2.5 mg/mL anesthetic in solution.

*Not recommend for children younger than 12 years. Usually supplied as a 0.25% solution.

TABLE 18-4.
Medications used for analgesia and sedation (titration recommended).

	Dose (mg/kg)	Route	Maximum Unit Dose (mg)	Precautions	Comments
Analgesic					
Morphine	0.05-0.1	IM/IV	10	Histamine release/respiratory depression	
Fentanyl	0.0005-0.002	IM/IV	0.05	Rigid chest	Decrease dose by one half in infants younger than 6 mo
	0.005-0.015	Transmucosal	400 µg	Vomiting may occur with higher dose	
Meperidine	1-2	IM/IV	100	Accumulation of toxic metabolite normeperidine	
Hydromorphone	0.015-0.02	Oral			
Hydrocodone	0.2	Oral	10		Combine with acetaminophen
Codeine	1-2	Oral	60	Gastrointestinal upset, vomiting	Combine with acetaminophen
Acetaminophen	10-15	Oral/rectal	1000		
Sedative					
Pentobarbital*	1-6	IV	100	CNS depression, porphyria	All barbiturates should be avoided in children with porphyria.
Methohexital*	0.5-1.0 18-25	IV Rectal	100	Respiratory depression	
Thiopental*	4-6 25	IV Rectal	300	Respiratory depression	
Midazolam	0.05-0.2 0.4-0.5 0.2-0.5	IM/IV Rectal Nasal/oral	6 6 6	Respiratory and CNS depression	May produce agitation rather than sedation
Chloral hydrate	50-100	Oral	2000	Liver and renal disease	
Propofol	1.5-2.5 0.025-0.15	IV bolus Continuous	100	Respiratory depression	
Other					
Ketamine	1-2 0.5-1.0 6-10	IM IV PO		Airway secretions, psychosis, increased ICP, hypertension, cardiac disease, younger than 3 mo	Pretreatment with atropine, 0.02 mg/kg (minimum, 0.1 mg; maximum, 0.5 mg) or glycopyrrolate. Do not use with head injury or increased intracranial or intraocular pressure.

*Therapeutic doses may vary.

appearing relatively quickly, this effect may be delayed up to 90 minutes after intramuscular or subcutaneous administration. Infants younger than 3 months are more sensitive to respiratory depressant effects and should be monitored more closely. The fact that these children are more sensitive is not a contraindication to the use of this drug in these patients, only an indication to administer it more cautiously. Morphine can cause histamine release, which may precipitate hypotension, itching, and wheezing. It should be used cautiously in asthmatics and potentially hypovolemic patients. Nausea, emesis, constipation, and myosis also are well-recognized side effects.

Fentanyl citrate is a synthetic narcotic that, unlike morphine, does not cause histamine release and has minimal adverse cardiovascular effects. Because of this profile, it is a good choice for both asthmatic and trauma patients. It has a much shorter onset of action than morphine but a much shorter duration of action, making it more attractive for brief procedures. In addition to respiratory depression, fentanyl can cause chest wall rigidity when given rapidly in high doses. Most chest wall rigidity is self-limited; however, in some instances, it may be reversed with naloxone or neuromuscular paralysis. Because of its potency, fentanyl is dosed in increments of micrograms per kilogram, so care should be taken when ordering or administering this drug.

Fentanyl also is the only agent currently administered as an oral transmucosal narcotic. It is available in a lollipop-type preparation containing 100 to 400 µg of fentanyl and is administered in a dose of 5 to 15 µg/kg with a maximum dose of 400 µg. Delivered in this manner, fentanyl is used more as a sedative than as an analgesic, and there is an increased risk of emesis.

Hydromorphone is a semisynthetic narcotic with analgesic properties similar to those of morphine. It is more potent than morphine, with a similar onset time and duration of action. This drug commonly is used for pain management in sickle cell patients and is frequently used as the analgesic in PCA devices.

Meperidine is another commonly used narcotic in children. It has few advantages and many disadvantages compared with morphine. It has a slightly shorter half-life and a steeper dose-response curve, making titration more difficult. Meperidine

seems to produce more of a euphoric state than morphine, which is why some patients will request it by name. The major disadvantage to meperidine use in children is the potential accumulation of normeperidine, a toxic metabolite associated with central nervous system excitation tremors, nausea, vomiting, dysphoria, and seizures. Normeperidine has a longer half-life than meperidine, and children given repeated doses of meperidine over a period of time may accumulate this metabolite and develop adverse reactions. Meperidine also can interact with certain monoamine oxidase inhibitors and should be avoided in patients receiving these drugs.

Hydrocodone is a synthetic narcotic that can be administered only orally. It is more effective and potent than codeine and produces fewer gastrointestinal complications. It is ideal as an oral analgesic for outpatient administration for painful conditions. Hydrocodone is available as an oral suspension with acetaminophen, making it useful for infants and small children.

Codeine is another agent that can be used both parenterally and orally, although it is most commonly combined with acetaminophen for oral administration. Codeine may produce vomiting and abdominal pain, which may limit its effectiveness.

Narcotic Antagonists. Inadvertent excessive narcotic administration can result in respiratory depression, central nervous system excitation, and hypotension. All of these effects are reversible through the use of narcotic antagonists such as naloxone or nalmefene. Naloxone is the standard opioid antagonist; it works through competitive inhibition of the µ- and κ-opioid receptors in the central nervous system. In children who have received overdoses, the recommended dose for antagonism is 0.1 mg/kg IV or IM. In larger children and adults, a standard dose of 2 mg may be administered. This dose can be repeated in 2 to 3 minutes if needed. The half-life of naloxone is ≈60 minutes, which is considerably less than that of most commonly used opioids. As a result, repeat doses for continual reversal of respiratory depression may be needed. A new alternative to naloxone is available; nalmefene has a duration of ≈10 to 12 hours. This drug has not been approved for use in children younger than 12 years, although anecdotal reports note that it has been used in children effectively with minimal side effects.

Non-Narcotic Analgesics

Aspirin, acetaminophen, and **nonsteroidal anti-inflammatory drugs** (NSAIDs) are effective analgesics that may be used in children with minor painful conditions. These drugs should not be used as a substitute for potent analgesics in children with acutely painful conditions that otherwise would require potent analgesics.

Other Analgesics

Ketamine hydrochloride is a dissociative agent that causes a functional electrophysiologic dissociation between the thalamocortical and limbic systems. The result of this dissociation is a trance-like cataleptic state with preservation of respiratory drive and protective airway reflexes. Ketamine also is a mild sympathomimetic that may induce a slight increase in blood pressure and intracranial and intraocular pressures. Children who receive ketamine appear to be awake with open eyes and may exhibit nonpurposeful movements and verbalizations, which sometimes will prompt parents to comment that the child actually is still awake and aware. Additional actions of ketamine include increased salivary and bronchial secretions as well as a mild increase in blood pressure and, occasionally, vomiting. The increase in airway secretions can be limited by pretreatment with either atropine (0.02 mg/kg; minimum, 0.1 mg; maximum, 0.5 mg) or glycopyrrolate (0.005 mg/kg; maximum, 0.25 mg). Transient laryngospasm has been reported but is usually self-limited and clinically inconsequential. Some children may have emergence reactions, including hallucinations and an unpleasant dream, as the drug wears off. This is uncommon in young children. The incidence can be reduced by the administration of midazolam with the ketamine.

Ketamine may be administered orally, intravenously, or intramuscularly. If given intramuscularly, the atropine can be mixed in the same syringe as the ketamine. One note of caution: ketamine is supplied as both a 10 and 100 mg/mL preparation. The lower concentration is used for intravenous administration, and the higher concentration is for intramuscular use. Anecdotal reports have noted that children have received 10 times the intended dose of ketamine when the higher concentration was inadvertently administered intravenously. Because of the safety profile of ketamine, these children had no adverse effects and only slept for an extended period of time. When given orally, ketamine is best mixed with a sugary syrup or provided as gelatin cubes.

Ketamine is most effective for use in acute painful procedures that cannot be effectively controlled through the use of regional anesthesia, including burns, wound debridement, repair of complex facial lacerations, difficult foreign body removals, incision and drainage of abscesses, and fracture repairs.

The pharmacologic actions of ketamine — reliable sedation and profound analgesia — in conjunction with its preservation of respiratory drive and protection of airway reflexes make it an ideal choice for the management of emergency department patients. In one report, only 19 possible complications were noted in >12,800 administrations of ketamine (0.2%). Oral, intramuscular, and intravenous doses for ketamine are given in Table 18-4. Contraindications to the use of ketamine include pulmonary infections, significant head injuries, increased intracranial pressure, glaucoma, acute ocular injuries, psychosis, thyrotoxicosis, and previous adverse reactions.

Nitrous oxide has been used effectively in older children and adolescents for analgesia in conditions such as burn debridement, laceration repair, and fracture reduction. It has dissociative amnesic effects and provides analgesia but not true anesthesia. It does not cause circulatory or respiratory depression, although it produces some skeletal muscle relaxation, drowsiness, euphoria, and a floating sensation. To be effective, an adequate amount of nitrous oxide must be used.

Most commercial delivery systems are fixed at a 50:50 mixture of nitrous oxide and oxygen. Some authors note this concentration is equivalent to 5 to 10 mg of morphine; others believe that, to be truly effective, a 70:30 mixture should be used.

Nitrous oxide should be used only in children old enough to self-administer this agent. Children must be able to hold a face mask in place for proper self-limited administration of this drug. When a deep state of sedation is achieved, the hand holding the mask in place falls away from the face, interrupting the delivery of the gas. Nitrous oxide is contraindicated in children with respiratory difficulty, pneumothorax, intestinal obstruction, altered level of consciousness, or significant facial injuries or chest injuries. When used in the emergency department, scavenger systems, which absorb any escaped gas, should be used to prevent passive inhalation by personnel.

Sedatives

In many children, a painful condition is not the problem; instead, the child is too excited or agitated to cooperate with a necessary part of treatment. Typically, these instances involve a child whose cooperation is required for a diagnostic study or an anesthetized surgical procedure. In these circumstances, a pure sedative is the pharmacologic agent of choice. Narcotic analgesics have sedation as a side effect, but their primary indication is relief from painful conditions. One exception to this generalization is **transmucosal fentanyl**, which is used primarily as a sedative. If sedation is what is required for a child, then an agent whose primary function is sedation should be the drug of choice. Similarly, if a child is agitated or uncooperative secondary to pain, then an analgesic and not a sedative is indicated.

Commonly used sedatives are listed in Table 18-4. The most commonly used sedatives include the **barbiturates** and **benzodiazepines**. Both of these drugs produce their effects by acting on the GABA receptors in the CNS. Both agents can stimulate the GABA receptor directly but also produce effects by enhancing the action of GABA itself.

Pentobarbital is a rapidly acting barbiturate of relatively short duration that typically is used parenterally for sedation for diagnostic studies. An excellent protocol with high efficacy and an proven safety profile is the use of progressive doses of pentobarbital in a stepwise fashion to produce somnolence in children undergoing CT scans. In this protocol, a child is administered 2.5 mg/kg IV of pentobarbital. If the child is not asleep 60 seconds after the administration of that dose, a dose of 1.25 mg/kg of pentobarbital is administered. If a child remains awake at 2 minutes after that dose, a final dose of 1.25 mg/kg is administered. This regimen is almost 100% effective in the induction of sleep for use in diagnostic radiography in children. As with all potent sedatives, appropriate monitoring

must be used, and the child must be observed for signs of respiratory depression.

Methohexital and **thiopental** most commonly are used to induce deep sedation for rapid sequence intubation of children. Both drugs also are used as sedatives for children. Administered rectally, both drugs are effective for sedation, although absorption can be erratic and close observation must be maintained. Intravenous methohexital has been used successfully in the emergency department for sedation of adults.

Midazolam is a benzodiazepine commonly used for the sedation of children. It has remarkable amnestic effects and a relatively rapid onset of action, with sedation occurring within 5 to 15 minutes. The half-life of midazolam is ≈1 to 2 hours, but there is wide individual variation. Midazolam may be administered intravenously, intramuscularly, intranasally, orally, and even rectally. Transmucosal absorption is erratic, and its efficacy is extremely variable. Occasionally, children administered midazolam will have a paradoxical reaction and become more agitated and combative. As with the barbiturates, these children should be monitored for respiratory depression. An advantage of the use of midazolam is that iatrogenic overdoses with respiratory depression can be reversed with the competitive antagonist **flumazenil**.

Propofol is a modified phenol with extremely potent sedative properties. Unlike the barbiturates and benzodiazepines, propofol does not work through any specific receptor site and instead seems to exhibit its action through infiltration directly into the cell membrane of the neurons. Propofol can be administered only intravenously. Its onset of action is extremely quick, generally within 10 to 15 seconds of intravenous administration, and its duration of action is extremely limited, generally dissipating within 8 to 15 minutes. These properties make propofol ideal for the sedation of patients on ventilators, those undergoing short procedures, or those in whom repeated neurologic examinations must be performed. Like other potent sedatives, propofol does induce respiratory depression and hypotension, and patients receiving propofol infusions should be monitored carefully.

Propofol may be administered as a bolus followed by a continuous infusion or a bolus followed by repeat smaller boluses to maintain sedation for a brief period of time.

Chloral hydrate is used primarily for sedation for diagnostic procedures and can be administered orally or rectally. Chloral hydrate is best given ≈30 to 60 minutes before a procedure, and its effects can last up to 12 to 24 hours. The duration of action limits its usefulness in emergency settings. Side effects consist of mild gastrointestinal symptoms, including nausea and possibly vomiting, as well as ataxia and disorientation.

Combination Drugs

Midazolam and fentanyl are used in combination intravenous doses for sedation and pain control. Extremely careful monitoring is essential, and single-agent dosing is preferred. If used, fentanyl should be given first at a dose of 0.5 to 2.0 µg/kg over 3 to 5 minutes. Midazolam then may be titrated slowly if needed at a dose of 0.05 mg/kg to a maximum total dose of 0.2 mg/kg.

ADDITIONAL READING

Acute Pain Management Guideline Panel. *Clinical Practice Guideline. Acute Pain Management: Operative or Medical Procedures and Trauma.* Rockville, Md: US Department of Health and Human Services; Public Health Service; Agency for Health Care Policy and Research; 1992.

American Academy of Pediatrics, Committee on Drugs. Guidelines for monitoring and management of pediatric patients during and after sedation for diagnostic and therapeutic procedures. *Pediatrics.* 1992;89:295-300.

American College of Emergency Physicians, Pediatric Emergency Medicine Committee. Rapid-sequence intubation of the pediatric patient. *Ann Emerg Med.* 1996;28:55-74.

American College of Emergency Physicians, Pediatric Emergency Medicine Committee. Pediatric analgesia and sedation. *Ann Emerg Med.* 1994;23:237-250.

American Society of Anesthesiologists, Task Force on Sedation and Analgesia by Non-Anesthesiologists. Practice guidelines for sedation and analgesia by non-anesthesiologists. *Anesthesiology.* 1996;84:459-471.

Dieckmann RA, Fiser DH, Selbst SM, eds. *Illustrated Textbook of Pediatric Emergency and Critical Care Procedures.* St Louis, Mo: Mosby; 1997.

Green SM, Clem KJ, Rothrock SG. Ketamine safety profile in the developing world: survey of practitioners. *Acad Emerg Med.* 1996;3:598-604.

Krause BS, Shannon M, Damian FJ, et al. *Guidelines for Pediatric Sedation.* Dallas, Tex: American College of Emergency Physicians; 1995.

Roberts JR. Intravenous regional anesthesia. In: Roberts JR, Hedges JR, eds. *Clinical Procedures in Emergency Medicine,* 2nd ed. Philadelphia, Pa: WB Saunders; 1991;499-503.

Schechter NL, Weisman SJ, Rosenblum M, et al. The use of oral transmucosal fentanyl citrate for painful procedures in children. *Pediatrics.* 1995;95:335-339.

Smith GA, Strausbaugh SD, Harbeck-Weber C, et al. Comparison of topical anesthetics without cocaine to tetracaine-adrenaline-cocaine and lidocaine infiltration during repair of lacerations: bupivacaine-norepinephrine is an effective new topical anesthetic agent. *Pediatrics.* 1996;97:301-307.

Terndrup TE. Pediatric pain control. *Ann Emerg Med.* 1996;27:466-470.

Terndrup TE. Establishing pain policies in emergency medicine. *Ann Emerg Med.* 1996;27:408-411.

Vinci RJ, Fish SS. Efficacy of topical anesthesia in children. *Arch Pediatr Adolesc Med.* 1996;150:466-469.

Chapter 19

Medication Use: Aids to Correct Dosing

OBJECTIVES

1. State the correct dose and dosage form for common medications used in pediatric emergencies.

2. Access authoritative reference material for checking common doses and identifying correct doses for less commonly used agents.

3. Calculate the correct volume of drugs for administration.

Knowledge of drug dosage does not ensure accurate dosing. The practitioner must know not only the correct dose but also the dosage form and must calculate the correct volume of drug to administer. In an emergency setting, calculation errors are frequent. Furthermore, correct calculation requires an accurate estimate of the child's weight, which is not always readily available. To improve dosing, the practitioner should use one or more of the following methods:

- Stock CPR carts and office, clinic, or other emergency carts with one preparation of each drug. These should be listed on the cart in clear view with accompanying dosage information.
- When possible, obtain a body weight on all children. In emergency situations, the estimates in Table 19-1 can be used.
- An emergency length-based drug tape can be used to more rapidly estimate dosages when weight is not known or cannot be determined (Figure 19-1). This system provides correct drug doses and volumes of commonly used emergency drug preparations. Alternatively, color-coded systems are available.
- Prepare dose-per-kilogram calculations for drugs (1 to 40 kg) on separate index cards kept on the CPR or emergency drug cart.
  Example: Patient with a weight of 15 kg
    Epinephrine (0.01 or 0.1 mg/kg)
       1:10,000   0.1 mg/mL = 1.5 mL
       1:1000   1.0 mg/mL = 1.5 mL
    Bicarbonate (1 mEq/kg)
       8.4%   1 mEq/mL = 15 mL
    Calcium chloride (20 mg/kg)
       10%   100 mg/mL = 3 mL
    Atropine (0.02 mg/kg)
       0.1 mg/mL (prefilled syringe) = 3 mL
       1 mg/mL (vial) = 0.3 mL

See Table 19-2 for aids in calculation.

Dose-per-kilogram calculations should not exceed adult doses. This maximum is reached at 25 kg for calcium (500 mg), 50 kg for atropine (1 mg) and bicarbonate (50 mEq). There is no upper limit for high-dose epinephrine.

Also remember that the minimum dose for atropine is 0.1 mg.

Dosages of commonly used resuscitation drugs and comments on their use are summarized in Table 19-3.

Preparation and dosages for intravenous infusion of resuscitation drugs are summarized in Table 19-4.

ADDITIONAL READING

American Academy of Pediatrics, Committee on Drugs. Drugs for pediatric emergencies. *Pediatrics*. 1998;101:1-11.

Laposata M. *SI Unit Conversion Guide*. Boston, Mass: NEJM Books; 1992.

Lubitz DS, Seidel JS, Chameides L, et al. A rapid method for estimating weight and resuscitation drug dosages from length in the pediatric age group. *Ann Emerg Med*. 1988;17:576-581.

Zaritsky A. Pediatric resuscitation pharmacology. *Ann Emerg Med*. 1993;22(pt 2):445-455.

FIGURE 19-1.
Section of length-based drug tape.

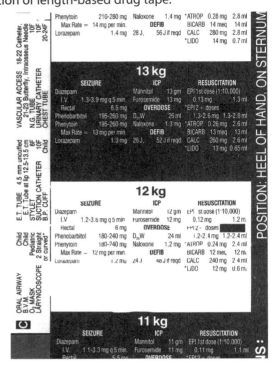

BROSELOW™ Pediatric Emergency Tape, Armstrong Medical Industries, Lincolnshire, Illinois. ©1993 Vital Signs, Inc. Reprinted with permission.

TABLE 19-1.
Body weight estimation guidelines.

Age	Weight (kg)	Estimated Weight
Term infant	3.5	Birth weight (BW)
5 mo	7	2 x BW
1 yr	10	3 x BW
4 yr	16	One fourth adult weight of 70 kg
10 yr	35	One half adult weight of 70 kg

TABLE 19-2.
Aids to drug calculations.

Percent Solutions
Percentage = number of grams per 100 mL, regardless of the substance

10% solution	= 10 g/100 mL
	= 0.1 g/mL
	= 100 mg/mL
$D_{10}W$	= 100 mg glucose/mL (10 g/100 mL)
10% $CaCl_2$	= 100 mg calcium chloride/mL

Serial Dilution

1:100, 1:1000, 1:10,000	= 1 g of any substance per 100, 1000, 10,000 mL
1:10,000 epinephrine	= 1 g/10,000 mL
	= 1 mg/10 mL
	= 0.1 mg/mL

Micrograms (µg)
1 µg = 1/1000 of a mg, or 1 mg = 1000 µg
Example: How many µg/mL are in a 1:10,000 solution of epinephrine?

1:10,000	= 1 g/10,000 mL
	= 1000 mg/10,000 mL
	= 1 mg/10 mL
	= 1000 µg/10 mL
	= 100 µg/mL

TABLE 19-3.
Intravenous push medications used in pediatric cardiopulmonary resuscitation and postresuscitation stabilization.

Drug	Dose	How Supplied	Remarks
Adenosine	0.1 mg/kg (0.03 mL/kg) Maximum dose is 12 mg	3 mg/mL	Give by rapid infusion† while monitoring ECG; successive doses of 0.1 and 0.15 mg/kg
Atropine sulfate	0.02 mg/kg (0.2 mL/kg)	0.1 mg/mL	Minimum dose of 0.1 mg (1 mL); use for bradycardia unresponsive to ventilation and due to heart block.
Bretylium tosylate	5 mg/kg (0.1 mL/kg)	50 mg/mL	Use if lidocaine is not effective. May be repeated with dose of 10 mg/kg if needed.
Calcium chloride	20 mg/kg (0.2 mL/kg)	100 mg/mL (10% solution)	Use only for ionized hypocalcemia, hyperkalemia, hypermagnesemia, and calcium blocker toxicity; give slowly.*
Diazepam	0.1-0.3 mg/kg (0.02-0.06 mL/kg)	5 mg/mL	May be repeated but give slowly; may cause respiratory depression.
Diazoxide	1-3 mg/kg (0.6-0.2 mL/kg)	15 mg/mL	Rapid IV bolus† in hypertensive crisis. Patient remains recumbent 30 min afte dose.
Epinephrine hydrochloride	0.01 mg/kg—initial (0.1 mL/kg of 1:10,000) 0.1 mg/kg—as needed subsequently (0.1 mL/kg of 1:1000)	1:10,000 (0.1 mg/mL) 1:1000 (1 mg/mL)	Most useful drug for cardiac arrest. Use subsequent high dose q3-5min if initial dose is not effective or initially if endotracheal tube is the only available route.
Fosphenytoin	10-20 mg PE‡/kg	50 mg/mL	Infuse at <3 mg PE‡/kg per minute.
Furosemide	1 mg/kg (0.1 mL/kg)	10 mg/mL	Give over at least 3 min but not faster than 4 mg/min.
Glucose	250-500 mg/kg (1-2 mL/kg of $D_{25}W$) or (2.5-5 mL/kg of $D_{10}W$)	0.5 g/mL (500 mg/mL of $D_{50}W$); dilute 1:1 for $D_{50}W$, dilute 1:4 for $D_{10}W$	May be important in infants. Infuse slowly* because it is hypertonic.
Lidocaine hydrochloride	1 mg/kg (0.1 mL/kg of 1%), (0.05 mL/kg of 2%)	10 mg/mL (1%), 20 mg/mL (2%)	May be bolused at 5-min intervals up to three times; if repeat boluses needed, begin an infusion.
Lorazepam	0.05-0.1 mg/kg	2, 4 mg/mL	Repeat twice at intervals of 10-15 min if needed; maximum dose of 4 mg
Midazolam	0.05-0.2 mg/kg (0.01-0.04 mL/kg)	5 mg/mL	Give slowly*; may cause respiratory depression.
Naloxone	0.1 mg/kg (0.25 mL/kg) Repeat in 2-5 min if needed	0.4, 1 mg/mL	A standard dose of 2 mg may be used if child is >5 years of age or >20 kg. Use to antagonize narcotic overdoses.
Phenobarbital	20 mg/kg	30, 60, 65, 130 mg/mL	Rate ≤100 mg/min
Phenytoin	10-20 mg/kg (0.2-0.4 mL/kg)	50 mg/mL	Infuse no faster than 1 mg/kg per minute; monitor cardiac rate and blood pressure.
Sodium bicarbonate	1-2 mEq/kg (1-2 mL/kg)	1 mEq/mL (8.4% solution)	Infuse slowly* and only when ventilation is adequate.

*Slow infusion usually means to give the drug over 1-3 min.
†Rapid push means to give the drug over 1-5 sec.
‡Phenytoin equivalents.

TABLE 19-4.
Intravenous infusion medications used in pediatric cardiopulmonary resuscitation and postresuscitation stabilization.

Drug (How Supplied*)	Dose	Preparation for Infusion†	Dosage Equivalents
Dopamine (40 mg/mL)	Begin at 10 µg/kg/min; titrate to desired effect up to 20 µg/kg/min.	6 x the body weight in kg is the number of milligrams to add to the diluent to make a final volume of 100 mL‡	Then, 1 mL/hr delivers 1 µg/kg per minute.
Dobutamine (12.5 mg/mL)	Begin at 10 µg/kg/min; titrate to desired effect up to 25 µg/kg/min.		
Nitroprusside (50 mg powdered vial)	Begin at 0.5 µg/kg/min; titrate to desired effect up to 10 µg/kg/min.		
Epinephrine 1:1000 (1 mg/mL)	Begin at 0.1 µg/kg/min and increase as needed to 3 µg/kg/min.	0.6 x the body weight in kg is the number of milligrams to add to the diluent to make a final volume of 100 mL.	Then, 1 mL/hr delivers 0.1 µg/kg per minute.
Norepinephrine 1:1000 (1 mg/mL)	Begin at 0.1-0.3 µg/kg/min and increase as needed to 1 µg/kg/min. Used in hypotensive septic shock.		
Prostaglandin E$_1$ (0.5 mg/mL)	Begin at 0.05-0.1 µg/kg/min; monitor for hypotension, apnea.		
Isoproterenol 1:5000 (0.2 mg/mL)	Infuse like epinephrine; carefully monitor heart rate and blood pressure.		
Lidocaine 2% (20 mg/mL)	Begin at 20 µg/kg/min and increase to maximum of 50 µg/kg/min as needed.	60 x the body weight in kg is the number of milligrams to add to the diluent to make a final volume of 100 mL.	Then, 1 mL/hr delivers 10 µg/kg per minute.

*Concentration listed is either the form available in prefilled syringes or the most commonly used concentration.
†The diluent should be a salt-containing solution (1/2 NS, NS, D5 1/2 NS, etc).
‡One of the advantages of the "Rule of 6" is that it can be used to calculate many infusions. It is also easy to determine the infusion rate being used for the patient.

Appendix 19-1. Conversion to SI Units.

In this volume, laboratory and pressure values are reported in the traditional units taught in most US medical schools and used in most medical and other scientific journals. A number of other nations and some journals use SI units as a means of reporting values for laboratory results and other items of scientific exchange, such as pressure, time, electric current, and temperature. The widespread use of SI units would standardize reporting for all such data throughout the world.

Adoption of SI units would result in the following changes in health care data:

- Conversion from mass (grams) to molecular units (moles)
- Use of the liter as the unit of volume
- In some instances, use of Pascal as the unit of pressure

The conversion from traditional units to SI units is relatively simple and involves multiplication by the conversion factor determined for each value. In many instances, the conversion factor is 1, so the value remains the same and only the nomenclature of the unit changes. Conversion from SI units to traditional units would involve division of the SI units by the same factor.

The conversion factors and the volume or molecular unit are listed in Table 19-5 for each of the laboratory tests or other measurements for which values are mentioned in this manual.

TABLE 19-5.
Conversion to SI units.

Traditional Unit	Constituent	SI Unit	Conversion Factor
U/L	Aspartate transferase (AST)	U/L	1
mg/dL	Glucose	mmol/L	0.05551
1 mEq/L	Potassium	mmol/L	1
mEq/L	Sodium	mmol/L	1
g/dL	Protein, serum	g/L	10
mg/dL	Protein, CSF	g/L	0.01
g/dL	Hemoglobin	g/L	10
%	Hematocrit	Fraction of 1.00	0.01
$10^3/mm^3$	WBC and RBC	$10^9/L$	1
mm Hg	PCO_2	kPa	0.1333
mm Hg	PO_2	kPa	0.1333
pH units	pH	pH units	1
% body weight	Blood volume	mL/kg	9.4

Chapter 20

Emergency Medical Services for Children: An Overview

OBJECTIVES

1. Explain the concepts of emergency medical services (EMS).

2. Recognize the particular needs of children in the EMS system — EMS-C.

3. Identify the communication and preparation necessary for interhospital transport.

It is important for practitioners to have an understanding of their EMS systems, which may be used to care for their patients. The term **EMS system** refers to a group of emergency health care delivery organizations that together allow for the appropriate delivery of out-of-hospital care and transport of children when suddenly ill or injured.

DEFINITIONS

Emergency medical services for children (EMS-C) refers to programs within EMS systems that provide for a specific focus on the emergency care needs of the pediatric patient. Measures to enhance EMS-C are clearly most effective when integrated into existing EMS systems. Table 20-1 lists five phases of the EMS-C continuum.

The **EMS-C continuum** encompasses all aspects of the care provided to an acutely ill or injured child. Caretaker recognition of an emergency, access to telephone-activated emergency 911 where available, ambulance dispatch, prehospital care and transport, emergency department and inpatient care, trauma centers, pediatric critical care networks, rehabilitation, and interfacility transfer are all included.

At the center of the EMS-C system, there is a **primary care physician.** Every child should have a medical home responsible for:

- Educating the family on prevention so the child does not have to use the system
- Appropriate recognition of acute illness or severe injury requiring the use of EMS-C
- Activation of the system

The primary care physician should follow the child through this illness or injury and, when possible, provide direct care and be responsible for recognition and management of psychological and physical conditions requiring rehabilitation. The primary care physician can play a central role in education directed at appropriate use of the system.

Emergency Medical Services. In most communities, the private and public safety agencies that provide ambulance service and prehospital care are referred to as EMS. The **EMS system** does not fall under the aegis of any one organization, agency, or specialty group. The individual components listed above often operate independently, may not interface well, or may not exist at all; this varies on a region-to-region basis. However, there usually is a lead agency, typically an EMS program within a state or county department of health or public safety agency.

Direct ("on-line") Medical Control. This refers to medical personnel based at a receiving facility, a central medical facility, or an EMS agency authorized to assist out-of-hospital personnel with medical and procedural decisions via telephone or radio while in the field.

Indirect ("off-line") Medical Control. This refers to physicians who provide input and collaborate on writing and modifying treatment protocols, triage criteria, and equipment lists, as well as assume responsibility for quality improvement. This input usually is provided by a committee of physicians who work with the EMS medical director. This is an excellent forum for physicians to become involved as advocates for the special needs of children.

PREHOSPITAL CARE ("PRIMARY TRANSPORT")

Prehospital care includes the entry and response phases, each of which involves several discrete

---

TABLE 20-1.
EMS-C continuum.

Illness and injury (prevention phase)
Entry phase (home/scene/professional office)
Response phase (prehospital)
Hospital phase (community/interfacility
    transport/definitive care)
Rehabilitation phase

From Dieckmann RA. *Pediatric Emergency Care Systems: Planning and Management.* Baltimore, Md: Williams & Wilkins; 1992. Adapted with permission.

actions. Most seriously ill children are transported for medical evaluation by their caretakers. A significant number of children, however, are assessed initially and transported by EMS personnel. Approximately 6% to 10% of all EMS calls are for patients younger than 19 years. Although most pediatric calls receive only basic life support (BLS) interventions, about one third receive advanced life support (ALS) responses. Children transported to emergency departments by EMS personnel are 5 to 10 times more likely to require admission than are those transported privately.

In most areas, pediatric EMS prehospital calls are divided more or less equally between traumatic and medical complaints. The most common mechanisms of injury are vehicular trauma (including a vehicle occupant, struck pedestrian, or struck bicyclist), falls, and burns. The most common medical complaints are seizures, respiratory distress, submersion, and poisonings. For children younger than 2 years, the majority of calls are for medical problems. Traumatic complaints predominate in children older than 2 years, with a peak in vehicular trauma among adolescents. This distribution of illnesses and injuries differs from that of adults.

Entry Phase

The entry phase requires that a **problem be identified** by the prospective patient or an observer, who then must activate the EMS system. In many areas of the United States, this is done via 911 telephone systems. Systems with **enhanced 911** capabilities can automatically trace caller location, thereby enabling medical assistance to be dispatched even if the caller is unable to provide that information. In areas without 911 service, access usually is provided through an emergency telephone number for the local law enforcement agency, fire department, or hospital. If medical assistance is required, the call is routed to a medical dispatcher. Using only the limited amount of information available by telephone, the medical dispatcher must be able to recognize and appropriately triage both adult and pediatric emergencies.

Based on the complaint and additional information, the **dispatcher** determines the required level of EMS response and activates the appropriate units. The dispatcher also may instruct the caller in the first aid and immediate BLS measures necessary for patient support until EMS units arrive. The dispatcher's actions usually are dictated by protocols. The development of specific pediatric dispatch protocols and dispatcher training are goals of EMS-C efforts.

EMS provider agencies have many organizational structures but are functionally divided into those providing BLS services, ALS services, or both. Although most pediatric cases receive only BLS support, many pediatric patients have a potential for deterioration and require constant reassessment by an ALS team.

Response Phase

In the response phase, EMS providers first perform a **scene assessment** for safety hazards and environmental/visual information that might influence patient assessment and care. Observation of a trauma scene can clarify the mechanism of injury by noting details such as the condition of a

car or bicycle or the presence of other victims and the nature of their injuries. Other scene details may help to assess the possibility of neglect or abuse or assist in the identification of a poison. Bystanders may provide historical information, such as initial level of consciousness or seizure activity, that may not be known by family members at the hospital.

The EMS provider then performs a rapid **patient assessment**. Emphasis is placed on early recognition of abnormalities in the airway and breathing because the majority of critically ill pediatric patients, including victims of serious blunt trauma, initially present with respiratory distress or failure. Precise determination of vital signs in the field, although important, is deemphasized due to the wide range of variability of normal pediatric vital signs and the difficulty of accurate measurement in the field. For these reasons, a key goal of EMS-C is to teach EMS providers to look for abnormalities in respiratory effort and peripheral perfusion in assessment of respiratory failure and shock.

TABLE 20-2.
Transport vehicle definitions.

Team	Definition
One-way transport	Transfer of patient using personnel, vehicles, and equipment — all of which are arranged and dispatched by a referring hospital
Two-way transport	Transfer of patient using personnel, vehicles, and equipment — all of which are arranged and dispatched by the receiving hospital
Acceptance time for transport	Time from request until decision to mobilize team
Response time	Elapsed time from transport request by referring hospital and/or physician until arrival of transport team at the referring hospital
Ready time	The elapsed time from request for a transport vehicle until vehicle is ready to depart on mission
Mobilization time	The elapsed time from requesting a transport team until the time the team departs hospital on its mission
Transit time	The elapsed time for travel between hospitals (referring or receiving)
Stabilization time	The amount of time spent by the transport team at the referring hospital, ie, from arrival of team until departure with patient

From American Academy of Pediatrics, Task Force on Inter-Hospital Transport. *Guidelines for Air and Ground Transport of Neonatal and Pediatric Patients.* Elk Grove Village, Ill: AAP; 1993. Used with permission.

Treatment and Triage

Patient assessment and treatment often occur simultaneously. The critically ill pediatric patient tends to deteriorate in a more progressive manner than a critically ill adult. Treatment therefore is conservative and stresses supportive measures such as maintenance of the airway, oxygen administration, prevention of hypothermia, and rapid transport to definitive care. ALS should be provided when necessary and available. Definitive airway management (ie, orotracheal intubation, spine immobilization, and vascular access when indicated) generally are the only ALS interventions performed at the scene. Other ALS treatments should be provided en route or if there is unavoidable transport delay due to an extrication problem or anticipated prolonged transport time.

The patient should be triaged to an appropriate destination on the basis of age, mechanism of injury or illness, and measures of acuity. Triage and treatment decisions may be dictated by protocol or made with the assistance of direct on-line medical control. Thus, another goal of EMS-C is to ensure that the physicians, nurses, and EMTs exercising this direct medical control be trained in special issues pertaining to the care of children in the field.

Once treatment and triage have been initiated, providers must make transport decisions. They must decide *how* (ground vehicle or air ambulance, ALS or BLS) and *when* to transport the patient. In general, trauma protocols specify that transport should begin within 10 minutes of arrival of the transportation team on the scene, with necessary interventions done en route, whereas patients with medical complaints usually receive emergency treatment in an effort to stabilize before transport.

Assessment and treatment are continued during transport. Requirements for radio or telephone contact with the receiving facility vary, but direct medical control is optimal. At the receiving hospital, the EMS crew should report the patient's status, pertinent information from the scene, interventions performed en route, and clinical course during transport. Responsibility for patient care is then transferred to the hospital staff, which initiates the next phase in the EMS-C continuum.

TABLE 20-3.
Evaluation of transport vehicles used for pediatric interfacility transfer.*

	Rotary-Wing Aircraft	Fixed-Wing Aircraft	Ground Ambulance
Safety	+ †	++ ‡	+++ ¶
Noise	– §	+	++
Vibration	–	++	++
Reliability	+	+	++
Costs	–	+	++
Divertability during transport	+	–	++
Patient transfer per trip	2-4	4	2
Availability	+	+	++
Transit time	+++	+++	+
Pressurization	Not available	+	Not available
Range (miles)	(3-4 hr) 200-400	800-1500	200-300
Space	±	+	++

*Table can be used to select the most appropriate vehicle type for region served and, when a combination of transport modes is used, to select the most appropriate vehicle for a specific transport. Other factors to be taken into account include availability, optimal response and transit times, current weather conditions, and team composition for a specific patient.
†Fair is indicated by +.
‡Good is indicated by ++.
¶Excellent is indicated by +++.
§ Poor is indicated by –.

From American Academy of Pediatrics, Task Force on Inter-Hospital Transport. *Guidelines for Air and Ground Transport of Neonatal and Pediatric Patients.* Elk Grove Village, Ill: AAP; 1993. Used with permission.

INTERFACILITY TRANSFER ("SECONDARY TRANSPORT")

Advances in pediatric prehospital, emergency, and critical care have led to great improvements in outcome for seriously ill and injured children. However, the fact that most serious illnesses or injuries do not occur in proximity to a pediatric tertiary care center means that the child may spend minutes or hours in a community hospital and require interfacility transport before reaching a pediatric intensive care unit (PICU).

This section presents an outline for choosing a mode of transport and transport team, transport triage, advance preparation for transport, preparing for the transport team, and communication.

Mode of Transport

Interfacility transport can be accomplished with private automobile, local ambulance, mobile intensive care unit ambulance from the receiving hospital, helicopter, or fixed-wing aircraft. The parameters outlined in Tables 20-2 and 20-3 are helpful in defining the choices.

Transport Team

Options for the team include public service or private EMS personnel, medical personnel from the referring hospital, hospital-based critical care teams that transport patients of all ages by ground or air ambulance, and dedicated pediatric or neonatal transport teams. Local EMS organizations rarely have the training, experience, or equipment for long-distance transport of a critically ill child. In addition, use of an area's only EMS personnel and vehicles for interfacility transport may deprive the local region of service in the event of other emergencies.

Use of a nurse or physician from the referring hospital may be the most rapid means of ground transport, requiring only a one-way travel time, but, again, may deprive the referring area of necessary resources. Reliable portable monitoring equipment may not be available. Expectations for care needed during transfer should never exceed the skills that would normally be provided by the accompanying caregiver unsupervised in the referring hospital.

Critical care transport teams that transport patients of all ages may or may not have appropriate training, experience, and equipment for optimal care of a critically ill or injured child.

When available, dedicated pediatric transport teams may be the preferred means of transport for critically ill children. Such teams are not available in all geographic regions, and a dedicated pediatric team may not have access to the appropriate type of transport vehicle. In the most critical cases, when a pediatric team is available, it should be used, *even if that team takes longer to arrive or to stabilize the patient.* This stands in contrast to the approach taken for pediatric prehospital transport, in which transport should not be delayed. However, for the child who needs immediate surgical intervention at a tertiary care center (eg, for multiple trauma or an epidural hematoma), the no-delay consideration applies to secondary as well as primary transport.

Transport Triage

There are no specific criteria that have been proved to predict need for a critical care transport team. Broad recommendations for use of a pediatric transport team include the following:

TABLE 20-4.
Advance preparation for interhospital transport.

List of pediatric tertiary care facilities with telephone numbers
List of transport systems with pediatric capabilities
List (or pack) of equipment and supplies that would be added to usual EMS equipment
Personnel training and experience
Administrative protocols

TABLE 20-5.
Preparing for the transport team.

Copy all records and radiographs
Obtain transport consent
Secure all lines and tubes
Stabilize cervical spine and fractures, if applicable
Prepare blood products, if appropriate
Obtain telephone number if pending laboratory results

- Any patient for whom PICU admission is anticipated at the receiving hospital. The patient who needs that level of monitoring and care on arrival will need it during transfer.
- Patients with respiratory distress that may progress during the time of transfer (ie, a patient with severe asthma or croup), who may not need PICU admission but whose condition may worsen sufficiently to require intervention during an hour-long ride.
- Patients with a recent life-threatening event, although stable at the time of transfer. This would include any patient who has required aggressive resuscitation (ie, seizure with apnea or shock) or neonates with a history of significant apnea.

Advance Preparation

It is important that all hospitals have policies and procedures for interfacility transport, including the type of patients to be transferred and tertiary facility transfer agreements (Table 20-4).

If local ambulance transport is an option, personnel should have specific training and ongoing experience in pediatric resuscitation. At a minimum, this can be accomplished by allowing EMS providers time to assist in the care of children in the emergency department. Ambulances should have at least the minimum equipment and supplies recommended by the National Emergency Medical Services for Children Resource Alliance.

Nurses who may accompany the patient during transport also should have training and experience in pediatric resuscitation. In addition, written protocols should be developed for the management of potential crises during transport (ie, respiratory failure or arrest, seizure activity, and cardiac arrest). All vehicles should carry appropriate equipment and supplies for pediatric resuscitation and critical care interventions.

Immediate Preparation

When a transport team from another hospital is used, the referring hospital can help ensure an efficient transfer (Table 20-5).

Communication

The initial call to transfer a patient should be from physician or other appropriate practitioner to physician. The referring physician should be able to provide specific details about vital signs, fluids administered, and timing of events. In a critical patient who requires expedited transport, a brief history of the illness/injury, interventions

TABLE 20-6.
Haddon matrix for injury prevention: motor vehicle.

	Host	Vector	Environment
Preevent	Graduated licensing	Brakes	Speed limit
Event	Use of safety belt	Automatic restraints	Guard rails
Postevent	Trauma center care	Fuel system repair	EMS

TABLE 20-7.
Anticipatory guidance for age <1 year.

Observation of parent-child interactions and addressing parenting skills

Notation of social supports for parents and referrals to social services for families under stress

Crib safety (removal of hanging mobile by 4 months of age, no plastic bags or other plastic material in or around the crib)

Age-appropriate toys and food

Transport issues (car seat, back seat placement of car seat to avoid air bag injury)

Supervision stressed

Fire safety (smoke detectors, advising against smoking in the home and especially in bed, access to fire extinguisher, practice family escape plan)

Water heater temperature lowered to 120°F

performed, and current clinical status will be sufficient information to allow for treatment recommendations and a decision about method of transport. The name of the accepting physician, the accepting hospital, and any advice received should be documented. In addition, nurse-to-nurse communication between the two facilities is important.

The referring physician should call the receiving hospital at any time during the transfer process if the patient's condition changes or consultation on patient management is needed. If a method of transport is chosen that does not involve the receiving hospital's transport team, a report should be called to that hospital immediately before the patient's departure. This report includes the patient's most recent vital signs, current clinical status, and estimated time of arrival at the receiving hospital. Two-way communication between the referring and receiving facilities is an important part of the transport process. The tertiary care center that accepts the patient has a responsibility to provide accessible telephone advice, and the transferring hospital has a responsibility to try to provide reasonable information needed to offer such advice.

INJURY PREVENTION

Injuries are the leading cause of death in the United States among children and adolescents. Injuries account for ≈20,000 deaths each year among those 0 to 19 years of age, a rate of 27.3:100,000. In 1992, injury rates were highest in the 15- to 19-year-age group at 67.4:100,000. The rates (per 100,000) for the other age groups are as follows: younger than 1 year, 29.6; 1 to 4 years, 18.9; 5 to 9 years, 9.8; and 10 to 14 years, 14. Office-based injury prevention activities must be guided by sound data on age-specific injury types, knowledge of the circumstances of injuries, and practical information for caretakers on ways to prevent injuries. Practitioners should be aware of geographic differences in injury types.

Definitions and Principles of Injury Prevention

Injury prevention can be defined as primary, secondary, or tertiary prevention. **Primary prevention** attempts to eliminate the hazard; **secondary prevention** reduces the severity of injury; and **tertiary prevention** involves treatment and rehabilitation of the injured. A framework for understanding prevention efforts was developed by

---

TABLE 20-8.
Anticipatory guidance for age 1 to 4 years.

Car seat and proper placement: special alert about the need for all children to be seated in the rear due to danger posed by inflation of air bags

Proper seating using booster seat

Reinforce use of smoke detector and checking batteries monthly; change batteries yearly

Use of four-sided pool fencing

Parental supervision is key

Secure medicines and cleaning supplies; poison control telephone number available

Continued vigilance regarding parent-child interaction and social supports for families under stress

---

TABLE 20-9.
Anticipatory guidance for age 5 to 9 years.

Seat belt use in the rear seat of the car

Pedestrian safety education (children younger than 10 years do not have the appropriate skills to cross streets safely. Parents should be reminded of this and be encouraged to walk children to school and to teach them the skills they will need to cross streets safely later. Avoidance of areas with high traffic density. Cross guards.)

Bicycle helmet use and teaching not to ride in the streets

Reinforce fire safety in the home

Supervision during swimming

Poisoning prevention education

Social supports

William Haddon, Jr. In the **Haddon matrix**, the epidemiologic triad of the host, vector, and environment is expanded to include the concepts of preevent, event, and postevent. Using this matrix, for example, the use of a safety belt serves to avoid or decrease the incidence of injury during a motor vehicle crash and represents an intervention at the host level during the event (Table 20-6).

Health practitioners who treat injured children have an opportunity to use the concepts exemplified by the Haddon matrix and in addition may use the advantage of the **teachable moment**. With this concept, the family of a child who has sustained a minor injury may be particularly open to injury prevention suggestions such as helmet use or protective gear to avoid more serious injury in the future. The injury prevention advice must be supportive of the family and practical.

Major Areas for Injury Prevention

A developmental and age-specific approach is necessary in injury prevention. In this section, each age-specific injury type is coupled with injury prevention anticipatory guidance (see Tables 20-7 through 20-11). The injury data presented below are derived from the National Center for Health Statistics. Only mortality data are presented for simplicity, but morbidity is equally important. The injury prevention strategies usually are applicable to both mortality and morbidity reduction.

Age of Younger than 1 Year

In the United States in 1992, 1186 children younger than 1 year died from injury. The specific causes were homicide (27%), suffocation (19%), motor vehicle traffic (13%), choking (9%), drowning (8%), and fire/flame (8%). Most of the homicide cases were due to child abuse. Death from suffocation occurs when the mouth and nose are covered, and one third of such deaths occurred in a crib or bed. Entrapment and strangulation are included in this category; the latter may be from a cord attached to a toy, pacifier, or clothing. Motor vehicle deaths were overwhelming (92%) occupant injuries.

Age of 1 to 4 Years

In the United States in 1992, 2931 children in this age group died from injury. The causes of deaths were motor vehicle traffic (25%), fire/flame (19%), drowning (18%), homicide (15%), pedestrian nontraffic (4%), and other (19%). Of the motor vehicle traffic deaths in this age group, 62% were occupant injuries. Pedestrian injuries due to motor vehicle traffic- and nontraffic-related causes represent special alerts for toddlers. Nontraffic injuries occurred in driveways, for example, when a toddler was run over by a car that was backing up.

Age of 5 to 9 Years

In the United States in 1992, 1796 children in

TABLE 20-10.
Anticipatory guidance for age 10 to 14 years.

Seat belt use for all, and for those younger than 12 years or shorter than 5'4", rear seating

Pedestrian safety stressed

Roller blading safety: helmets, wrist guards

Bicycle helmet use

Gun safety (support for handgun ban; discuss with parents the hazards of owning a gun, especially in homes with adolescents; proper storage of guns, ie, unloaded and separate from bullets)

Supervision when swimming

Fire safety education reemphasized and fire escape plan in place

TABLE 20-11.
Anticipatory guidance for age 15 to 19 years.

Promote passage of graduated licensing laws for adolescents and urge parents to adopt the principles of graduated licensing (stages of driving privileges to allow time for skills training and social support to maintain good driving behavior; begin by driving only with an adult and no night driving; zero tolerance for alcohol use)

Promote nonownership of guns to parents; for owners, review the risks of homicide and suicide for adolescents and proper training, use, and storage this age group died from injury. Motor vehicle injuries accounted for 48%; fire/flame, 12%; drowning, 11%; homicide, 8%; and other, 21%. In this age group, motor vehicle injuries could be classified as occupant, pedestrian, and pedal cyclist. Occupant injuries represented 51% of deaths; pedestrian injuries, 38%; and pedal cyclist, 11%.

Age of 10 to 14 Years

In the United States in 1992, 2538 children in this age group died from injury. The specific injury causes were motor vehicle traffic (38%), firearms (21%), drowning (9%), fire/flame (4%), and other (28%). Among motor vehicle traffic injuries in this age group, 60% were occupant; 22%, pedestrian; 15%, pedal cyclist; and 3%, motorcycle. Firearm deaths were included as a separate category, regardless of intent, due to their severity and the need for specific preventive strategies.

Age of 15 to 19 Years

In the United States in 1992, 11,520 adolescents in this age group died from injury. The specific injury causes were motor vehicle traffic (41%), firearms (36%), other intentional (9%), and other unintentional (14%). The majority of motor vehicle deaths were occupant deaths (86%). The rest were due to pedal cycling (7%), motor cycling (6%), and pedestrian injures (1%). Behavioral risk hazards in this age group included alcohol and drug use while driving, risk taking such as speeding, and relative inexperience of young drivers. Firearm injuries were the second leading cause of death in this age group; due to developmental issues, firearm prevention (eg, safe storage) is relatively ineffective. Primary prevention, including nonownership and legislative ban of handguns, offers the most effective means of decreasing morbidity and mortality from firearms.

Role of the Acute Care Specialist and Resources Available

The acute care specialist can play a extremely important role in the primary, secondary, and tertiary prevention of child injury. The specialist must be alert to new types of injury and varying circumstances and focus on the mechanisms of injury to better intervene. The specialist is in the unique position of using the concept of the teachable moment to alert parents of ways of preventing or reducing the severity of injuries. The specialist must form alliances with parents, community groups, and organizations, such as the American Academy of Pediatrics and Safekids of America, that have developed age-specific educational materials to be used by both professionals and parents.

SUMMARY

The concept of the EMS-C continuum stresses the integration of all components from the preinjury (educational and prevention) phase through rehabilitation while acknowledging the unique nature and contributions of each. The EMS-C concept encourages increased interaction between EMS personnel and other medical professionals. Pediatric medical, surgical, and emergency medicine professionals can play a vital role in enhancing the pediatric care capabilities of EMS providers through educational programs and involvement in all aspects of medical direction, including direct medical control, protocol development, equipment selection, and quality assurance.

Because EMS systems vary in both organization and capabilities, all primary and emergency care and other subspecialty practitioners should have a working understanding of how their local systems function. It is important for the patient (family) and professional personnel to know how to access the system and what level of care is available. This knowledge will enable physicians to provide patients and families with better anticipatory guidance for emergencies, thereby participating in the first phase of the EMS/EMS-C continuum. It also may assist in the decision-making process in cases of office-to-hospital and interfacility pediatric transports.

ADDITIONAL READING

American Academy of Pediatrics. Policy Reference Guide of the American Academy of Pediatrics: *A Comprehensive Guide to AAP Policy Statements Issued through December 1995*. Elk Grove Village, Ill: American Academy of Pediatrics; 1996.

American Academy of Pediatrics, Committee on Injury and Poison Prevention and Committee on Adolescence. The teenage driver. *Pediatrics*. 1996;98:987-990.

American Academy of Pediatrics, Committee on Injury and Poison Prevention. Firearm injuries affecting the pediatric population. *Pediatrics*. 1992;89:788-790.

American Academy of Pediatrics, Committee on Injury and Poison Prevention. *Injury Prevention and Control for Children and Youth*, 3rd ed. Elk Grove Village, Ill: American Academy of Pediatrics; 1997.

American Academy of Pediatrics, Task Force on Interhospital Transport. *Guidelines for Air and Ground Transport of Neonatal and Pediatric Patients*. Elk Grove Village, Ill: American Academy of Pediatrics; 1993.

Aoki BY, McCloskey K, eds. *Evaluation, Stabilization and Transport of the Critically Ill Child*. St Louis, Mo: Mosby–Year Book; 1992.

Baker SP, Fingerhut LA, Higgins L, et al. *Injury to Children and Teenagers: State-by-State Mortality Facts*. Vienna, Va: The National Maternal and Child Health Clearinghouse; February 1996.

Barkin RM, Seidel JS, Schiffman MA, et al. Pediatrics in the emergency medical services system. *Pediatr Emerg Care*. 1990;6:72-77.

Committee on Ambulance Equipment and Supplies, National Emergency Medical Services for Children Resource Alliance. Guidelines for pediatric equipment and supplies for basic and advanced life support ambulances. *Ann Emerg Med*. 1996;28:699-701.

Committee on Pediatric Emergency Medicine, Singer JS, Ludwig S. *Emergency Medical Services for Children: The Role of the Primary Care Provider*. Elk Grove Village, Ill: American Academy of Pediatrics; 1992:69-87.

Day S, McCloskey K, Orr R, et al. Pediatric interhospital critical care transport: consensus of a national leadership conference. *Pediatrics*. 1991;88:696-704.

Dieckmann RA. The EMS-EMSC continuum. In: Dieckmann RA, ed. *Pediatric Emergency Care Systems: Planning and Management*. Baltimore, Md: Williams & Wilkins; 1992:3-17.

Hunt RC, Bryan DM, Brinkley VS, et al. Inability to assess breath sounds during air medical transport by helicopter. *JAMA*. 1991;265:1982-1984.

Johnston C, King WD. Pediatric prehospital care in a southern regional emergency medical service system. *South Med J*. 1988;81:1473-1476.

Macnab AJ. Optimal escort for interhospital transport of pediatric emergencies. *J Trauma*. 1991;31:205-209.

McCloskey KAL, Orr RA, eds. *Pediatric Transport Medicine*. St Louis, Mo: Mosby; 1995.

Meador SA. Age-related utilization of advanced life support services. *Prehosp Disaster Med*. 1991;6:9-14.

National Committee for Injury Prevention and Control. *Injury Prevention: Meeting the Challenge*. New York, NY: Oxford University Press; 1989.

Pon S, Foltin G, Tunik M, et al. Utilization of prehospital care by pediatric patients in New York City. *Pediatr Emerg Care*. 1989;5:286. Abstract.

Seidel JS. EMS-C in urban and rural areas: the California experience. In: Haller JA Jr, ed. *Emergency Medical Services for Children: Report of the Ninety-Seventh Ross Conference on Pediatric Research*. Columbus, Ohio: Ross Laboratories; 1989:22-30.

Seidel JS. Emergency medical services and the pediatric patient: are the needs being met? II. Training and equipping emergency medical services providers for pediatric emergencies. *Pediatrics*. 1986;78:808-812.

Seidel JS, Hornbein M, Yoshiyama K, et al. Emergency medical services and the pediatric patient: are the needs being met? *Pediatrics*. 1984;73:769-772.

Tsai A, Kallsen G. Epidemiology of pediatric prehospital care. *Ann Emerg Med*. 1987;16:284-292.

Chapter 21

Preparedness for Pediatric Emergencies in the Emergency Department of a General Hospital

OBJECTIVES

1. Assist in preparing the general hospital emergency department for care of children.

2. Access an authoritative list of equipment needed for the care of children in the general emergency department.

The generally accepted "gold standard" for pediatric emergency care is that which is practiced by subspecialists in pediatric emergency medicine in facilities with immediate access to a wide variety of pediatric specialists and services. However, it also is recognized that >90% of pediatric emergency care is delivered in physician offices and emergency departments of general hospitals. Although texts and pediatric emergency care courses teach individual practitioners to provide optimal care, it is essential that an institutional and office commitment to the care of the child with an illness or injury exists.

PEDIATRIC EMERGENCY AREA WITHIN THE GENERAL HOSPITAL

Care of children in the general hospital emergency department can be as separate or integrated as the specific situation allows. Many resources can be shared among different subsections of the emergency department, including patient care space (eg, casting or ENT room), facilities (eg, staff lounge, storage rooms), and staff (eg, cross-trained medical and nursing personnel). Fiscal realities demand that these adaptations be considered. By assessing the needs and resources of a specific department and patient population, the proper balance between providing a special "pediatric experience" and resource sharing can be achieved.

A separate dedicated entrance to the pediatric area of the emergency department is preferable and should be clearly marked when viewed from the street. Prompt greeting, triage, and registration are top priorities. Curbside assistance, if possible, and convenient provisions for short-term parking are important because parents will be uncomfortable if unable to accompany their child into the hospital as care is initiated. Optimally, a separate path is followed by pediatric patients so exposure to frightening sights and sounds is minimized. Similarly, it is preferable to have separate paths for children with serious or traumatic illness.

Waiting areas in the pediatric emergency department reflect the orientation of the facility to the child and family unit. Play areas, telephones, access to food, and educational experiences for parents and children can enhance the waiting period. Efforts should be made to separate children with suspected contagious disease. Bedside registration, although more staff intensive, is a great convenience to the parent desiring to be with the patient at all times and should be available if the condition of the patient and unavailability of family members make central registration impractical. Initial care of the acutely ill patient, however, should not be delayed for the collection of demographic information.

If possible, the creation of a visually and acoustically isolated space for pediatric procedures is desirable so patients can perceive their emergency department bed as a relatively safe haven. In addition, a dedicated procedure room allows central stocking of medications, syringes, needles, and other supplies. A dedicated pediatric resuscitation room is imperative. It should be supplied with all essential pediatric equipment and drugs, including a readily available dose and size chart.

Atmosphere of the pediatric area is difficult to evaluate objectively, yet it is crucial in providing an optimal environment for nurturing health. The use of light and color, as well as familiar graphics and symbols, helps shift the patient's focus away from illness. However, smiling faces, playful behavior, and demeanor conveying warmth, efficiency, and caring are immeasurably more important than decorative walls. The overall effort should be to convey to children and families that they are in an appropriate place for a child.

The importance of safety cannot be overemphasized. Inherent dangers in the emergency department environment and the normal curiosity of children create a high-risk situation. Inspection of the facility for possible sources of injury should be undertaken from a child's perspective.

Ideally, care is rendered to children by physicians with specific interest, training, and experience in pediatric emergencies. Patient volume may not support full-time dedicated pediatric coverage, but a review of patient flow studies by age will determine appropriate times for such coverage. The evening hours usually are the busiest in terms of pediatric visits. Nurses with emergency medicine and pediatric experience are an important resource for the orientation and continuing education of other staff members. Adult and pediatric nurses should be able to assist each other as patient volume dictates, thereby maximizing efficiency. Triage must be accomplished accurately and without delay. This critical post should be staffed by highly trained persons. When volume peaks are anticipated, provisions should be made for additional triage staff.

Blood collection from infants and small children can be emotionally taxing and technically difficult. It is imperative that phlebotomists be experienced in pediatrics. Specific pediatric training, interest, and experience should be a minimum requirement for the respiratory therapy staff as well. Optimally, the respiratory therapist will accomplish or assist in administration of nebulized treatments, preparation for intubation, ventilator management, and the drawing of blood gases. A carefully planned and frequently reiterated in-service training program must be initiated for all those managing the care of children.

The most competent pediatric emergency care providers are ineffective without proper equipment (Table 21-1). *A dedicated pediatric code cart is a necessity.* The contents should be clearly organized and restocked after each use. Pediatric monitoring capabilities are essential and will in a large part determine the ability to care for critically ill children. Correct-sized endotracheal tubes, microsample blood containers, and small-gauge cannulation devices can contribute to improved pediatric care in specific situations. Appropriate sizes of all equipment should be stocked in the pediatric area. Suture materials, syringes, needles, monitoring leads, orthopedic supplies, defibrillator paddles, airway equipment, oximetry adaptors, and low-dose defibrillators are examples.

TABLE 21-1.
Pediatric equipment and supplies, guidelines for the general emergency department.

Monitoring
Cardiorespiratory monitor with strip recorder
Defibrillator (0 to 400 J capability) with pediatric and adult paddles (4.5 and 8 cm)
Pediatric and adult monitor electrodes
Pulse oximeter with sensors, newborn through adult
Sphygmomanometer
Doppler blood pressure device
Thermometer/rectal probe (temperature capability 25° to 44°C)
Hypothermia thermometer
Blood pressure cuffs (neonatal, infant, child, adult, and thigh)
End-tidal CO_2 detector or other method to monitor endotracheal tube placement

Vascular Access
Seldinger technique vascular access kit (with 3, 4, and 5 French catheters)
Catheter-over-needle devices (14 to 24 gauge)
Butterfly needles (19 to 25 gauge)
Intraosseous needles (16 and 18 gauge) or bone marrow aspiration needles (13 or 15 gauge)
IV tubing
Arm boards (infant, child, and adult)
IV fluid/blood warmer
Infusion device (to regulate rate and volume)
Umbilical vein catheters (3.5 and 5 French) (available in the hospital)

Airway Management
Bag-valve-mask resuscitator, self-inflating (450 and 1000 mL sizes)
Laryngoscope handle (pediatric and adult)
Laryngoscope blades
  Curved (sizes 2 and 3)
  Straight (sizes 0 to 3)
Magill forceps (pediatric and adult)
Endotracheal tubes
  Uncuffed (sizes 2.5 to 8.5)
  Cuffed (sizes 5.5 to 9)
Stylets (pediatric and adult)
Tracheostomy tubes (sizes 00 to 6)
Oral airways (sizes 00 to 5)
Nasopharyngeal airways (12 to 30 French)
Clear oxygen masks (preterm, infant, child, and adult)
Nonrebreathing masks (infant, child, and adult)
Nasal cannulae (infant, child, and adult)
Flexible suction catheters (5 to 16 French)
Yankauer suction tip
Nasogastric tubes (6 to 14 French)
Chest tubes (8 to 40 French)

Resuscitation Medications
See Table 21-2

Miscellaneous
Infant and standard scales
Heating source (infrared lamps or overhead warmer)
Towel rolls/blanket rolls or equivalent
Pediatric restraining devices
Resuscitation board
Sterile linen for burn care (available in hospital)
Medical photography capability (desirable)
Infant formula and oral rehydrating solutions

Specialized Pediatric Trays
Tube thoracostomy with water seal drainage
Surgical airway kit (may include tracheostomy tray, cricothyrotomy tray, transtracheal jet ventilation setup)
Venous cutdown
Lumbar puncture (spinal needles, 20, 22, and 25 gauge)
Obstetric pack
Newborn kit
  Umbilical vessel cannulation supplies
  Meconium aspirator
Urinary catheterization (Foley 5 to 16 French)

Fracture Management
Cervical immobilization equipment (infant to adult)
Extremity splints
Femur splints (child and adult)

From Committee on Pediatric Equipment and Supplies for Emergency Departments, National Emergency Medical Services for Children Resource Alliance. Guidelines for pediatric equipment and supplies for emergency departments. *Ann Emerg Med.* 1998;31:54-57. Adapted with permission.

TABLE 21-2.
Resuscitation medications.

	Concentration	Quantity per Container
Adenosine	3 mg/mL	2 mL
Atropine	0.1 mg/mL	5 mL, 10 mL
Bretylium	50 mg/mL	10 mL, 20 mL
Calcium chloride	100 mg/mL	10 mL
Dextrose	25%, 50%	10 mL
Dobutamine	12.5 mg/mL	20 mL
	25 mg/mL	10 mL
Dopamine	40 mg/mL	5 mL, 10 mL
Epinephrine	1:1000, 1 mg/mL	1 mL, 2 mL, 30 mL
	1:10,000, 0.1 mg/mL	3 mL, 10 mL
Isoproterenol	0.2 mg/mL	5 mL
Lidocaine	2 mg/mL	500 mL, 1000 mL
	4 mg/mL	250 mL, 500 mL
	8 mg/mL	250 mL, 500 mL
	10 mg/mL	5 mL, 20 mL, 30 mL, 50 mL
	20 mg/mL	5 mL, 10 mL, 20 mL, 30 mL, 50 mL
	40 mg/mL	5 mL, 10 mL, 25 mL, 50 mL
	100 mg/mL	10 mL
	200 mg/mL	5 mL, 10 mL
Naloxone	0.4 mg/mL	1 mL, 10 mL
	1 mg/mL	2 mL
Sodium bicarbonate	8.4%, 1 mEq/mL	10 mL, 50 mL
	4.2%, 0.5 mEq/mL	10 mL

Also, medication chart, tape, or other system to ensure ready access to information on proper per-kilogram doses for resuscitation drugs and equipment sizes (length-based with color codes or other predetermined kg/dose method).

From Committee on Pediatric Equipment and Supplies for Emergency Departments, National Emergency Medical Services for Children Resource Alliance. Guidelines for pediatric equipment and supplies for emergency departments. *Ann Emerg Med.* 1998;31:54-57. Adapted with permission.

Quality monitoring is a joint responsibility of all health care providers and administration. Leadership in this area is best undertaken by a small group; the administrative, nursing, and physician directors should collaborate closely with pediatric participation. In addition to reviewing charts, procedures, mortality, and admissions, this group should creatively solve problems relating to patient and staff satisfaction for the maximum positive gain.

A general hospital emergency department that opens its doors to children must have a commitment from its administration and board. Acceptance of the responsibility of providing care to a sick or injured child is not an activity to be taken lightly. Personnel, programs, and procedures must be appropriate for children, not considered as an afterthought. If the administration does not actively support pediatrics, the staff will find itself floundering for needed equipment, skills, and educational endeavors, impairing their ability to care for the seriously ill child.

Emergency care systems and providers unable to support appropriate care for children should make necessary arrangements for the stabilization and orderly transfer of the ill child to a facility with suitable commitment and ability.

ADDITIONAL READING

Committee on Pediatric Equipment and Supplies for Emergency Departments, National Emergency Medical Services for Children Alliance. *Ann Emerg Med.* 1998;31:54-57. http://www.acep.org/POLICY/P0004112.HTM

Nelson DS, Walsh K, Fleisher GR. Spectrum and frequency of pediatric illness presenting to a general community hospital emergency department. *Pediatrics.* 1992;90:5-10.

Santamaria JP. Design considerations in pediatric emergency care. In: Riggs LM, ed. *Emergency Department Design.* Dallas, Tex: American College of Emergency Physicians; 1993:199-206.

Santamaria JP. Pediatric emergency department integrated into a general hospital ED. In: Riggs LM, ed. *Emergency Department Design.* Dallas, Tex: American College of Emergency Physicians; 1993:265-268.

Chapter 22

Preparing for Office Emergencies

OBJECTIVES

1. Explain the importance of preparedness for common pediatric emergencies in the office setting.

2. Discuss the importance of physician and staff education in the basic principles of handling emergencies.

3. Recognize the value of periodic practice sessions for major emergency interventions, such as resuscitation.

4. Select equipment and supplies needed for basic and advanced treatment of emergencies.

5. Assess the stabilization and transport priorities for patients with major trauma presenting in the office setting.

6. Manage minor surgical procedures in the office setting.

A wide spectrum of emergencies can be encountered in a pediatric or family medicine office setting. Physicians and their staffs who do not encounter emergencies on a regular basis understandably will feel a certain level of discomfort when faced with life-threatening situations. Anticipation of the types of emergencies that are likely to be seen and preparation of the staff and office environment for handling these situations will alleviate much of this natural discomfort and greatly facilitate the provision of appropriate, early intervention. The process of preparedness begins with ensuring that the physicians and office staff are trained in the performance of resuscitation and emergency intervention. Office settings also must be stocked with the correct, appropriately sized equipment to allow maximum effectiveness of trained personnel. Once a patient is stabilized to the degree that is possible in the office setting, the office staff must be prepared to arrange rapidly for emergency transportation to the most appropriate definitive care facility.

It is recommended that an ambulatory site caring for pediatric patients should, at a minimum, be prepared to handle the emergencies cited in Table 22-1. Specific evaluation and management of these problems are discussed in other sections of this manual. This chapter provides a review of issues related to general office preparedness for handling medical and traumatic emergencies and discusses certain office activities, such as telephone triage and education, that have an impact on the prevention, identification, and appropriate handling of potential emergencies.

STAFF EDUCATION

Initial training and periodic practice drills require dedication of staff time to the process of developing preparedness. Training in basic life support (BLS) and pediatric advanced life support (PALS) is recommended. BLS training typically requires 1 day, and PALS is a 2-day course. All staff should be trained in BLS, and all physicians and at least one nurse should be trained in PALS. APLS is a 2-day pediatric emergency medicine course that is desirable for physician, nursing, and other health care personnel who work in sites in which a substantial amount of emergency care is delivered. The course concentrates on the initial evaluation and management of life-threatening pediatric illnesses and injuries. In the majority of cases, early appropriate intervention will prevent deterioration to cardiorespiratory arrest. Once initial training is complete, no more than a few hours per month is required to maintain a reasonable state of preparedness. The American Heart Association recommends annual re-recognition for BLS and biannual re-recognition for PALS (Table 22-2).

Once training is completed, periodic practice drills are required to avoid deterioration of newly acquired knowledge and skills. This is especially important in environments in which emergency cases are rare. Such drills also assist the staff in maintaining the ability to locate and assemble emergency equipment quickly.

Not each drill must be a full mock code. Simply locating and preparing equipment and medications as though they were going to be used for an emergency and then discussing what would be done in the event of a real emergency can provide a useful experience for the staff with a minimal input of resources and time. One physician and one nurse can work together to plan the sessions, and it is a good idea to involve as many of the staff as possible in conducting the sessions. When the mock code format is used, it is a good idea to assign one or two individuals to observe and to share their observations constructively with the group. An important part of the wrap-up is ensuring that all participants have had an opportunity to share their observations as well. The involvement of community emergency physicians and EMS personnel can facilitate the conduct of practice sessions and build relationships that further help the staff to function effectively under true emergency conditions.

Practice sessions should be conducted regularly, preferably on at least a monthly basis, to maintain a reasonable degree of staff readiness, confidence, and comfort.

EQUIPMENT AND MEDICATIONS

The equipment and medications listed in Tables 22-3 and 22-4 can be assembled easily without a major investment of time or money and are sufficient for most pediatric or family medicine offices. Table 22-5 provides an expanded equipment list that is more appropriate for a large, busy, or remote site or one seeing high-risk children. The following considerations are important in deciding on the equipment needs of a specific office:

- Frequency and type of emergencies seen
- Proximity to a hospital emergency department
- Response time for EMS
- Level of training of EMS personnel

Emergency equipment should be stored in a specific location that is easily accessible in the emergency situation. Storage cases can be used to organize emergency equipment and make it readily available. Ready-made kits are available. The Broselow/Hinkle Pediatric Emergency System contains seven color-coded nylon packs that correspond to the size ranges on the Broselow tape. This system is relatively expensive but provides the greatest degree of convenience.

Checking and restocking, although not particularly time consuming, must be completed on a regular basis. For medications with expiration dates, an arrangement for exchange with a hospital pharmacy or emergency department may assist in keeping costs down. Responsibility for periodically checking and updating equipment and medications preferably should be assigned to one person. An equipment checklist should be completed and reviewed regularly by the physician in charge.

TABLE 22-1.
Pediatric emergencies encountered in physicians' offices.

Anaphylaxis
Respiratory distress (asthma, airway obstruction)
Seizures/status epilepticus
Sepsis/shock
Sickle cell crisis
Trauma
(Cardiac arrest, but rarely)

TABLE 22-2.
Courses.

Course	Sponsoring Organization	Duration (days)	Recommended Update
BLS	AHA	1	Annually
PALS	AHA/AAP	2	Biannually (1 day)
APLS	AAP/ACEP	2	Every 4 years

EMERGENCY TRANSPORT

Staff in a physician's office must be knowledgeable with regard to accessing emergency transportation services. In ≈60% of the United States, the emergency response system is contacted by simply dialing 911. If the office is not located in an area served by a 911 system, the specific seven-digit emergency number or numbers should be posted prominently in the clinic area.

MAJOR TRAUMA

The outcome after major trauma is related directly to the interval between the precipitating event and the initiation of therapy. Although the majority of severely injured pediatric patients are appropriately routed to an emergency department or a trauma center, it is not rare for children with very significant injuries to be brought to the office of a pediatrician or family physician.

MINOR TRAUMA

Minor emergencies account for large numbers of unscheduled urgent care visits not only to the emergency department, but also to the physician's office. Emergency physicians as well as office-based pediatricians and family practitioners therefore require a working knowledge of management of such conditions. The management of frequently encountered minor emergencies is summarized in the following sections.

Minor Head Trauma

The incidence, severity, external causes, nature, clinical course, and early outcomes of severe brain injuries in children have been well defined through population-based studies. Such data are not available for minor head trauma in children because most such events are not reported. However, it is known that head injury is involved in 51% of patients admitted to pediatric trauma centers, and head injury is the primary diagnosis in 25% of such patients.

Minor head trauma may be defined as closed-head injury without traumatic brain injury. The severity of intracranial injury can be classified as outlined in Table 6-3. Mild head injury includes closed-head injury with:

- No loss of consciousness
- Brief loss of consciousness (<1 minute)
- Glasgow Coma Scale score of 15
- Normal neurologic examination

Head injuries more severe than those listed above and injuries occurring in children with suspected child abuse or a history of preexisting neurologic or hematologic illness should be considered potentially severe and generally warrant complete evaluation in the emergency department. The occurrence of an impact seizure is not, by itself, a reason to consider a head injury potentially more severe.

Children who sustain blunt trauma to the head

TABLE 22-3.
Basic equipment and supplies.

Airway
Pulse oximeter
Oxygen source with flowmeter (tank, wheel, and regulator)
Nebulizer for inhalation treatments
Oxygen masks for infants and children
Suction apparatus, catheters, and Yankauer suction tip
Oral airways (sizes 0-5)
IV
Over-the-needle IV catheters, 24-gauge and IV tubing
IV boards, tape, and tourniquets
Lactated Ringer's or normal saline, 2 L
Miscellaneous
Nasogastric tubes
BROSELOW™ Pediatric Emergency Tape

TABLE 22-4.
Emergency medications.

Activated charcoal, 125 g
Albuterol, 0.5% nebulization solution, 20 mL
Atropine, 500 µg/mL, five 1-mL vials
Bicarbonate, 4.2%, five 50-mL vials
Ceftriaxone, 5 g
Corticosteroid
Dextrose 25% or 50%, 200 mL
Diphenhydramine, 50 mg/mL, 1-mL vial
Epinephrine, 1:1000, 10 amp of 1 mg/mL
Epinephrine, 1:10,000, 10 mL
Epinephrine, racemic, 2.25%, 15-mL vial
Lidocaine, 1%, 50-mL vial
Lorazepam
Naloxone, 1 mg/mL, 2-mL vial
Phenytoin
Tetanus toxoid, 0.5 mL

with no retrograde amnesia or loss of consciousness are extremely unlikely to deteriorate and rarely have any abnormality on computed tomography (CT) scan. For this reason, a CT scan rarely is necessary after mild head injury with no loss of consciousness. Treatment should consist of careful history and thorough physical and neurologic examination, looking for evidence of associated injuries, as well as the findings listed in Table 6-1. If the history reveals nothing to suggest the possibility of child abuse or preexisting neurologic or hematologic illness and the physical examination is otherwise normal, the child may be discharged to the observation and care of a competent adult who has been instructed to examine the child at frequent intervals for the ensuing 24 hours, according to the instructions given in Table 6-4.

Children who sustain blunt trauma to the head with retrograde amnesia or brief loss of consciousness (≤1 minute) should generally be referred to the emergency department for repeat evaluation, consideration of CT scanning, and observation by medical personnel. Even if physical and neurologic examinations are normal on arrival in the emergency department or physician's office, there is a small but significant chance of subsequent deterioration. A common approach is to obtain a CT scan and, if normal, observe the child in the emergency department for 4 to 6 hours; then, if no sign of deterioration is detected, the child can be discharged for continued observation by a competent adult for the ensuing 24 hours. Other practitioners use observation alone without CT scanning in this situation, and currently available data do not establish one approach or the other as superior.

TABLE 22-5.
Expanded equipment list.

Accucheck
Blood glucose oxidase reagent strips
ECG with defibrillator
Endotracheal tubes (10)
Intraosseous needles, 15 or 18 gauge
Laryngoscope blades of various sizes
Laryngoscope handle
Lumbar puncture kit
Magill forceps

The need for skull radiographs after minor head trauma has been much debated and studied in recent years. Skull radiographs are realized to be of little use in conscious patients and no longer are ordered routinely or for medicolegal reasons. A skull fracture, by itself, is a poor marker of brain injury. The CT scan is the diagnostic modality of choice.

Physiologic sequelae, such as headache and behavioral disturbances, are rare after mild head trauma. Persistent headache is the most common complaint, reported to occur in 7% of children 1 month after injury. Interventions designed to decrease parental anxiety have been shown to decrease the incidence of behavioral problems.

Minor Torso Trauma

In children with blunt trauma to the chest or abdomen, the absence of symptoms or signs of serious injury and the presence of normal vital signs for age should reassure the examining physician that internal injury is unlikely. However, abnormalities in vital signs must be taken seriously. In a recent study of patients admitted to pediatric trauma centers, abnormal vital signs for age were associated with startlingly high mortality rates. Accordingly, children who present with abnormal vital signs for age after seemingly trivial trauma warrant immediate evaluation in the hospital by physicians familiar with the initial management of major trauma in the pediatric population.

Certain physical findings also warrant immediate evaluation. Children who present with significant chest pain, noisy or rapid breathing, respiratory insufficiency, or blood in the mouth are candidates for potentially serious intrathoracic injuries. Children who present with significant abdominal pain, swelling, tenderness, distention, abdominal wall contusions, or vomiting may have potentially serious intra-abdominal injuries. Vomiting is particularly significant when associated with blood or bile. Children who present with mild, localized, superficial chest or abdominal wall tenderness are not likely to have significant injuries, especially if such tenderness is limited to soft tissues located over bony prominences, such as the ribs or pelvis, and is accompanied by superficial abrasions and there is no associated bony point tenderness or adjacent deep soft tissue tenderness. All children with chest wall injury require careful evaluation for decreased or absent breath sounds and palpation for subcutaneous emphysema, either of which points toward the diagnosis of pneumothorax.

There are, however, certain mechanisms of blunt injury that require more detailed evaluation. A child who sustains a sharp blow to the epigastrium, particularly from a handlebar during a fall from a bicycle, is at higher than usual risk for hepatic, splenic, and pancreatic injury. A child who sustains a sharp blow to the flank, particularly during contact sports, also is at high risk of renal injury and should be referred to an emergency department for evaluation.

Hematuria also is an important indicator of intra-abdominal injury, so a urine dipstick test for occult blood should be performed in any child with a history of blunt abdominal trauma. Although significant renal injury is unlikely to have occurred unless there are >20 red blood cells per high power field on microscopic examination, patients with any degree of hematuria should have a reevaluation within 2 days. If even a few red blood cells persist, a sonogram should be obtained because renal abnormalities frequently are heralded by microscopic hematuria after trivial trauma. Evaluation in the emergency department and CT scan of the abdomen are indicated if gross or significant microscopic hematuria is found.

Soft Tissue Injuries

Soft tissue contusions are treated by elevation of the affected part to the extent possible. Ice packs may retard swelling in the immediate postinjury period but may cause hypothermia in small children. After the acute period, warm showers, baths, and soaks or application of a carefully monitored heating pad several times daily may promote more rapid reabsorption of blood. Aspirin-containing analgesics should be avoided because they may interfere with platelet function and promote hematoma development.

A common soft tissue injury that may require specific treatment is the **subungual hematoma**. The technique for evacuation of a subungual hematoma is discussed in Appendix 22-1.

Closure of lacerations may present special technical problems in children, chiefly because the child usually is moving or thrashing about. The use of passive restraints such as the Papoose board and involvement of the parent or parents for

psychological support of the child during suturing may facilitate the repair. The use of topical anesthetic agents, such as tetracaine-epinephrine (adrenaline)-cocaine (TAC) or lidocaine-epinephrine-tetracaine (LET), infiltrative anesthetic agents buffered with sodium bicarbonate to reduce pain, and appropriate sedative agents, also may be useful in reducing the anxiety and discomfort traditionally associated with suturing of lacerations in children. No techniques of suturing are required in children that are different from those used in adults (Appendix 22-2, Tables 22-6 through 22-10), but it is wise to remember the following points:

- The suture material chosen should be strong enough to withstand reinjury, especially when the laceration is on an extremity. Sutures of thin diameter and low reactivity are used in highly visible areas such as the face.
- Sutures should be large enough, placed far enough apart, and tied loosely enough so they are easy to remove and there is not enough tension to cause unsightly cross-hatching.
- Given the uncanny ability of children to reinjure the involved areas, sutures should not be removed from the extremities until it is clear that complete healing has occurred. This may require up to 2 to 3 weeks after injury over joints.

Many minor wounds can be closed with the use of a tissue adhesive; this technique is discussed in Appendix 22-3.

Most experts believe that systemic antibiotics are of little use, and of potential harm, in patients with blunt trauma, even if extensive. Systemic antibiotics also have no proven role in patients with clean lacerations, especially those of the face and scalp, provided they are closed promptly, within 4 to 6 hours of injury. Older wounds and tetanus-prone wounds should be treated with systemic antibiotics as well as aggressive local care, including debridement of devitalized tissue. Patients with such wounds also require tetanus prophylaxis, including tetanus immune globulin if the immunization series has been deficient.

The importance of timely and appropriate wound care in the prevention of wound infection cannot be overemphasized. Wounds must be debrided thoroughly and irrigated before closure. This may require surgical consultation for jet lavage or pulse irrigation if wounds are extensive. For wounds involving penetration of a body cavity, surgical consultation is mandatory.

HUMAN AND ANIMAL BITES

Bites inflicted by humans and animals result in grossly contaminated wounds due to the plethora of microorganisms that reside in oral cavities. *Staphylococcus* and both aerobic and anaerobic streptococci are found in all species, and *Pasteurella* species are prominent in the oral cavity of cats. Bite wounds should routinely be cleaned thoroughly, debrided meticulously, and irrigated liberally. Most can be left open, but if closure is necessary, the wound edges should be only loosely approximated. With the exception of deep puncture wounds, bite wounds of the head and face can be closed in the usual manner. Tetanus immunization status must be determined, and appropriate measures should be taken if the immunization series is incomplete. The risk of rabies also should be considered based on the type of animal, circumstances of the attack, and treatment instituted in appropriate cases.

Antibiotics are not necessary for meticulously cleaned, superficial human and dog bite wounds. However, puncture wounds and other deep, irregular or extensive bite wounds should be treated with antibiotics, as should all wounds involving the hands, wrists, feet, and ankles. All cat bites should be treated with antibiotics. Amoxicillin/clavulanic acid, in a dose of 30 to 50 mg/kg per day of amoxicillin, divided into three doses, is a good choice. An alternative is penicillin VK (25 to 50 mg/kg per day) divided into four doses, plus dicloxacillin (50 mg/kg per day) also divided into four doses.

Penicillin-allergic patients may be treated with a cephalosporin unless the penicillin allergy history is consistent with anaphylaxis, shock, or airway compromise. Erythromycin may be used when cephalosporins are contraindicated. After cleansing or closure, the wound should be elevated, immobilized, and observed frequently for signs of cellulitis. At the first sign of infection, immediate hospitalization is required.

FOREIGN BODIES

Most subcutaneous and subungual foreign bodies and loose foreign bodies of the eye, ear, or nose in children can be removed in the emergency department or physician's office if they can be seen clearly or felt and the patient is of an age that infiltrative anesthesia will be tolerated (Appendices 22-4 through 22-8; Figures 22-3 through 22-9). Conscious sedation may facilitate management of such problems but should be undertaken only

FIGURE 22-1.
Rule of nines. A, Infants. B, Toddlers. C, Adolescents.

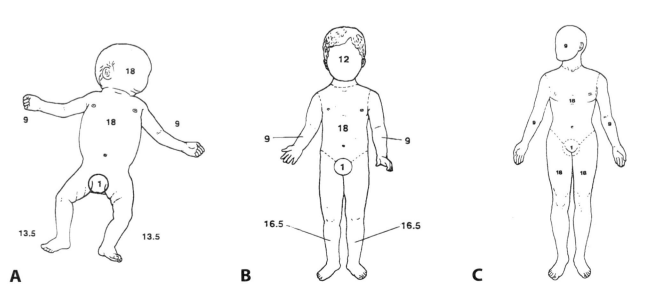

A   B   C

under circumstances in which the treating physician is experienced in its use and proper monitoring is available. Foreign bodies of the gastrointestinal tract usually will pass spontaneously and should be allowed to do so, except when an alkaline battery has been ingested, for which endoscopic or surgical removal may be required. Patients with foreign bodies of the gastrointestinal tract that do not reach the stomach or are excessively delayed in transit and all tracheobronchial foreign bodies should be referred promptly to a qualified specialist for definitive management. A hand-held metal detector can be used to determine passage of metallic foreign bodies into the stomach, thus eliminating the need for routine radiographs.

The techniques for removal of a fish hook from skin and a ring from a swollen digit and for releasing penile zipper entrapment are discussed in Appendices 22-9 through 22-11 (Figures 22-10 through 22-12).

FIGURE 22-2.
Rule of palms for burns.

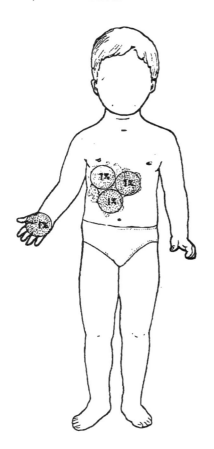

MINOR BURNS

Minor burns may be defined as burns not requiring inpatient or burn center care. Most sunburns and scald and contact burns, which involve <10% of total body surface area, may be considered minor. Children with scald or contact burns involving >10% of total body surface area or any burns involving the eyes, ears, face, hands, feet, or genitalia and those crossing a joint space require inpatient or burn center treatment. Children with electrical burns and burns associated with inhalation injury or major trauma also are candidates for burn center treatment. Burn size may be estimated using the rule of nines modified for use in pediatric patients (Figure 22-1) or the rule of palms, which states that the size of any child's palm is equal to ≈1% of his or her body surface area (Figure 22-2).

Outpatient management of minor burns begins with gentle cleansing of burned skin with mild soap or detergent, preferably dilute povidone-iodine scrub or chlorhexidine scrub. Once the wound has been cleansed, large and small bullae that have broken or are expected to break are debrided carefully with clean instruments. Finally, a thin layer of silver sulfadiazine cream is applied to the wound and covered with nonadherent gauze. This process is repeated twice daily in the emergency department or physician's office or, if possible, in the home. Follow-up is arranged at least twice weekly in the emergency department or physician's office. Daily rechecks may be indicated initially for more complex wounds. Prophylactic antibiotics are avoided because they may promote the emergence of resistant organisms. Tetanus immunization status is confirmed, and toxoid is administered as indicated. Oral fluids are encouraged to replace transepidermal water losses that occur when skin is not intact.

IMMOBILIZATION OF INJURED EXTREMITIES

When a fracture of an extremity is suspected, the extremity should be splinted to include the joints above and below the area of injury. Immobilization will reduce pain and reduce the likelihood of further injury to soft tissues as a result of movement of fracture fragments.

MONITORING OF THE WAITING AREA

Early intervention is key to optimal outcome. The staff should be vigilant to periodically check the waiting area for the possibility of deterioration of patients. Parents may be less vigilant once they have reached the health care facility and may miss signs of deterioration.

TELEPHONE TRIAGE

The staff answering the telephone in the physician's office should be proficient in telephone triage. They must be able to determine which patients are in need of immediate referral to an emergency department, which patients need to be seen immediately but can be evaluated in the office, and which can be scheduled for a routine appointment. Parents often are in need of advice and reassurance. To be able to accomplish all of these requirements, proper training is essential. The physician should conduct periodic training sessions to cover the common and important problems that are likely to be the basis of parental calls.

PATIENT AND PARENT EDUCATION

Education of parents and patients in regard to preventive measures is a key role of the pediatrician or family physician. Effective injury prevention training programs include those that cover the use of infant car seats, seat belts, and bicycle helmets, as well as the use of poison control centers. Early recognition of age-appropriate signs and symptoms of serious illness is another area of educational need for parents, and this topic leads logically to the discussion of how to proceed when an emergency occurs.

Aftercare instruction is an important adjunct to an office visit. Specific questions can be responded to and parents can be given guidelines to follow and instructions regarding what to anticipate, what to be concerned about, and when to call the office or go to an emergency department.

SUMMARY

Preparation of an office for handling pediatric emergencies need not be overly time consuming nor expensive. Proper matching of training and stocking of supplies and equipment with the number and type of emergencies seen will lead to improved staff confidence and allow the facility to effectively meet the emergency care needs of its patient population.

ADDITIONAL READING

Applebaum JS, Zalut T, Applebaum D. The use of tissue adhesion for traumatic laceration repair in the emergency department. *Ann Emerg Med*. 1993;22:1190-1192.

Bell RS, Loop JW. The utility and futility of radiographic skull examination for trauma. *N Engl J Med*. 1971;284:236-239.

Bonadio WA. TAC: a review. *Pediatr Emerg Care*. 1989;5:128-130.

Casey R, Ludwig S, McCormick MC. Minor head trauma in children: an intervention to decrease functional morbidity. *Pediatrics*. 1987;80:159-164.

Casey R, Ludwig S, McCormick MC. Morbidity following minor head trauma in children. *Pediatrics*. 1986;78:497-502.

Coren CV. Burn injuries in children. *Pediatr Ann*. 1987;16:328-332.

Cristoph RA, Buchanan L, Begalia K, et al. Pain reduction in local anesthetic administration through pH buffering. *Ann Emerg Med*. 1988;17:117-120.

Davis RL, Hughes M, Gubler KD, et al. The use of cranial CT scans in the triage of pediatric patients with mild head injury. *Pediatrics*. 1995;95:345-349.

Dietrich AM, Bowman MJ, Ginn-Pease ME, et al. Pediatric head injuries: can clinical factors reliably predict an abnormality on computed tomography? *Ann Emerg Med*. 1993;22:1535-1540.

Dire DJ, Welsh AP. A comparison of wound irrigation solutions used in the emergency department. *Ann Emerg Med*. 1990;19:704-708.

Edlich RF, Thacker JG. Wound irrigation. *Ann Emerg Med*. 1994;24:88-90. Editorial.

Flowerdew R, Fishman IJ, Churchill BM. Management of penile zipper injury. *J Urol*. 1977;117:671.

Gausche M. Genitourinary surgical emergencies. *Pediatr Ann*. 1996;25:458-464.

Gausche M. Genitourinary trauma. In: Barkin RM, ed. *Pediatric Emergency Medicine: Concepts and Clinical Practice*, 2nd ed. St Louis, Mo: Mosby; 1997:355-370.

Gausche M, Seidel J. Releasing penile foreskin trapped in a zipper. *Pediatr Rev*. 1993;14:140.

Hahn YS, McLone DG. Risk factors in the outcome of children with minor head injury. *Pediatr Neurosurg*. 1993;19:135-142.

Hennes H, Lee M, Smith D, et al. Clinical predictors of severe head trauma in children. *Am J Dis Child*. 1988;142:1045-1047.

Kanegaye JT, Schonfeld N. Penile zipper entrapment: a simple and less threatening approach using mineral oil. *Pediatr Emerg Care*. 1993;9:90-91.

Kraus JF, Fife D, Conroy C. Pediatric brain injuries: the nature, clinical course, and early outcomes in a defined United States' population. *Pediatrics*. 1987;79:501-507.

Kraus JF, Fife D, Cox P, et al. Incidence, severity, and external causes of pediatric brain injury. *Am J Dis Child*. 1986;140:687-693.

Lescohier I, DiScala C. Blunt trauma in children: causes and outcomes of head versus extracranial injury. *Pediatrics*. 1993;91:721-725.

Lieu TA, Fleisher GR, Mahboubi S, et al. Hematuria and clinical findings as indications for intravenous pyelography in pediatric blunt renal trauma. *Pediatrics*. 1988;82:216-222.

Masters SJ, McClean PM, Arcarese JS, et al. Skull x-ray examinations after head trauma. Recommendations by a multidisciplinary panel and validation study. *N Engl J Med.* 1987;316:84-91.

Mitchell KA, Fallat ME, Raque GH, et al. Evaluation of minor head injury in children. *J Pediatr Surg.* 1994;29:851-854.

Mizrahi S, Bickel A, Ben-Layish E. Use of tissue adhesives in the repair of lacerations in children. *J Pediatr Surg.* 1988;23:312-313.

Morton RJ, Gibson MF, Sloan JP. The use of histoacryl tissue adhesive for the primary closure of scalp wounds. *Arch Emerg Med.* 1988;5:110-112.

Noordzij JP, Foresman PA, Rodeheaver GT, et al. Tissue adhesive wound repair revisited. *J Emerg Med.* 1994;12:645-649.

O'Neill JA. Burns in children. In: Artz CP, Moncrief JA, Pruitt BA, eds. *Burns: A Team Approach.* Philadelphia, Pa: WB Saunders; 1979:341-350.

O'Shea C. Cyanoacrylate tissue adhesive and facial lacerations. *BMJ.* 1989;299:1217-1218. Letter.

Product monograph. Histoacryl Blue Tissue Adhesive. Davis+Geck. Wayne, NJ.

Quinn JV, Drzewiecki A, Li MM, et al. A randomized, controlled trial comparing a tissue adhesive with suturing in the repair of pediatric facial lacerations. *Ann Emerg Med.* 1993;22:1130-1135.

Rivara F, Tanaguchi D, Parish RA, et al. Poor prediction of positive computed tomographic scans by clinical criteria in symptomatic pediatric head trauma. *Pediatrics.* 1987;80:579-584.

Rosenthal BW, Bergman I. Intracranial injury after moderate head trauma in children. *J Pediatr.* 1989;115:346-350.

Saraf P, Rabinowitz R. Zipper injury of the foreskin. *Am J Dis Child.* 1982;136:557-558.

Schaffer DJ. Clinical comparison of TAC anesthesia solutions with and without cocaine. *Ann Emerg Med.* 1985;14:1077-1080.

Schilling CG, Bank DE, Borchert BA, et al. Tetracaine, epinephrine (adrenaline), and cocaine (TAC) versus lidocaine, epinephrine, and tetracaine (LET) for anesthesia of lacerations in children. *Ann Emerg Med.* 1995;25:203-208.

Schunk JE, Rodgerson JD, Woodward GA. The utility of head computed tomographic scanning in pediatric patients with normal neurologic examination in the emergency department. *Pediatr Emerg Care.* 1996;12:160-165.

Teasdale GM, Murray G, Anderson E. Risks of acute traumatic haematoma in children and adults: implications for managing head injuries. *BMJ.* 1990;300:363-367.

Trott A. *Wounds and Lacerations.* St Louis, Mo; Mosby-Year Book; 1991.

Watson DP. Use of cyanoacrylate tissue adhesive for closing facial lacerations in children. *BMJ.* 1989;299:1014.

Wyatt JP, Scobie WG. The management of penile entrapment in children. *Injury.* 1994;25:59-60.

Appendix 22-1. Subungual Hematoma Drainage.

Subungual hematomas, which are exquisitely painful, can be decompressed easily using the following method.

1. Prepare the nail with an antiseptic such as an iodophor.
2. Unfold a standard paper clip and hold one end for several seconds in a flame until the tip becomes red hot.
3. Immediately apply the hot tip to the nail overlying the center of the hematoma using gentle pressure until it burns a hole in the nail. Then disengage the paper clip.

This permits sufficient decompression of the subungual hematoma to relieve the pain as the remainder of the subungual hematoma spontaneously resorbs.

Appendix 22-2. Step-by-Step Guide to Suturing.

Basic wound management begins with wound assessment (Table 22-6), followed by the application of local anesthesia (Table 22-7), wound preparation (Table 22-8), and selection of appropriate suture material (Table 22-9). Most wounds are closed with either a simple interrupted stitch or a horizontal mattress stitch.

Simple Interrupted Stitch

1. Select appropriate suture material.
2. In a sterile fashion, remove suture material from packet and arm tip of needle holder one third of the way from the swage (needle-suture junction). To prevent needlestick, do not use fingers to adjust needle.
3. Enter the skin ≈5 mm from the laceration with the needle at 90 degrees to the skin surface.
4. Following the curvature of the needle, complete the stitch by exiting the opposite side of the wound at the same depth and distance from the wound edge as the entrance bite.
5. Tie a surgical knot with the instrument tie. Use five knots for nylon, six for coated nylon, and three for polyglactin absorbable or silk. Cut the suture with a 3-mm tail.
6. Place the next stitch ≈5 mm from the first stitch.
7. Arrange all knots symmetrically on the same side of the wound (preferably the side least susceptible to ischemia or cosmetic problems).
8. Apply a dressing; a simple band-aid is acceptable.

Horizontal Mattress Stitch

1. The horizontal mattress stitch is useful when a wound is under slight (not extreme) tension. It **should not** be used in areas of cosmetic importance (eg, face or hands).
2. Begin with the first stitch as above. Instead of tying this simple stitch, continue to the second half of the horizontal mattress suture by identifying the location you would have placed your next simple stitch (5 mm away). Do not cut suture!
3. Rearm the needle holder and enter the skin in the same manner from the **second side to the first side**. This is the simple stitch going back to the first side of the wound.
4. Tie the stitch on the first side of the wound parallel to the wound. It should look like a little box, with sides parallel to the laceration.

Instruct the patient to return for suture removal at the appropriate time based on the site of the laceration (Table 22-10).

TABLE 22-6.
Wound assessment.

Mechanism of injury	Sharp versus blunt trauma, bite
Time since injury	Suture up to 12 hr; 24 hr on face
Foreign body	Explore and obtain radiograph for metal or glass
Functional examination	Neurovascular, muscular, tendons

TABLE 22-7.
Types of anesthesia.

Agent	Route of Administration	Dose	Onset	Duration
EMLA*	Topical to intact skin	A thin layer of cream	45 min	1 hr
TAC[†]/TAC gel	Topical: **never** on mucous membranes	2-3 mL on a cotton ball; use latex glove.	15 min	1 hr
LAT/LET[‡]	Topical	5-10 mL	15 min	1 hr
Lidocaine Lidocaine plus epinephrine[§]	Injectable	4.5 mg/kg, maximum 7 mg/kg, maximum	10 min	1 hr
Bupivacaine Bupivacaine plus epinephrine[§]	Injectable	1.5 mg/kg 2.5 mg/kg	20 min	4 hr

Note: Sedation also may be necessary to achieve optimal patient compliance.

*Eutectic mixture of local anesthetics.
[†]Tetracaine/epinephrine/cocaine.
[‡]Lidocaine/adrenaline/tetracaine or lidocaine/epinephrine/tetracaine.
[§]Epinephrine should not be used in wounds on digits, ears, nose, or penis.

TABLE 22-8.
Wound preparation.

Remove excess dirt/debris by simple washing in sink (if possible).

Cleanse anesthetized wound by irrigation with ≥200 mL of normal saline solution using a 30-mL syringe and 18-gauge angiocatheter or splash shield to achieve optimal water pressure.

Do not use iodine-based solution, hydrogen peroxide, or hexachlorophene **inside** an open wound. **Intact** skin edges may be cleansed carefully with these agents if desired.

Hemostasis: A wound should not be sutured until proper hemostasis has been achieved.

TABLE 22-9.
Suture material.

Suture Type	Examples	Anatomic Area
External skin sutures		
Nylon	Ethilon, Dermalon	Body,* face
Nylon coated with polypropylene glycol	Prolene, Surgilene	Body, face*
Rapidly degrading absorbable suture material	Vicryl *rapide*	Body, lips
Surgical staples		Scalp,* noncosmetic areas
Wound closure strips	SteriStrips, ProxiStrips	Superficial epidermal closure
Silk (not recommended unless others are not available)		
Absorbable "deep" sutures		
Polyglactin	Vicryl, Dexon	Most commonly used
Catgut (plain or coated)		Not commonly used anymore
Monofilament	Monocryl	Newer variety

*Primarily indicated suture type.

TABLE 22-10.
Suture removal guidelines (may vary in individual cases).

Anatomic Area	Days Until Removal	External Suture Size
Face	3-5	6-0
Scalp	7-10	4-0, staples
Upper body	7-10	4-0
Hand	7-10	5-0
Lower body	10-14	4-0
Over joint (recommend splint)	14-21	4-0

Appendix 22-3. Technique for Tissue Adhesive Application.

1. Clean wound.
2. Achieve hemostasis.
3. Wear tight-fitting gloves.
4. Ensure that parents and patients are aware of procedure, including possibility of heat sensation with application.
5. Approximate the wound edges for good cosmetic result.
6. "Spot weld": place a bead of glue and allow to run as far as possible on the surface of the laceration and repeat until complete laceration has been glued.
7. Dab up excessive glue with cotton-tipped applicator or gauze.
8. Hold laceration for ≈30 seconds to 1 minute.
9. Release patient, and give instructions to parents relating to complications, such as infection, allergic reaction, and dehiscence.
10. Instruct parents that glue will fall off by itself.
11. Keep area as clean and dry as possible.

Notes
- This technique should be used in low-tension areas.
- Avoid contact with mucosal or conjunctival surface.
- Do not place inside the wound.
- Anticipate development of new applicators and higher viscosity tissue adhesives in the near future.

Appendix 22-4. Ocular Foreign Body Removal.

Superficial ocular foreign bodies that cannot be dislodged through repetitive blinking, washing the foreign body toward the medial canthus, usually can be removed with the following methods.

1. For loose foreign bodies, press the eyelashes against the superior orbital rim. Locate the foreign body and gently brush it downward with a moistened cotton-tipped applicator (Figure 22-3).
2. If the foreign body cannot be located, evert the eyelid by grasping the eyelashes, pressing downward in the center of the dermal surface of the eyelid with the cotton-tipped end of an applicator (Figure 22-4A) to rotate the tarsal plate (Figure 22-4B) and proceed as above.
3. The use of a topical anesthetic, such as proparacaine, may facilitate foreign body removal.
4. Loose and superficially embedded foreign bodies that cannot be removed with these simple measures and all partially or fully embedded foreign bodies should be removed by an ophthalmologist.

FIGURE 22-3.
Ocular foreign body removal.

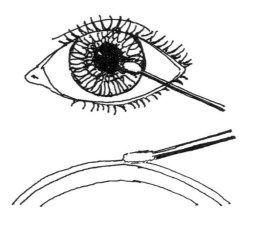

FIGURE 22-4.
Lid eversion.

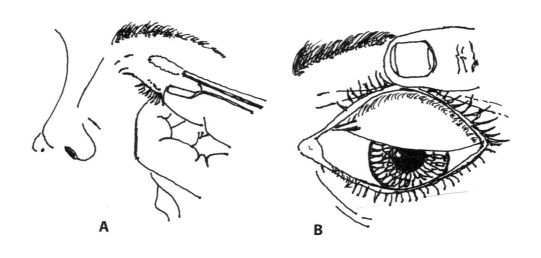

A   B

Appendix 22-5. Cerumen/Aural Foreign Body Removal.

Impacted cerumen and loose foreign bodies usually can be removed with the following methods (Figure 22-5).

1. Retract the pinna posteriorly, exposing the external auditory canal.
2. Insert the operating head of a functioning otoscope into the external auditory canal if necessary to expose the impacted cerumen or foreign body.
3. For soft cerumen or foreign bodies, such as food matter, pass a long, narrow, cylindric, thin-walled Frazier-type suction device into the external auditory canal until it makes contact with the entrapped matter. Occlude the side port of the suction device and then gently extract the suction device and entrapped matter as a unit.
4. Repeat as necessary.
5. For hard cerumen or hard foreign bodies, pass a cerumen spoon or foreign body extractor into the external auditory canal along its outer circumference, opposite the impacted cerumen or foreign body, until the tip of the instrument has passed beyond it. Rotate the cerumen spoon or foreign body extractor until its spatulated or angulated tip engages the entrapped matter and then gently extract the instrument, pulling the entrapped matter ahead of it. Avoid scraping the outer circumference of the external auditory canal with the instrument because it is exquisitely sensitive to pain.

Entrapped matter that cannot be removed with these simple measures should be removed by an otorhinolaryngologist.

FIGURE 22-5.
Cerumen/foreign body removal techniques.

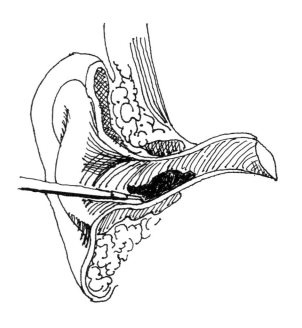
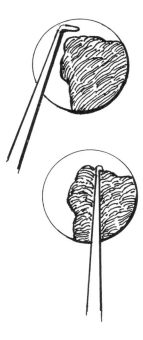

Appendix 22-6. Nasal Foreign Body Removal.

1. Explain the procedure to the parent and child.
2. Assess the need for sedation and administer medications as indicated.
3. Ensure adequate immobilization with a sheet or papoose board along with assistants as needed.
4. Instill a topical vasoconstrictor, such as phenylephrine, cocaine, or epinephrine, to reduce nasal mucosal tissue.
5. With a good headlight for visualization, insert a nasal speculum and open it vertically to avoid injury to the nasal septum.
6. Depending on the shape and size of the foreign body, use one of the following techniques:
   • Using alligator forceps, grasp the foreign body and extract it.
   • Place a wire loop or curette behind the foreign body and extract the foreign body and loop as a unit.
   • Attach a suction apparatus to the foreign body and extract it.
   • Apply an adhesive, such as Super Glue, to a cotton-tipped applicator. Once the foreign body has adhered to the applicator, it can be extracted.
   • Pass a Foley or Fogarty catheter (size 8) beyond the object, then inflate the balloon and withdraw it along with the foreign body.
7. Once a foreign body is removed, check for additional objects.
8. If removal is unsuccessful, immediate ENT consultation can be sought. If immediate removal is not essential, the child can be started on antibiotics and referred to an otorhinolaryngologist for removal.

Appendix 22-7. Nail Bed Splinter Removal.

Splinters of the nail bed usually can be removed with the following method (Figure 22-6).
1. Use of a digital block may facilitate splinter removal.
2. Pass a straight mosquito hemostat longitudinally along the underside of the nail directly adjacent and parallel to the splinter, just past its tip on each side of the splinter, with the jaws of the hemostat closed.
3. Slightly open the jaws of the hemostat and pass each blade along the underside of the nail, straddling the splinter.
4. Close the jaws of the hemostat over the splinter and gently extract the hemostat and splinter as a unit.

FIGURE 22-6.
Nail bed splinter removal.

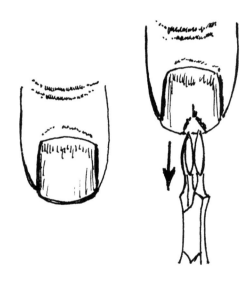

Appendix 22-8. Subcutaneous Foreign Body Removal.

Subcutaneous foreign bodies often can be removed with simple methods appropriately suited to the type of foreign body that has been retained.

1. Obtain anterior-posterior and lateral radiographs of the affected part to localize a metallic foreign body.
2. Prepare the site adjacent to the entrance wound with an antiseptic such as an iodophor.
3. For a long, sharp, metallic foreign body, such as a needle, pin, or nail:
   - Anesthetize the skin adjacent to the entrance wound and along the shaft of the foreign body with a short-acting local anesthetic, such as lidocaine.
   - Slightly enlarge the entrance wound.
   - Press gently over the deep end of the foreign body to elevate the superficial end into the entrance wound.
   - Pass a straight mosquito hemostat into the entrance wound until it makes contact with the foreign body (Figure 22-7).
   - Open the jaws of the hemostat, grasp the foreign body and remove the hemostat and foreign body as a unit.
4. For a pencil point (Figure 22-8):
   - Anesthetize the skin adjacent to the entrance wound with a short-acting local anesthetic, such as lidocaine.
   - Grasp the skin directly adjacent to the entrance wound with a towel clip, gently retract the towel clip to slightly elevate the entrance wound, and make a small, elliptical incision around the entrance wound (Figure 22-8A-D). Deepen the incision, extending it into a V that cuts just below the tip of the pencil point.
   - Remove the excised tissue and pencil point as a unit (Figure 22-8E) and then close the skin.
5. For a horizontally embedded wooden splinter (Figure 22-9):
   - Anesthetize the skin along the entire length of the splinter with a short-acting local anesthetic, such as lidocaine.
   - Incise the skin over the splinter starting over the entrance wound and extend as far as necessary to expose the end of the splinter and then remove the splinter with a straight mosquito hemostat.
   - Loosely close the skin if necessary.
6. For a vertically embedded wooden splinter:
   - Anesthetize the skin adjacent to the entrance wound with a short-acting local anesthetic, such as lidocaine.
   - Incise the skin longitudinally, and press down on the wound edges to expose the superficial end of the splinter, and then remove the splinter with a straight mosquito hemostat.
   - Convert the longitudinal incision into an elliptical incision if the splinter is eccentrically located.
   - Loosely close the skin if necessary.

Foreign bodies that cannot be removed easily with these simple measures should be removed by an emergency physician or general surgeon.

Appendix 22-8. Subcutaneous Foreign Body Removal (continued).

FIGURE 22-7.
Subcutaneous foreign body removal.

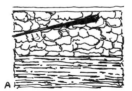
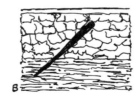
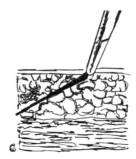

FIGURE 22-8.
Removal of subcutaneous pencil point.

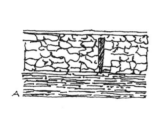
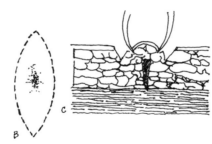
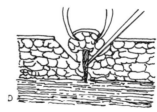
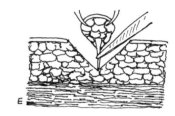

FIGURE 22-9.
Horizontal splinter removal.

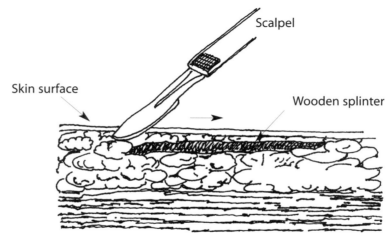

Scalpel

Skin surface

Wooden splinter

Appendix 22-9. Fish Hook Removal.

Fish hooks usually can be removed with either of the following methods (Figure 22-10).

1. Prepare the skin adjacent to the entrance wound with an antiseptic, such as an iodophor.
2. Anesthetize the skin overlying the barb with a short-acting local anesthetic, such as lidocaine (Figure 22-10A).
3. Advance the fish hook following the curve of the belly until the barb passes outside the skin, piercing through from inside the skin (Figure 22-10B).
4. Cut the barb from the hook with wire cutters (Figure 22-10C) and then retract the hook, following the cure of the belly until completely removed (Figure 22-10D).
5. **Alternatively**, lever the hook using the shaft so the barb is elevated to a point just beneath the skin Figure 22-10E) and slightly enlarge the entrance wound using a hypodermic needle (Figure 22-10F), with the beveled tip facing the barb, by passing it through the skin alongside the barb on its inner aspect (Figure 22-10G). Then, advance the needle so the beveled tip engages the sharp end of the barb; extract the needle and hook as a unit (Figure 22-10H).

FIGURE 22-10.
Fish hook removal techniques.

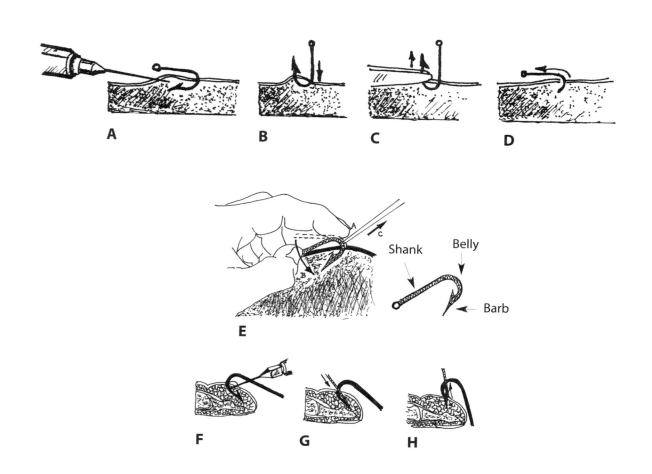

Appendix 22-11. Ring Removal.

Rings entrapped by soft tissue swelling of the digit distal to the ring that cannot be removed with lubricant, after elevation of the digit and immersion in cold water, often can be removed with the following method (Figure 22-11).

1. Use of a digital block may facilitate ring removal.
2. Place the proximal end of a piece of string beneath the ring.
3. Wrap the distal end tightly around the digit in a spiral manner, from a point just distal to the ring to a point beyond the distal interphalangeal joint, laying each turn so it touches the other and in such a way that the outer circumference of each turn is slightly less than the inner circumference of the entrapped ring.
4. Grasp the proximal end of the string and pull gently but firmly toward the distal end of the digit.
5. The string will lift the ring off the finger as it unravels circumferentially.

FIGURE 22-11.
Ring removal.

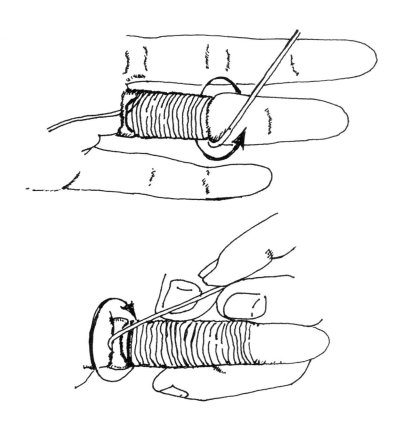

Appendix 22-11. Management of Penile Zipper Injury.

Young, uncircumcised males, usually between the ages of 3 and 6 years, entrap the foreskin in the zipper mechanism when attempting to zip pants. Splitting the median bar of the zipper mechanism with a bone cutter (or wire cutter) can be accomplished without local or general anesthesia as long as the patient remains cooperative (Figure 22-12).

1. Infiltrate the skin locally with lidocaine without epinephrine and douse the zipper and foreskin with mineral oil, then use gentle traction to disengage the zipper.
2. If the foreskin is caught between the teeth of the zipper only and not in the zipping mechanism, then simply cut the zipper below the entrapment and pull apart the teeth.

If none of these strategies is successful, then consultation with a urologist and circumcision may be needed, but this is rare.

FIGURE 22-12.
Bone cutter shown cutting the median bar of the zipper, releasing the foreskin entrapment.

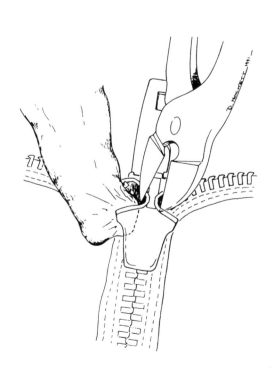

From Gausche M. Genitourinary trauma. In: Barkin RM, ed. *Pediatric Emergency Medicine: Concepts and Clinical Practice*, 2nd ed. St Louis, Mo: Mosby; 1997: 355-370. Adapted with permission.

Chapter 23

Neonatal Emergencies

OBJECTIVES

1. Describe the transition from intrauterine to extrauterine circulation that takes place over the first few days to weeks of extrauterine life.

2. List and explain the significance of the signs and symptoms of distress in the neonate.

3. Describe the diagnosis, management, and disposition of specific diseases of the newborn who is likely to present to the emergency department or pediatrician's office.

In medicine, few patients present a challenge as daunting as the neonate. Newborns with a wide range of congenital and acquired diseases tend to present with the same nonspecific signs and symptoms (Table 23-1), making diagnosis perplexing and management difficult.

The neonatal age group is considered to extend from the moment of birth to 28 days. This chapter focuses on problems likely to be encountered by the emergency physician or office-based practitioner. Diseases usually encountered in the neonatal intensive care unit, such as respiratory distress syndrome, are beyond the scope of this discussion. For a discussion of emergency delivery, refer to the *Pediatric Advanced Life Support* course or the Neonatal Resuscitation Program of the American Academy of Pediatrics.

NEONATAL PHYSIOLOGY

At delivery, ligation of the umbilical cord initiates the neonate's transition from reliance on the placenta for the delivery of nutrients and oxygen and the removal of waste products to complete dependence on an intact cardiopulmonary system. Systemic vascular resistance rises, and the neonate's first few breaths initiate a fall in pulmonary vascular resistance and an increase in pulmonary blood flow. The ductus arteriosus begins to close, eliminating the conduit that has allowed 90% of blood to bypass the lungs. In the normal neonate, the ductus is functionally eliminated within 15 hours of birth. Complete transition from the intrauterine to the extrauterine circulation takes days to weeks. Functionally, the transition is largely completed within the first postnatal day.

The neonate is more vulnerable to physiologic stress than the older infant. A large surface area-to-body weight ratio and poor thermoregulation can result in rapid cooling and hypothermia, which are poorly tolerated by neonates. The neonatal myocardium contains limited contractile elements. Cardiac output and tissue oxygen delivery primarily are dependent on heart rate rather than on stroke volume. Pulmonary vascular resistance is relatively labile; vasoconstriction and right-to-left shunting can result from stresses such as hypoxia, hypercarbia, and acidosis. A large tongue, high larynx, small nares, and poor muscle control can make it difficult to maintain a patent airway in the unconscious neonate. Limited alveolar space and a tendency to atelectasis can adversely affect gas exchange. High glucose requirements despite low glycogen reserves can rapidly result in hypoglycemia, especially during periods of physiologic stress.

SIGNS AND SYMPTOMS

Lethargy

When awake, most neonates are alert and interact with their mothers (**bonding**) and the environment. The neonate who is lethargic or listless should be considered critically ill until proved otherwise. In the absence of other signs and symptoms, lethargy usually implies an acute metabolic disorder, infectious disease, or neurologic injury or anomaly.

The lethargic neonate should be assessed for compromise in oxygenation, ventilation, and cardiovascular stability. Poor perfusion of the extremities as indicated by diminished peripheral pulses or delayed capillary refill may be an ominous finding. A complete neurologic examination is undertaken.

The normal awake neonate will appear alert and will interact with the environment. Examination of the skull is carried out, looking for evidence of macrocephaly, microcephaly, or craniosynostosis. The fontanel is palpated for size and pulsations. Pupils should be checked for their response to light. A number of primitive reflexes may be elicited to demonstrate muscle tone (Table 23-2). Responses should be symmetrical and demonstrate good muscular tone.

TABLE 23-1.
Common presenting complaints in neonates.

Cardiorespiratory Symptoms
  Rapid breathing
    Pneumonia
    Bronchiolitis
    Congenital diseases
  Cough
  Nasal congestion
  Noisy breathing/stridor
  Apnea/periodic breathing
  Blue spells/cyanosis
  Sudden death

Crying/Irritability/Lethargy
  Testicular torsion
  Traumatic conditions
    Battered child syndrome (fractures, burns, etc.)
    Falls (skull and extremity fractures)
    Open diaper pin
    Strangulation of digit or penis
    Corneal abrasion or foreign body
  Infections
    Meningitis
    Generalized sepsis
    Otitis media
    Urinary tract infection
    Gastroenteritis

Eye Symptoms
  Discharge
  Redness

Fever

Gastrointestinal Symptoms
  Feeding difficulties
  Regurgitation
  Vomiting
  Diarrhea
  Abdominal distention
  Constipation
  Intestinal colic
  Incarcerated hernia
  Anal fissure

Skin Symptoms
  Jaundice
    ABO/Rh incompatibility
    Sepsis
    Congenital infections
    Bruising
    Physiologic
    Bile duct atresia
    Hepatitis
    Hemolytic anemias
    Hypothyroidism
    Breast milk jaundice
  Diaper rash/oral thrush

From Kissoon N. Common neonatal problems. In: Tintinalli JE, Ruiz E, Krome RL, eds. *Emergency Medicine: A Comprehensive Study Guide*, 4th ed. New York, NY: McGraw-Hill; 1996:591. Adapted with permission.

An appropriate evaluation includes a complete blood count with differential and platelet count, serum glucose, electrolytes, blood urea nitrogen, creatinine, calcium, phosphate, serum ammonia, and blood pH. A septic work-up is indicated, including cultures of the blood, urine, and cerebrospinal fluid. A chest radiograph also is necessary.

Management includes transfer to an intensive care environment. If cardiorespiratory compromise is present, intubation and mechanical ventilation may be required, and aggressive fluid resuscitation may be indicated. Metabolic abnormalities such as hypoglycemia require correction. Empiric therapy with broad-spectrum antibiotics is indicated until sepsis is eliminated as an etiology. An elevated serum ammonia may mean an inborn error of metabolism and warrants an emergent endocrinology consultation.

Apnea

Many parents bring neonates to the emergency department with the complaint, "My baby stopped breathing." It is important to try to distinguish true apnea from normal periodic breathing. Many normal full-term neonates have episodes during which regular breathing is interrupted by short pauses, especially during sleep. Premature infants are especially likely to have such episodes, lasting 5 to 10 seconds, followed by a period of rapid respirations. In premature babies, periodic breathing usually resolves around 36 weeks of gestation.

Pathologic apnea (>20 seconds) always is a cause for concern, especially if associated with pallor, mottling of the skin, cyanosis, desaturation, or bradycardia. Apnea that recurs frequently or develops in a neonate older than 2 weeks also warrants urgent investigation. Detailed history should include whether episodes occur when the infant is awake or asleep, and whether they resolve spontaneously and, if not, what intervention is required to restore breathing.

Metabolic abnormalities, seizures, medications, and severe anemia may cause apnea. The most likely cause is a serious infection, such as bacterial sepsis associated with meningitis. Respiratory syncytial virus (RSV) is a likely cause of apnea, even in neonates without the pulmonary manifestations of bronchiolitis.

The evaluation of the neonate with apnea is similar to that of the lethargic neonate. During appropriate times of the year, nasopharyngeal washings should be sent for RSV antigen.

In cases of pathologic apnea, admission to a pediatric intensive care unit is desirable. Admission to a general pediatric floor is acceptable when careful monitoring can be ensured. In the emergency department, it is essential that the patient is on a cardiac monitor. Neonates with recurrent apnea may require intubation and ventilatory support. Any metabolic abnormality

TABLE 23-2.
Neonatal reflexes.

Reflex	Performance	Response	Disappearance (mo)
Moro	Supine, elevate head 30° and allow head to fall back into examiner's hand	Extension and abduction of shoulders, followed by adduction of the arms	1-3
Palmar grasp	Stroke the palm	Grasp	4
Root response	Stroke the cheek	Mouth turns to stimulus	3-4
Tonic neck	Turn head to side	Extension of ipsilateral arm and leg; flexion of contralateral arm and leg	5-6
Babinski	Stroke the sole	Dorsiflexion of big toe and fanning of toes	12-30

From Fuchs S. Age-specific neurologic examination. In: Strange GR, Ahrens W, Lelyveld S, et al, eds. *Pediatric Emergency Medicine: A Comprehensive Study Guide.* New York, NY: McGraw-Hill; 1996:219. Adapted with permission.

should be corrected, and empiric antibiotic therapy should be considered.

Cyanosis

Cyanosis may be peripheral or central. **Peripheral cyanosis (acrocyanosis)** is common in neonates and usually involves the hands, feet, and circumoral area. It most often occurs when the baby is undressed and exposed to a cool environment and usually does not indicate serious disease. Peripheral cyanosis that persists after the baby has warmed up can indicate poor peripheral perfusion and is a cause for concern.

Central cyanosis involves the trunk as well as the extremities. The mucous membranes also may appear blue. It can result from pulmonary insufficiency, congenital heart disease, or hypoventilation from a central nervous system lesion. A PaO_2 that does not rise above 100 mm Hg, despite the administration of 100% oxygen, suggests cyanotic heart disease, with a fixed right-to-left shunt.

Any neonate without a known cause for central cyanosis should be admitted to an intensive care unit. The workup is directed toward determining the underlying cause and may include an evaluation for sepsis, chest radiograph, ECG, echocardiogram, upper and lower body pulse oximetry, arterial blood gas, and "hyperoxia test." Treatment depends on etiology.

Irritability

It is essential to distinguish the truly irritable neonate from one who simply cries more than usual. Irritability implies that the baby is in pain. Rocking or cuddling may not console because it hurts. The differential diagnosis is wide and includes meningitis, shaken baby syndrome, urinary tract infection, septic arthritis, and abuse. The irritable baby must be undressed completely and examined from head to toe. Traumatic lesions, such as occult fractures or corneal abrasions, are possible. Abdominal tenderness may indicate peritonitis. The fingers, toes, and genitalia must be inspected carefully to exclude strangulation by a hair or piece of thread. Scrotal examination should be conducted and include an evaluation for incarcerated hernia.

In the absence of another explanation, the irritable neonate requires a full evaluation for sepsis, trauma, and meningitis. Admission is prudent until a diagnosis is reached.

Grunting

Grunting is a short sound that occurs during expiration when the neonate expels air against a closed glottis. Physiologically, this serves to maintain positive end-expiratory pressure and prevent alveolar collapse. Grunting most commonly is seen in premature newborns with hyaline membrane disease. When it occurs in older neonates, it virtually always signals significant respiratory distress, which may result from primary pulmonary pathology or be secondary to systemic illness, especially sepsis. The presence of grunting always mandates a thorough evaluation to determine the underlying pathology, which frequently is infectious.

Vomiting

Vomiting is a common complaint in neonates. The forceful expulsion of stomach contents must be distinguished from **regurgitation**, which occurs to some extent in virtually all babies. Regurgitation usually can be managed by reducing the volume of each feeding and increasing the frequency with which the baby is "burped." It is essential to characterize true vomiting as bilious or nonbilious. Bilious emesis never is normal and always signifies an obstructive lesion, commonly a malrotation. Persistent, forceful, or bile-stained vomiting within the first 24 hours of life also is suggestive of obstruction. Often, there is a maternal history of polyhydramnios. In the older neonate, projectile emesis is characteristic of pyloric stenosis. Vomiting is a common finding in neonates with increased intracranial pressure and may be the presenting sign in sepsis and meningitis.

The evaluation of the neonate with vomiting depends on the specific details elicited in the history and physical.

Constipation

More than 90% of normal newborns pass meconium within the first 24 hours, and virtually all of the remainder do so within the first 36 hours after delivery. From then on, the pattern of bowel movements varies widely. Breast-fed infants may pass 8 to 12 stools a day or have stool intervals as much as every 48 hours or more. Formula-fed infants usually pass stool 1 or 2 times a day, but this also varies, and a infant who passes stool every 48 hours probably is normal. Constipation occurs when stools become dry, hard, or difficult to pass. Delayed stooling associated with abdominal distention, discomfort, or vomiting is not normal and is cause for concern. Medical causes of constipation include dehydration, opioids, congenital hypothyroidism, and infant botulism. The most common surgical lesion presenting to the emergency department with constipation is Hirschsprung's disease.

The vast majority of neonates with constipation do not have serious disease. Those who passed stool normally within the first 24 hours of life and have a normal physical examination do not require laboratory or radiographic evaluation. Failure to pass stool within the first 24 hours after delivery should raise concern regarding the possibility of cystic fibrosis or Hirschsprung's disease.

Diarrhea

Diarrhea is present when there is an increase in the frequency and water content of the stools. In many neonates, especially breast-fed babies, frequent stools are normal, and it is a change in the pattern that is significant. Diarrhea can result from overfeeding or the use of a formula with a high osmotic content or one of the carbohydrate malabsorption syndromes. For the neonate, infectious etiologies cause the most concern, especially when the pathogen is bacterial. *Salmonella* gastroenteritis may be associated with bacteremia. Rotavirus is a common cause of profuse watery diarrhea and can result rapidly in significant dehydration. Diarrhea can be a nonspecific manifestation of systemic illness, such as a urinary tract infection.

It is important to try to determine the frequency of bowel movements and character of the stools. Blood in the stools can be due to structural abnormalities such as intussusception or anal fissure but may result from a bacterial infection. The physical examination focuses on the general appearance of the neonate and state of hydration. In the febrile neonate with diarrhea, stool microscopy is indicated to assess the presence of fecal leukocytes or red blood cells (both are common in *Salmonella* gastroenteritis). If bacterial enteritis is suspected, stool cultures are indicated. In the febrile patient, cultures of blood, urine, and cerebrospinal fluid also should be considered. Hospital admission and empiric antibiotic therapy are prudent. An enzyme-linked immunosorbent assay for rotavirus is indicated during periods of expected epidemics.

Fever

In the first few days of life, elevated temperature (≥38°C, 100.4°F) may be due to environmental factors, but in neonates beyond the first few days of life, fever virtually always signals an acute infectious disease. The majority of these result from viruses and are self-limited illnesses. However, a significant number of febrile neonates have bacterial infections. It is axiomatic that any bacterial infection in a neonate is a serious illness. An immature immune system that cannot localize and eliminate a bacterial focus makes the neonate vulnerable to hematogenous dissemination and the development of devastating illness, such as meningitis or sepsis. These problems can originate from sites of infection, such as the middle ear, that in older infants and children would be unlikely sources for the development of systemic infection. Even neonates with an obvious focus of infection such as cellulitis, may have positive blood cultures.

The general appearance of the febrile neonate is of paramount importance. Irritability is a cause for concern, and lethargy is ominous. Any febrile neonate with apnea or cyanosis is gravely ill. The patient should be assessed for signs of cardiovascular instability, such as mottled extremities, diminished peripheral pulses, or delayed capillary refill. These patients require aggressive fluid resuscitation and may require intubation and artificial ventilation (see Chapter 14). For the well-appearing febrile neonate, complete blood cell count should be determined, and cultures should be done of the blood, urine, and cerebrospinal fluid. Because a viral illness presumes exclusion of a bacterial etiology, febrile neonates usually are hospitalized and treated with parenteral antibiotics until cultures are definitively negative.

SPECIFIC DISEASES AND DISORDERS

There are several diseases and disorders for which neonates are likely to present to emergency departments or other outpatient facilities for treatment, as described in the following sections.

Cardiac Disease

Congenital heart disease usually is classified into lesions that result in cyanosis and those that do not. In many cases of significant disease, the newborn will manifest symptoms within hours of birth, during transition from the uteroplacental circulation. These patients are unlikely to be discharged from the nursery. This section focuses on lesions that are likely to be seen by the emergency physician or office-based practitioner.

Cyanotic heart disease results when there is a right-to-left shunt. Diseases in which there is complete obstruction to pulmonary blood flow, such as tricuspid or pulmonary atresia, usually result in severe cyanosis within hours after birth. In cases in which there is mild or moderate obstruction to pulmonary flow or mixing of arterial and venous blood, presentation may be somewhat delayed. Failure of PaO_2 to rise above 100 mm Hg despite treatment with 100% oxygen (**hyperoxia test**) increases the likelihood of a fixed shunt secondary to cyanotic heart disease. Cyanotic neonates can present with respiratory distress, irritability, poor feeding, or lethargy. Cyanosis may not be obvious on physical examination.

Acyanotic heart disease usually presents with signs and symptoms of congestive heart failure or cardiogenic shock, often due to severe obstruction of the left ventricular outflow tract. The clinical picture is dominated by respiratory distress, with tachypnea and occasionally grunting. Babies may have a history of respiratory difficulty and sweating during bottle feeding or nursing. Auscultation of the lungs may reveal wheezing, but rales are uncommon in all congenital heart diseases other than critical left-sided obstructive lesions. Hepatomegaly may be present. Cardiac enlargement and signs of congestive heart disease may be present on chest radiograph.

Congenital heart disease that becomes symptomatic in the first few postnatal days usually is associated with closure of the ductus arteriosus. Considering the possibility of a "ductal-dependent" lesion is important because prostaglandin E_1, a potent dilator of the ductus, is available for infusion. During the first few postnatal weeks, prostaglandin E_1 can be used to reopen or maintain patency of a closing ductus and reestablish flow to the lower half of the body or provide sufficient pulmonary blood flow to permit oxygenation adequate for survival. Prostaglandin infusion should be considered, as a temporizing measure, for right-sided obstructive lesions in which pulmonary blood flow is dependent on left-to-right shunting (pulmonary atresia, pulmonary stenosis, tetralogy of Fallot, transposition of the great vessels, tricuspid atresia, Ebstein's anomaly) and left-sided obstructions in which systemic blood flow is dependent on right-to-left shunting (coarctation of the aorta, aortic stenosis, hypoplastic left heart). It is a temporizing measure until a corrective or palliative surgical procedure is performed. Prostaglandin-induced apnea may require intubation and mechanical ventilation.

Cyanotic Heart Disease

Tetralogy of Fallot consists of obstruction to pulmonary outflow, a ventricular septal defect, right ventricular hypertrophy, and dextroposition of the aorta. The right-to-left shunt usually results in an oxygen saturation of 75% to 85%, which shows minimal improvement despite supplemental oxygen. Physical examination usually reveals normal pulses and a characteristic harsh systolic murmur at the left sternal border that may be accompanied by a thrill. An ECG reveals right ventricular hypertrophy, whereas a radiograph may reveal a characteristic "boot-shaped" heart, occasionally with a right-sided aorta. Echocardiography is extremely helpful in reaching a diagnosis.

Although it is uncommon for a neonate to present with tetralogy of Fallot, neonates suspected of having tetralogy of Fallot require transport to a center with expertise in pediatric cardiac surgery. Supplemental oxygen is indicated and temperature control must be maintained because hypothermia can produce acidosis and exacerbate the right-to-left shunt by increasing pulmonary vascular resistance. Prostaglandin E_1 can be used to reopen the ductus arteriosis and improve oxygenation in patients with significant pulmonary outflow tract obstruction. A **Blalock-Taussig shunt**, in which the subclavian artery is anastomosed to the pulmonary artery, can provide palliation until a definitive repair is possible.

In **transposition of the great arteries**, the aorta arises from the right ventricle, and the pulmonary artery arises from the left ventricle. Thus, oxygenated blood returning from the lungs is recirculated through the right heart rather than being ejected to the systemic circulation, which instead receives recirculated venous blood. Some mixing occurs at the foramen ovale. In simple transposition, the ventricular septum is intact; in patients with a ventricular septal defect, some mixing can occur and cyanosis may not be severe. The condition is much more common in boys.

Most infants with this condition present with cyanosis and tachypnea. Hypoxemia can be severe, and metabolic acidosis can result. Congestive heart failure is not present. Neither ECG nor chest radiography is often helpful, but echocardiography should be diagnostic.

Arterial oxygenation can be improved if the ductus arteriosis is opened with an infusion of prostaglandin E_1. Hypothermia, hypoglycemia, and acidosis should be corrected. Transfer to a center with expertise in pediatric cardiology is essential because palliative therapy consists of a Rashkind balloon septostomy, a procedure in which a catheter-directed balloon is used to create a large atrial septal defect that permits mixing of systemic and venous blood. Ultimately, corrective surgery is necessary.

Acyanotic Heart Disease Resulting in Congestive Heart Failure or Cardiogenic Shock

In **coarctation of the aorta**, there most often is a constriction distal to the left subclavian artery, usually at the site of the insertion of the ductus arteriosus. In neonates, this lesion often is found in conjunction with other cardiac anomalies, especially patent ductus arteriosus and ventricular septal defect. Some associated anomalies are quite complex.

Coarctation can be diagnosed anytime in childhood. In neonates, acute congestive heart failure, which in some cases can be severe, is the common presentation. A systolic murmur audible in the back may be present, as may hepatomegaly. Careful examination will reveal that femoral pulses are diminished compared with those in the upper extremities, and there is a discrepancy in blood pressure between the arms and the legs. Chest radiography may reveal congestive heart failure. Echocardiography can be diagnostic.

Infusion of prostaglandin E_1 can reopen the ductus and improve blood flow to the lower extremities to neonates in extreme distress. This may improve tissue oxygenation and acidosis. Diuretics may help relieve symptoms of congestive heart failure. Urgent pediatric cardiology consultation is indicated.

Patients with severe coarctation are candidates for immediate surgical repair, especially if prostaglandin infusion fails to improve lower extremity perfusion.

In an **interrupted aortic arch**, there is discontinuity between the ascending and descending aortas. Clinical manifestations are similar to those of coarctation. Signs of severe congestive heart failure predominate. Physical examination reveals diminished pulses and blood pressure in the lower extremities. Improvement may follow infusion of prostaglandin E_1. Emergent surgical repair is indicated.

Hypoplastic left heart syndrome includes a devastating group of disorders that result in a small and severely dysfunctional left ventricle. Systemic circulation depends on the ductus arteriosis. Patients usually develop early signs of congestive heart failure and can be extremely ill on presentation. Pulses are diffusely diminished. The chest radiograph may show pulmonary congestion. A variety of surgical procedures, including cardiac transplant, has been tried with mixed results.

The most common congenital cardiac anomaly, **ventricular septal defect (VSD)**, can occur as an isolated lesion or in combination with other lesions. Most VSDs are defects in the membranous septum.

The manifestations of a VSD depend on its size. Small defects, although audible early, can remain asymptomatic. Large VSDs can be silent at birth but as pulmonary vascular resistance falls in the first few weeks, signs and symptoms of congestive heart failure ensue. It is thus characteristic for a significant VSD to manifest within the first few postnatal weeks. Dyspnea and perspiration during feeding are characteristic, as is poor weight gain. Physical examination may reveal a prominent apical impulse with a thrill and systolic murmur. Peripheral pulses are normal. The chest radiograph may reveal pulmonary vascular congestion, and the ECG may reveal biventricular hypertrophy. Echocardiography is diagnostic.

Patients with congestive heart failure secondary to a large VSD usually respond to diuretics. If their symptoms can be managed and adequate growth maintained, they can be treated conservatively. Most VSDs close spontaneously, but some infants will require surgery.

In **truncus arteriosus**, a solitary arterial vessel arises from the left ventricle and supplies the pulmonary and arterial circulations. All patients also have a VSD. In most patients, greatly increased pulmonary blood flow results in congestive heart failure, which may be severe. Cyanosis usually is not clinically significant. The precordium is hyperactive, and there is a systolic ejection murmur. The chest radiograph may show increased pulmonary vascularity, and in some cases a right-sided aortic arch. Echocardiography can be helpful in diagnosis. Management is medical until surgical correction can be performed.

Pulmonary Disorders

Congenital Laryngeal Stridor

Stridor with onset in the neonatal period usually is due to an abnormality involving or adjacent to the larynx and most commonly is due to laryngomalacia or tracheomalacia. Collapse of the abnormally weak airway during inspiration results in stridor. Stridor may increase during feeding or when the baby cries, but characteristically, infants do not experience respiratory distress and continue to feed well. Expiratory stridor should not occur, and when present, it suggests a more serious disorder. The vast majority of patients do well with no treatment. Stridor accompanied by respiratory distress should be evaluated with laryngoscopy, bronchoscopy, or both.

Tracheoesophageal Fistula

Approximately 95% of tracheoesophageal fistulas are characterized by an interruption of the esophagus and are diagnosed within the first 24 hours after delivery. In a few cases, the abnormality is characterized by an H-type fistula, in which there is a connection between the esophagus and trachea. Affected neonates may present with choking, gagging, or cyanotic episodes during feeding. Aspiration pneumonia can occur. In suspected cases, referral to a pediatric surgeon is indicated. Diagnosis is confirmed with bronchoscopy or contrast study.

Vascular Ring

Abnormalities of the aortic arch can result in the formation of vascular rings that can obstruct or encircle the trachea and cause significant obstruction. The most common is a double aortic arch. Affected patients may have wheezing or biphasic stridor that is worse during feeding or flexion of the neck. Barium swallow may show indentation of the esophagus. Definitive diagnosis is made with aortography. Surgical correction usually is necessary.

Pneumonia

Bacterial pneumonia is fairly uncommon in healthy neonates discharged from the nursery. Group B *Streptococcus* can cause pneumonia within the first 24 hours after delivery. A late-onset form of group B *Streptococcus* disease has been observed up to 30 days of age. In most cases, respiratory distress begins within hours of birth, and affected patients are gravely ill. In neonates with acquired pneumonia, bacterial etiologies include *Staphylococcus aureus, Escherichia coli, Haemophilus influenzae, Streptococcus pneumoniae,* and *Klebsiella.*

Neonates with pneumonia present with cough, tachypnea, and grunting. They may or may not have fever. Auscultation of the chest may or may not be helpful. The chest radiograph may show a consolidation and, in the presence of *Staphylococcus,* a pleural effusion. Cultures of blood and cerebrospinal fluid are indicated. All neonates with pneumonia require admission for intravenous antibiotics.

Chlamydia trachomatis is a well-known cause of interstitial pneumonitis in neonates. Onset is usually 3 to 4 weeks of age. The predominant symptom is a staccato cough. Fever is uncommon. Affected patients often have slight wheezing or dry rales on auscultation and may have significant retractions. An eye discharge may be present. If respiratory distress is mild and oxygenation is adequate, the baby can be treated as an outpatient with erythromycin.

Gastrointestinal Problems

Surgical Lesions

Malrotation of the intestine results when the embryonic intestine fails to rotate to its normal position. In general, the cecum does not migrate into the right lower quadrant. Adhesive bands (**Ladd's bands**) may obstruct the duodenum, and a narrow mesenteric pedicle renders the bowel vulnerable to midgut volvulus and strangulation.

Neonates with malrotation with or without volvulus often present during the first postnatal week with emesis that is bilious. All cases of bilious emesis in a neonate should be considered a surgical emergency until proved otherwise. Abdominal distention or peritoneal findings suggest the presence of volvulus, which may be intermittent. Bloody or heme-positive stools indicate bowel ischemia secondary to volvulus. Diagnosis is made with upper gastrointestinal series. An emergency pediatric surgical consultation is indicated because delayed repair of a volvulus can result in bowel infarction, short gut syndrome, and life-long disability. Interim management includes withholding oral intake, passing a nasogastric tube, and providing intravenous fluids.

Hypertrophic **pyloric stenosis** is a fairly common condition that affects males much more often than females. Muscular hypertrophy of the stomach antrum causes outflow tract obstruction. Most patients become symptomatic around 2 to 3 weeks of age, when they develop nonbilious vomiting that may be projectile. In severe cases, significant dehydration can develop, accompanied by a characteristic hypochloremic, hypokalemic metabolic alkalosis. In milder, more chronic cases, babies may become significantly malnourished. Typically, they will act hungry and drink vigorously.

Physical examination may reveal a palpable "olive" just to the right of the epigastrium, especially immediately after vomiting. However, the examination often is normal. Diagnosis can be made with ultrasonography or an upper gastrointestinal series. Surgery is curative. Interim management includes withholding oral intake, passing a nasogastric tube, providing intravenous fluids, and correcting metabolic abnormalities.

Hirschsprung's disease, also known as **congenital megacolon**, results from absence of ganglion cells in the bowel wall; most commonly, the lesion is at the rectosigmoid area, at which an area of functional obstruction is created. The large bowel proximal to the obstruction can become extremely dilated. In extreme cases, toxic megacolon can occur, which is life threatening.

Most cases of Hirschsprung's disease are diagnosed in the nursery, when a baby fails to pass stool within the first 24 hours. Occasionally, constipation develops later. At times, it is associated with overflow diarrhea. In severe cases, vomiting and abdominal distention may be present, which is virtually never the case with nonpathologic constipation. The abdominal examination may reveal a fecal mass, and due to obstruction at the rectosigmoid junction, digital examination reveals an empty rectum.

Presumptive diagnosis can be made with barium enema, which shows colonic dilatation above the aganglionic stricture. Definitive diagnosis requires rectal biopsy, which confirms the absence of ganglion cells. Surgery is necessary. In an ill-appearing infant suspected of having Hirschsprung's disease, toxic megacolon is likely, and admission to an intensive care unit is advisable. Coverage with broad-spectrum antibiotics is indicated.

If not associated with toxic megacolon, Hirschsprung's disease is not a surgical emergency, and the patient can be stabilized with hydration and transferred nonemergently for biopsy and surgery as indicated.

Nonsurgical Gastrointestinal Problems

Infectious gastroenteritis in the neonate results in vomiting and diarrhea. **Rotavirus** is a common etiology. Less commonly, bacteria are implicated, including *Salmonella*, enterotoxic and enterinvasive *E. coli*, and, rarely, *Shigella*. Bacterial gastroenteritis is likely to result in bloody or heme-positive stools and fecal leukocytes.

Neonates with vomiting and diarrhea as part of a febrile illness require cultures of blood, urine, and cerebrospinal fluid. In patients with fecal blood or leukocytes, stool cultures are indicated.

The major risk in neonates with gastroenteritis is dehydration and electrolyte abnormality because they are particularly vulnerable to fluid loss. Their hydration status must be assessed carefully. Afebrile patients who are well hydrated can be managed as outpatients with clear liquids instead of formula for 24 hours. Caretakers should be instructed regarding the signs and symptoms of dehydration. Close follow-up is necessary and should include weight checks. For any neonate who appears dehydrated, hospitalization and intravenous fluid therapy should be considered. Febrile neonates with gastroenteritis require hospitalization for antibiotic therapy because bacterial pathogens, especially *Salmonella,* can cause bacteremia.

Significant **gastrointestinal bleeding** is rare in the neonate. However, hematemesis and hematochezia are fairly common presenting complaints. It is first essential to determine whether the bleeding arises from the baby or the mother. Newborns can swallow blood during delivery, which can appear in vomitus or stool. Women who breastfeed can develop cracks and fissures in their nipples, which can result in the baby swallowing small amounts of blood. If an adequate sample can be obtained, maternal and neonatal blood can be differentiated with the **Apt test.** Neonatal blood is composed mainly of fetal hemoglobin, which is alkali resistant, whereas maternal hemoglobin A is denatured and will change color when exposed to an alkaline solution.

A likely cause of significant upper gastrointestinal bleeding in the first postnatal week is **hemorrhagic disease of the newborn.** This is secondary to a deficiency in vitamin K-dependent clotting factors. Deficiency can be especially severe in neonates whose mothers were treated with phenobarbital or phenytoin during pregnancy. Bleeding also can occur from the nose, intracranially, or from a circumcision. Hemorrhagic disease in the newborn is averted in large part with the empiric administration of vitamin K immediately after delivery.

Neonates with active bleeding and a prolonged prothrombin time (PT) are treated with vitamin K. Normal PT values vary among laboratories, and normal values differ for neonates. Vitamin K can be administered orally, subcutaneously, intramuscularly, and intravenously, but the intravenous route is preferred with severe prolongation of the PT. The intravenous dose is 1 to 5 mg, diluted in normal saline and given at a rate not to exceed 5% of the total dose per minute. The major adverse effect of intravenous administration is **anaphylaxis.** Close observation is required for 1 to 2 hours after administration. With subcutaneous and intramuscular administration, **hematoma formation** may be a problem.

In severe cases, fresh frozen plasma is indicated to help reverse the coagulopathy.

A fairly common cause of mild hematochezia in the neonate is **rectal fissure,** a small tear in the anal

mucosa. No treatment is usually necessary, beyond reassuring the parents that the condition is not serious.

Neonates who are **allergic to cow's milk protein** may develop bloody diarrhea, which may be accompanied by vomiting. The clinical picture is that of colitis. The babies usually appear well. If fever is present, bacterial enteritis is more likely, and a full septic workup, including stool cultures, is indicated. Because many patients intolerant of cow's milk protein also are intolerant of soy-based formulas, an elemental formula may be necessary.

Neurologic Disorders

Neonatal Seizures

Neonatal seizures are fairly common. The immaturity of the nervous system is such that seizures result in a wide variety of nonspecific symptoms. Focal convulsions are common and can be limited to one extremity or to the muscles of the face, especially the eyes. They may be accompanied by spells of apnea or bradycardia, often associated with cyanosis. Occasionally, it is extremely difficult to distinguish seizure activity from the normal tremulousness many neonates exhibit.

Seizures that occur within the first 24 hours after delivery most often are secondary to perinatal hypoxic ischemic disease, birth trauma, metabolic disease, or congenital malformations of the central nervous system. The baby is likely to be extremely ill. Seizures occurring after the second postnatal day are more commonly due to central nervous system infection and, in the preterm infant, intracranial hemorrhage. Rarely, neonatal seizures are due to inborn errors of metabolism. An extremely rare but treatable metabolic cause of neonatal seizures is pyridoxine dependency. In cases of intractable seizures, 50 to 100 mg pyridoxine is given intravenously.

The evaluation of neonatal seizures includes serum glucose, electrolytes, calcium, phosphate, and magnesium; complete blood cell count; and cultures of the blood, cerebrospinal fluid, and urine. If no metabolic or infectious etiology of the seizures is discovered, intracranial ultrasonography or computed tomography is indicated.

Acutely, seizures usually can be controlled with benzodiazepines (see Chapter 17). Phenobarbital is useful for chronic control. The prognosis of neonatal seizures depends on the etiology.

Narcotic Withdrawal Syndrome

Neonates born of narcotic-addicted mothers can experience narcotic withdrawal syndrome. The usual signs include tremulousness, tachypnea, vomiting, diarrhea, and irritability. Convulsions are uncommon but more likely when the mother is addicted to methadone than to heroin. Symptoms usually appear within 24 to 48 hours of birth but can be delayed.

The diagnosis most often is made by obtaining a history of maternal drug abuse. Hypoglycemia, hypocalcemia, and central nervous system infection must be excluded. Hospitalization for parenteral fluids and controlled withdrawal with the use of sedatives or narcotics is necessary.

Metabolic Disorders

Early Hypocalcemia

Early hypocalcemia most commonly occurs in premature babies, very ill newborns, and infants of a diabetic mother during the first 3 days after delivery. As such, it is unlikely to be diagnosed in the emergency department or office setting.

Late Hypocalcemia

Late hypocalcemia can occur in neonates fed with formulas containing a high phosphate content, including human milk. The elevated serum phosphate level that results can depress serum calcium, especially because the neonate's parathyroid glands are immature and unable to compensate. The most common manifestation of significant hypocalcemia is **seizure**, although **irritability** and **tremulousness** can occur. The ECG may demonstrate a prolonged corrected QT interval. Serum calcium is <7 mg/dL. Acute treatment consists of 10% calcium gluconate at a dose of 2 mL/kg. The high-phosphate diet must be eliminated.

Hypoglycemia

In full-term infants, blood glucose is usually 50 to 60 mg/dL by 72 hours of age. Before this, the normal level may be as low as 30 mg/dL. Low glycogen stores can result in hypoglycemia during periods of physiologic stress, especially in premature infants or neonates with intrauterine growth retardation, who have significantly reduced body fat. Severe hypoglycemia can occur in neonates with Beckwith syndrome, which is characterized by large size, macroglossia, and visceromegaly. Nesidioblastosis, characterized by proliferation of pancreatic islet cells and hyperinsulinemia, can result in severe neonatal hypoglycemia. Infants of diabetic mothers are especially vulnerable to hypoglycemia, but this usually develops within the first 24 hours after delivery.

Hypoglycemic neonates may be jittery or irritable or experience lethargy, intermittent cyanosis, or convulsions. Treatment of symptomatic patients is with 2.5 to 5 mL/kg 10% glucose IV, followed by an infusion. For persistent severe hypoglycemia, an infusion of ≥8 mg/kg per minute of 10% to 12.5% glucose is indicated. In the event that intravenous access is not possible, glucagon at a dose of 0.025 mg/kg IM is administered (maximum dose is 1 mg). Glucagon is not indicated in infants who are small for gestational age. It is essential to determine the underlying cause of hypoglycemia.

Unconjugated Hyperbilirubinemia

Unconjugated hyperbilirubinemia is extremely common in neonates, especially during the first week after delivery, when the immature liver assumes the role of conjugating and excreting bilirubin. Particularly in the preterm, septic, or acidotic infant, unconjugated bilirubin can cross the blood-brain barrier and result in **kernicterus**, a potentially devastating neurologic disorder. The serum level at which unconjugated bilirubin is toxic to the central nervous system is controversial, but in otherwise well term infants, kernicterus is rare when levels are <25 mg/dL. Excessive levels of unconjugated bilirubin are managed with phototherapy or exchange transfusion.

Physiologic jaundice is the most common cause of unconjugated hyperbilirubinemia in the well neonate. Jaundice usually peaks at 3 to 4 days of age and rarely exceeds 10 to 12 mg/dL. The typical neonate with physiogic jaundice is mildly icteric, feeds well, and has normal stools. Serum bilirubin can be followed as an outpatient.

Unconjugated hyperbilirubinemia can develop in breast-fed infants, usually after the fourth day. Cessation of breast feeding results in a decline in bilirubin, which does not rise after the reintroduction of breast milk. In cases in which breast milk jaundice is suspected, consultation with the patient's pediatrician is advisable.

Unconjugated hyperbilirubinemia that does not fit the patterns of physiologic or breast milk jaundice may be pathologic. A variety of congenital metabolic and hemolytic conditions are possible. A thorough physical examination, searching for a collection of blood, such as a cephalohematoma, that may have resulted in excess blood breakdown is indicated. The hemolysis can occur from a maternal-fetal blood group incompatibility that exceeds the conjugating ability of the liver. The laboratory evaluation includes a complete blood cell and reticulocyte count. Blood typing and Coomb's testing of both mother and infant is essential. The patient should be evaluated for a source of infection. Urinary infection is a common finding. When serum bilirubin is >15 mg/dL or rapidly rising, admission for phototherapy generally is recommended.

Direct Hyperbilirubinemia

Direct or mixed hyperbilirubinemia virtually always is pathologic. It often develops in the first few postnatal days. A variety of **intrauterine infections**, including syphilis, toxoplasmosis, and rubella, can cause mixed hyperbilirubinemia. **Congenital hepatitis** is a possibility, as is **biliary atresia**. **Urinary tract infection** and **sepsis** also are possible.

The neonate with mixed hyperbilirubinemia always requires a through evaluation. Consultation with a pediatric gastroenterologist may be helpful.

Infectious Diseases

The neonate has a predictable vulnerability to certain infections. The invasive nature of these organisms makes it imperative to exclude hematogenous spread to the meninges, even in apparently localized infections. For example, septic arthritis is a common bacterial infection often associated with meningitis.

Group B *Streptococcus* is a common cause of sepsis in the first 24 hours after delivery. Premature infants are at higher risk than term infants. There may be a history of prolonged rupture of membranes or maternal fever. Respiratory distress often is the initial symptom; the clinical picture often is similar to that of hyaline membrane disease. Most affected newborns are gravely ill. In its "late-onset" form, group B *Streptococcus* is a highly invasive organism, and patients often present with a combination of sepsis and meningitis. It also can cause septic arthritis. Affected neonates usually are between 2 to 4 weeks of age. Symptoms include lethargy, apnea, and poor feeding. The baby may be febrile and have signs of cardiovascular instability. Antibiotic coverage in neonates should always be directed at the possibility of group B *Streptococcus*.

Gram-negative organisms, especially *E. coli,* are common causes of bacterial infections in neonates. Other Gram-negative organisms include *Klebsiella* and *Enterobacter*. The usual focus of infection is the **urinary tract**. Unlike urinary tract infections (UTIs) in older infants and children, UTIs in neonates occur through hematogenous spread of the offending organism. Symptoms of a UTI are nonspecific and include vomiting, diarrhea, and poor feeding. Fever often is present and can be the sole manifestation. It is imperative that urinalysis and culture are obtained through suprapubic aspiration or catheterization. Blood and cerebrospinal fluid cultures also are essential. Hospitalization and parenteral antibiotic therapy are indicated in the neonate with a UTI. Due to a high incidence of associated anomalies, follow-up imaging studies of the urinary tract are indicated.

Staphylococcus aureus can cause septic arthritis, cellulitis, and breast abscess in neonates. *Salmonella* has a predilection to cause bacteremia in neonates with infectious gastroenteritis and can result in septic arthritis or meningitis. *Listeria monocytogenes* is an uncommon but potentially lethal cause of sepsis and meningitis in neonates. Like group B *Streptococcus,* it tends to occur in an early and a late form, and the signs and symptoms are similar to those seen with group B *Streptococcus* infection.

Although most viral infections in neonates are self-limited, Herpes simplex can cause devastating infection. Usually acquired during delivery, infection often becomes apparent during the first week after delivery, with symptoms identical to those of bacterially mediated sepsis. Many affected neonates present with skin vesicles or mouth ulcerations. Localized disease usually progresses to systemic illness involving the central nervous system. Diagnosis depends on isolation of the virus, but treatment should not be delayed pending results. Treatment with 500 mg/m² acyclovir IV every 8 hours for 10 days, or 15 mg/kg adenine arabinoside IV daily for 10 days has proved helpful in lowering mortality.

Umbilical Disorders

Parents frequently become concerned about the appearance of the **umbilical cord stump**, which normally undergoes necrosis during the early neonatal period. Varying amounts of granulation tissue may develop after separation of the umbilical remnant and present as a red, raw mass of tissue. One or more topical treatments with silver nitrate are indicated.

On rare occasions, the umbilical remnant and surrounding tissues can become infected, resulting in purulent drainage and erythema. This condition is known as **omphalitis** and, if untreated, can progress rapidly to sepsis.

Brown or yellow drainage from the umbilicus can result from remnants of the omphalomesenteric duct or the urachus. Such remnants may or may not communicate with the small bowel or bladder. These remnants require surgical excision.

Umbilical hernias are common, especially in African-American infants. They usually close spontaneously during the first few years of life. Incarceration is rare. If spontaneous closure does not occur, surgical closure is recommended before the child begins elementary school.

Traumatic Disorders

The vast majority of trauma involving the neonate occurs during delivery, although the possibility of abuse always must be considered.

The **clavicle** may be fractured during delivery; this is a benign injury that heals rapidly. Treatment is with a figure-of-eight bandage or a sling. Humeral fractures also can occur during delivery and are managed in a sling.

Mild degrees of **head trauma** and **head molding** are extremely common during the birth process, particularly in the macrosomic infant. The most common injury is a cephalohematoma, a subperiosteal hemorrhage always limited to one bone. There usually is localized swelling that may feel somewhat firm and does not cross suture lines. No treatment is necessary. **Subgaleal hemorrhage** also can occur, usually after forceps or vacuum extraction, and can acutely result in significant blood loss or later cause hyperbilirubinemia as extravasated blood is broken down. Unlike cephalohematoma, bleeding from subgaleal hemorrhage is diffuse and crosses suture lines. In patients with subgaleal hemorrhage, it is prudent to obtain a hematocrit and baseline serum bilirubin and begin volume replacement. **Subconjunctival hemorrhage** is a common finding that can cause parental anxiety but is benign and does not require treatment.

On occasion, a difficult delivery can result in **peripheral nerve injury** involving the brachial plexus. In Erb-Duchenne paralysis, the injury involves cervical nerves 5 and 6, and the affected arm is held in adduction and internal rotation. In Klumpke paralysis, cervical nerves 7 and 8 are affected, along with the first thoracic nerve. Affected neonates can present with a paralyzed hand and occasionally ptosis and miosis. Prognosis varies.

SUMMARY

A physician likely to encounter a critically ill infant should be familiar with the anatomic and physiologic differences that predispose neonates to particular diseases and with the diversity and significance of the signs and symptoms of neonatal illness. Perhaps the most important function of the emergency physician or office practitioner is to recognize and appropriately manage the neonate with imminent respiratory or circulatory failure. Resuscitative efforts should consist of airway control, oxygenation, ventilation, stabilization of the circulation, and temperature control. In addition, the physician should be aware of the conditions that require urgent medical or surgical subspecialty evaluation.

ADDITIONAL READING

American Academy of Pediatrics, Provisional Committee for Quality Improvement, Subcommittee on Hyperbilirubinemia. Practice parameter: management of hyperbilirubinemia in healthy term neonates. *Pediatrics.* 1994;94:558-565.

American Academy of Pediatrics and American Heart Association. *Textbook of Neonatal Resuscitation.* Elk Grove Village, Ill: American Academy of Pediatrics; 1994.

Baraff LJ, Bass JW, Fleisher GR, et al. Practice guideline for the management of infants and children 0 to 36 months of age with fever without source. Agency for Health Care Policy and Research. *Ann Emerg Med.* 1993;22:1198-1210.

Behrman RE, Kliegman RM, Arvin AM. *Nelson Textbook of Pediatrics,* 15th ed. Philadelphia, Pa: WB Saunders; 1996.

Chameides L, Hazinski MF, eds. *Pediatric Advanced Life Support.* Dallas, Tex: American Heart Association; 1997:9-1 to 9-10.

Dillon PW, Cilley RE. Newborn surgical emergencies. Gastrointestinal anomalies, abdominal wall defects. *Pediatr Clin North Am.* 1993;40:1289-1314.

Gerardi M. Neonatal emergencies. *Pediatr Emerg Med Rep.* 1996;1:113-124.

Seashore MR, Rinaldo P. Metabolic disease of the neonate and young infant. *Semin Perinatol.* 1993;17:318-329.

Stafstrom CE. Neonatal seizures. *Pediatr Rev.* 1995;16:248-255.

.

Index

Page numbers followed by f indicate figures; page numbers followed by t indicate tables.

W